Donald N. Ross · Terence A. H. English
Roxane McKay

Principles of Cardiac Diagnosis and Treatment

A Surgeons' Guide

Second Edition

With 169 Figures by Barbara Hyams

Springer-Verlag
London Berlin Heidelberg New York
Paris Tokyo Hong Kong
Barcelona Budapest

Donald N. Ross, FRCS, DSc, FACS
Consultant Surgeon Emeritus, National Heart Hospital London,
25 Upper Wimpole Street, London WIM 7TA, UK

Sir Terence A. H. English, KBE, PRCS, FRCS
Consultant Cardiac Surgeon, Papworth Hospital, Cambridge CB3 8RE, UK

Roxane McKay, MD, FRCS
Consultant Paediatric Cardiothoracic Surgeon, The Royal Liverpool Children's Hospital, Liverpool L12 2AP, UK

ISBN 3-540-17494-X Springer-Verlag Berlin Heidelberg New York
ISBN 0-387-17494-X Springer-Verlag New York Berlin Heidelberg

British Library Cataloguing in Publication Data
Principles of cardiac diagnosis and treatment.–2nd. ed.
1. Humans. Heart. Therapy
I. English, Terence 1932– II. McKay, Roxane 1944–
616.12
ISBN 3-540-17494-X

Library of Congress Data available

Typeset by Best-set Typesetters Ltd, Hong Kong
Printed by Henry Ling, The Dorset Press, Dorchester
2128/3830 543210 Printed on acid-free paper

Preface to the Second Edition

This book was first published in 1962 with a second volume added in 1967, at a time when cardiac surgery was progressing quite rapidly and exploring new fields. This progress was the result of a number of technological advances in allied techniques, particularly those involving increasingly complex investigational methods.

At that time clinical cardiology was largely in the hands of cardiologists of the 'presurgical' era! It was clear that there was a need to bridge the gap between cardiac surgery and traditional cardiology and, logically, the onus was on surgeons to learn some of the more basic diagnostic skills of this well-established medical specialty.

Brock had already begun to close this gap within his small group of trainees and Zenker was the catalyst who saw the need to present the somewhat obscure cardiological jargon of the day in a more readily assimilable form to a wider audience, including the new group of cardiac surgeons. With his stimulus and encouragement the original books were produced.

Since that time clinical and particularly specialised diagnostic methods have become increasingly sophisticated and are widely used by both physicians and surgeons working in this field. Thus a new need arises to bridge an ever-widening gap between the 'student' (pre- and postgraduate) and an increasingly remote group of medical and surgical specialists. It is our hope that this revised and enlarged book will help to provide the link. Moreover, allied health professionals in nursing, physiotherapy and radiology now require a basic understanding of the diagnosis and treatment of cardiac disease.

As far as possible the original format and simple illustrations of the first edition have been used while some of the newer techniques such as echocardiography and coronary angiography have been included. Again no attempt has been made to provide detailed operative techniques, which are outside the scope and aim of this book. Only principles of treatment are given.

The work is by no means fully comprehensive but aims to include the common conditions encountered in the practice of cardiac surgery. By retaining current developments in complex congenital heart surgery we hope to emphasise the concept of a broadly based and well-rounded knowledge of established principles which can be applied to any aspect of cardiac surgical practice.

Acknowledgements

We gratefully acknowledge the contributions of Tricia Part, Sheila Critchley, Jill Davies, Barbara Hyams, Paul Hetherington, and Dr Raymond Galloway to the preparation of this volume

February 1991

Donald N. Ross
Terence A. H. English
Roxane McKay

materials and microsurgical techniques achieved the ideal of direct operation upon the coronary arteries themselves.

More recent advances have reflected progress in related disciplines. Studies of myocardial biochemistry have begun to elucidate mechanisms of ischaemic damage to the heart, leading to the use of cardioplegic techniques and other specific measures during open heart surgery to preserve cardiac function. Mechanical support of the circulation for longer periods of time has become safer as the result of improved devices for oxygenating and circulating the blood, as well as better understanding of the physiology of cardiopulmonary bypass. The development of special types of apparatus now permits partial support of the heart or lungs for periods of several days or weeks, giving time for organ recovery or replacement. Transplantation of the heart, lungs, or heart and lungs has become a practical treatment for end-stage or inoperable disease, just as methods for myocardial preservation have made possible the transport of donor organs over long distances. Spectacular advances in immunology and the control of organ rejection, continue to revolutionise the entire field of transplantation.

In addition, non-surgical techniques that complement and extend operative procedures have been introduced by the development of balloon catheters capable of dilating stenosed vessels or valves.

And, finally, the rigorous application of statistical analysis to the results of cardiac surgery is beginning to provide surgeons with objective yardsticks by which to measure their achievements, as well as the means to identify causes of surgical failure and to quantitate success.

Further Reading

Kirklin JW. The science of cardiac surgery. Eur J Cardiothorac Surg 1990; 4: 63–71

McNamara DG, Manning JA, Engle MA, Whittemore R, Neill CA, Ferencz C. Helen Brooke Taussig: 1898–1986. J Am Coll Cardiol 1987; 10: 662–671

Sealy WC. Hypothermia: Its possible role in cardiac surgery. Ann Thorac Surg 1989; 47: 788–791

Selzer A. Fifty years of progress in cardiology: A personal perspective. Circulation 1988; 77: 955–963

Chapter 2

Anatomical and Physiological Considerations

A sound anatomical knowledge is one of the three pillars upon which an accurate diagnosis must rest, the other two being physiology and pathology. Brock's first principle in diagnosis, whether relating to the abdomen, chest or heart, was to establish initially the precise anatomical site of the lesion. Having determined this, he then asked 'taking into consideration the history, age and sex of the patient, what is the most likely diagnosis?' Using this simple approach, the diagnosis often became obvious, and these ground rules are equally applicable today.

Anatomical Features

The detailed gross anatomy of the heart and its relationship to the lungs and other intrathoracic structures, while of fundamental importance, is outside the scope of this work. Similarly, cardiac embryology, a fascinating subject in its own right, is here considered only where it facilitates understanding of pathology

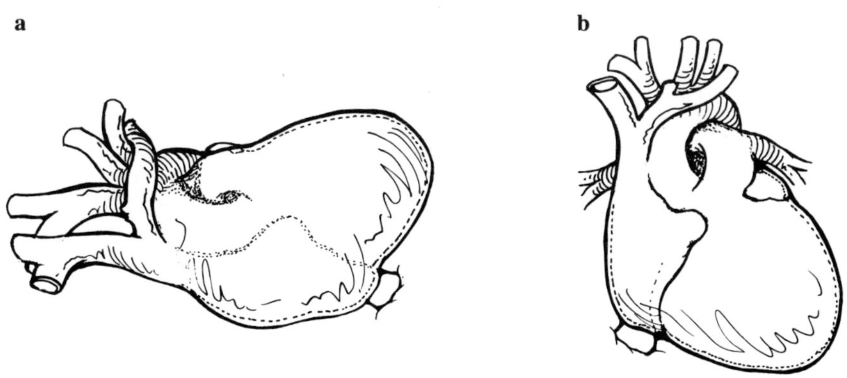

Fig. 2.1. Surgical (**a**) and anatomical (**b**) orientations of the heart.

and surgical management. One point worth emphasising is that the living anatomy of the heart as observed by the surgeon often bears little resemblance to the formalin-hardened post-mortem specimens seen in museums or illustrated in textbooks. Also, the appearance of the heart viewed by the surgeon standing on the patient's right side is very different from that in the standard anatomy textbook, where the heart is presented in an upright, anatomical position.

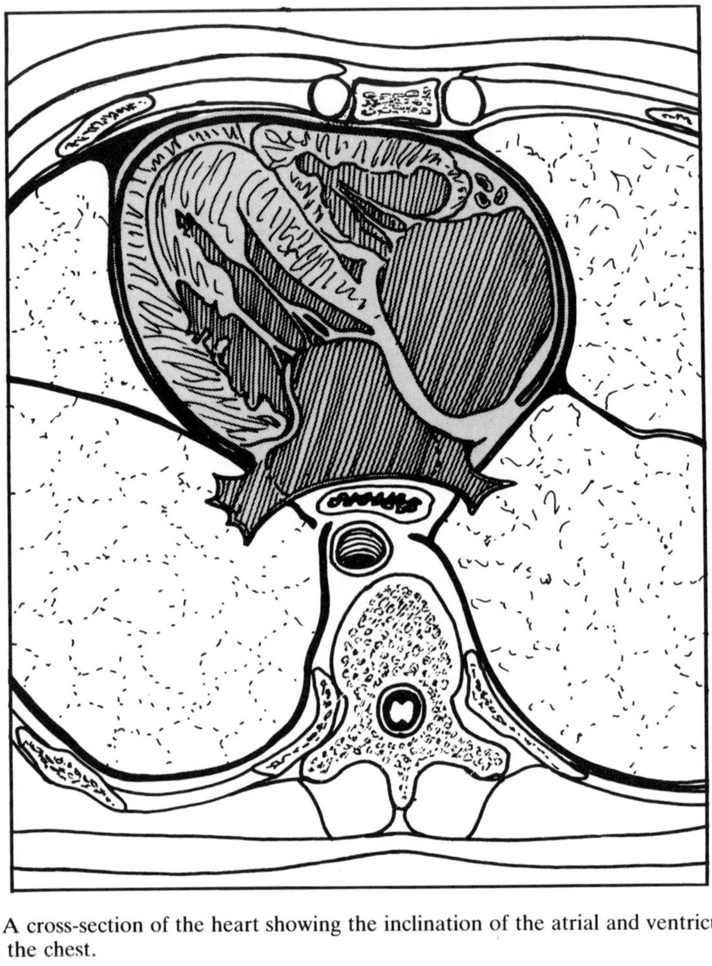

Fig. 2.2. A cross-section of the heart showing the inclination of the atrial and ventricular septa in relation to the chest.

Of primary concern to the surgeon planning intracardiac access is the position of the heart within the chest. Normally, the apex lies to the left ('levocardia'), and the septa are obliquely inclined, as demonstrated by the anatomist Walmsley. The left atrium and left ventricle are thus relatively less accessible than the right, and the mitral valve may be visualised more easily from the patient's right side, through either the atrial septum or an incision in front of the pulmonary veins. When the cardiac apex points to the right ('dextrocardia'), the left ventricle rotates in front of the right atrium and right ventricle, but the latter chambers are still approached as before. This is in contrast with 'situs inversus', where a morphological right atrium receives the systemic venous return on the patient's left side and most intracardiac procedures are performed with the surgeon working from the opposite side of the operating table.

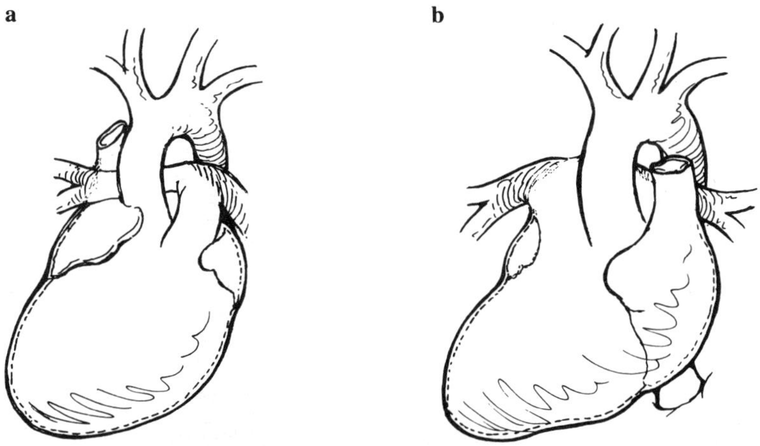

Fig. 2.3. Dextrocardia (**a**) indicates that the apex of the heart is rotated towards the right chest, in contrast to situs inversus. (**b**) where all the cardiac chambers are in a mirror-image position.

Wedged between the mitral and tricuspid valves, the aortic root and left ventricular outflow tract occupy a central position within the heart. Each sinus of the aortic valve has important relations to at least one cardiac chamber and to several subvalvar structures. The right coronary sinus is adjacent to the infundibular septum of the right ventricle, and the commissural angle between right and non-coronary cusps lies above the membranous septum, the central fibrous body and the penetrating atrioventricular bundle of the conduction system. Aneurysms or infective lesions of this sinus may extend into the interventricular septum, causing disturbances of heart rhythm or a fistula

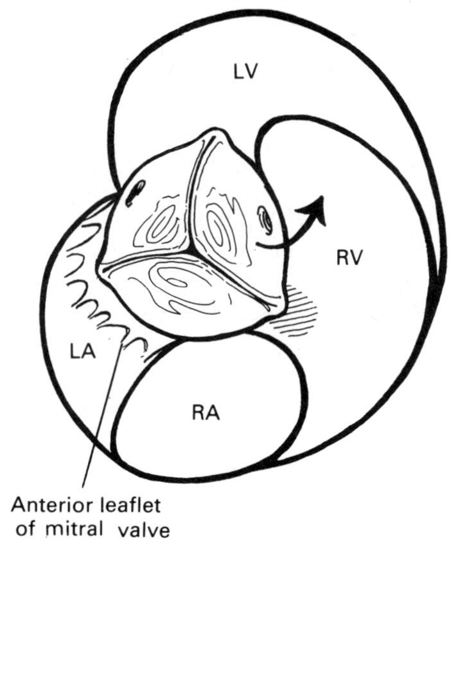

Fig. 2.4. Relationship of the aortic valve sinuses to the cardiac chambers. LA, Left atrium; LV, left ventricle; RA, right atrium; RV, right ventricle.

between the aorta and right ventricle. The vulnerability of the conduction system must be respected in dealing with calcification of the septum associated with aortic valve disease. With ventricular septal defects, prolapse of an unsupported right coronary cusp into a subjacent defect of membranous or infundibular septum may produce incompetence of the aortic valve.

The non-coronary sinus is related primarily to the right atrium and forms the aortic mound above the atrioventricular node. A suture placed too deeply during closure of an atrial septal defect may impale the non-coronary cusp, while aneurysms of this sinus tend to rupture above the tricuspid valve into the right atrium. Below the commissure between the left and non-coronary cusps lies the posterior wall of the left ventricular outflow, consisting of the anterior leaflet of the mitral valve separated from the aortic annulus by a variable length of fibrous tissue. Infections of the aortic valve may spread directly to the mitral valve by this route or by a jet lesion from aortic regurgitation. The adjacent portions of the left and non-coronary sinuses are closely related to the left atrium. Only the lateral part of the left coronary sinus lacks immediate relations to a cardiac chamber.

Because of this, the left coronary sinus may rupture into the pericardium, and a left coronary artery which originates anomalously from the pulmonary artery may be transferred directly through the transverse sinus to the aorta for reimplantation in its anatomical position. These relationships acquire particular importance in the surgery of subaortic stenosis and have been demonstrated beautifully by Walmsley with longitudinal sections through the human heart.

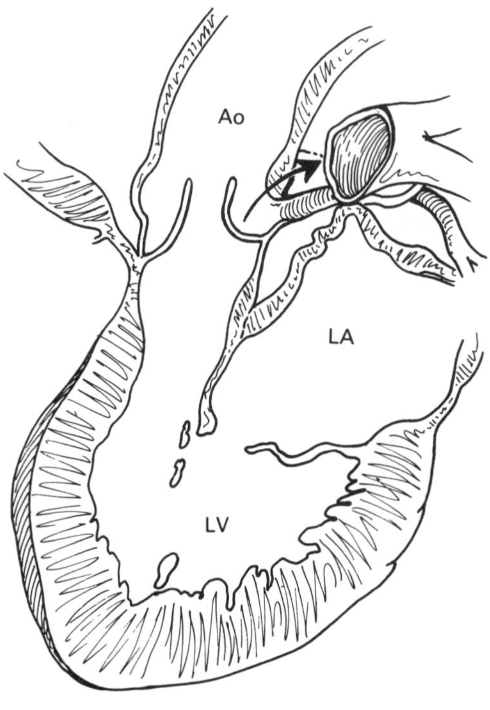

Fig. 2.5. Longitudinal section through the intact heart, demonstrating the relationships of the left coronary artery and sinus of Valsalva to the tranverse sinus and left atrium. Ao, Aorta.

The size of each cardiac valve in the normal heart reflects the velocity and volume of the blood passing throught it, for the total cardiac output flows sequentially through each chamber of the heart. The tricuspid and pulmonary valves on the low-pressure, right side of the heart are thus larger than their mitral and aortic counterparts on the left side, and the atrioventricular valves (tricuspid and mitral) have a much greater diameter than the semilunar valves (pulmonary and aortic). It is useful to remember this fact in selecting a prosthesis for cardiac valve replacement, assessing adequacy of a stenotic orifice after valvotomy or repairing complex congenital heart defects.

Supported by the muscular right ventricular outflow tract, the pulmonary valve is the only cardiac valve which is not incorporated in the fibrous skeleton of the heart. For this reason, it may be removed intact and used to replace a diseased valve in the aortic position of the same patient.

The outflow tract of the right ventricle consists of the relatively smooth, funnel-shaped portion between the large trabeculated inflow and the pulmonary annulus. Enlargement of muscle bundles in this region commonly contributes to the narrowing or infundibular stenosis present in Fallot's tetralogy. Ventricular septal defects of the supracristal and perimembranous type may be approached through an incision in the infundibulum of the right ventricle.

The left and right sides of the ventricular septum are distinctly asymmetrical. On the right side, the septum is trabeculated and gives rise to chordae and papillary muscles of the tricuspid valve. The smooth, left side is void of mitral valve attachments but has the important left bundle branch of the conduction system fanning out across its surface from the membranous septum. Defects in the trabecular portion of the ventricular septum may appear to be single on the left side and yet communicate with the right ventricle by several openings between these trabeculations or muscle bundles. Because the mitral valve is attached more proximally than the tricuspid, a portion of both the membranous and muscular septum lies between the left ventricle and right atrium, the 'atrioventricular' septum. Malformations in this part of the heart produce a spectrum of surgically important defects involving the mitral and tricuspid valves as well as the adjacent atrial and ventricular septal structures.

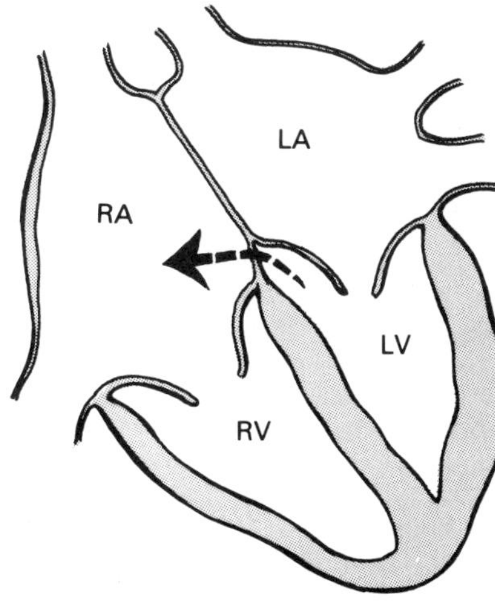

Fig. 2.6. Offsetting of the mitral and tricuspid valves results in a portion of septum which lies between the left ventricle and the right atrium of the normal heart.

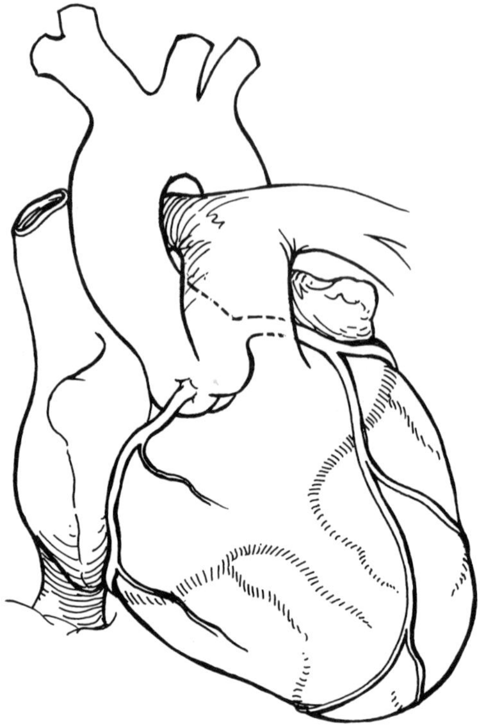

Fig. 2.7. Distribution of the major coronary arteries on the surface of the heart.

The anatomy of the coronary circulation assumes paramount importance in planning cardiac incisions, understanding and preventing ischaemic injury to the myocardium, and performing operations directly upon the coronary arteries themselves. The left and right coronaries usually arise independently from the two sinuses of the aortic valve which face the pulmonary artery. They then follow the atrioventricular or interventricular grooves in their epicardial distribution. Whichever vessel supplies the crux of the heart by a branch in the posterior interventricular groove (usually the right) is said to be 'dominant', although this is not necessarily the larger or more important of the two vessels. A dominant left coronary artery is commonly found in association with a bicuspid aortic valve, and because of its close relationship to the posterior mitral annulus, may be at risk of injury during mitral valve replacement. Although the entire length of the right coronary is surgically accessible, exposure of the left main coronary behind the pulmonary annulus and its circumflex branch in the atrioventricular groove is difficult and generally avoided by using more distal branches for revascularisation procedures. Anomalous origin of a coronary artery may predispose the myocardium to ischaemic damage, or, in the case of a left anterior descending branch arising from the right coronary, prevent a standard right ventriculotomy incision.

Elementary Haemodynamics

The pressure and flow in the pulmonary and systemic circulations are dependent upon the output of each ventricle and the resistance encountered by the ejected blood. Since the two circulations work in series it follows that, under normal circumstances, the output of both ventricles must be the same. As a result of the ventricles discharging their contents into progressively narrowing tubes, the pressure of the blood in the tubes rises to a point at which resistance to forward flow is overcome. The blood pressure (BP) is, therefore, a reflection of the cardiac output (CO) and the peripheral resistance (PR):

$$BP = CO \times PR.$$

The blood pressure in the pulmonary artery is only about 20 mmHg, while that in the aorta is around 100 mmHg. Since the output of each ventricle is the same, it follows that the peripheral obstruction (or resistance) met within the systemic vascular bed is much greater than that in the pulmonary vascular bed.

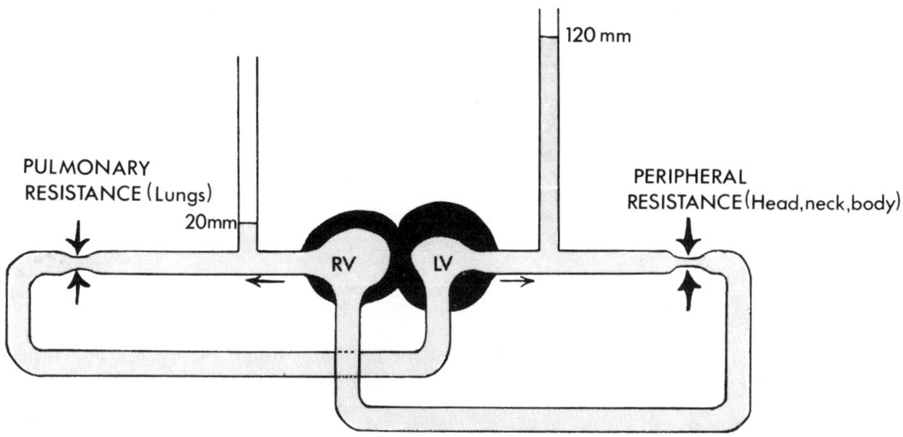

Fig. 2.8. The high pressure generated in the systemic bed is the result of the high peripheral resistance.

Just as there can be factors that increase the systemic vascular resistance and give rise to a high systemic blood pressure, so there can be changes in the pulmonary circulation that increase the peripheral resistance in the lungs and result in raised pulmonary artery pressure, 'pulmonary hypertension'.

Pulmonary Hypertension

This term is often used loosely and without an adequate understanding of the underlying mechanisms or their implications. It simply means a pulmonary artery pressure in excess of the normally accepted systolic value of 20–30 mmHg. There are a number of possible causes of a raised pulmonary artery pressure, but for simplicity, these can be classified as follows:

1. Primary pulmonary hypertension
2. Secondary pulmonary hypertension
   - Passive
   - Active
     - Secondary to increased flow
     - Secondary to increased resistance
3. Non-cardiac pulmonary hypertension

So-called 'primary pulmonary hypertension' is a disease of the vessels within the lung and might be more accurately designated 'unexplained' pulmonary hypertension. Although the pathological findings may be identical to those produced by cardiac disease, the heart is anatomically normal or shows only changes secondary to the increased pulmonary arterial pressure. All other non-cardiac causes of raised pulmonary artery pressure, such as chronic hypoxia from generalised lung disease, multiple pulmonary emboli and parasitic infection, must also be excluded to make this diagnosis. Surgically, the only possible treatment is transplantation of the heart and lungs, or possibly the lungs alone.

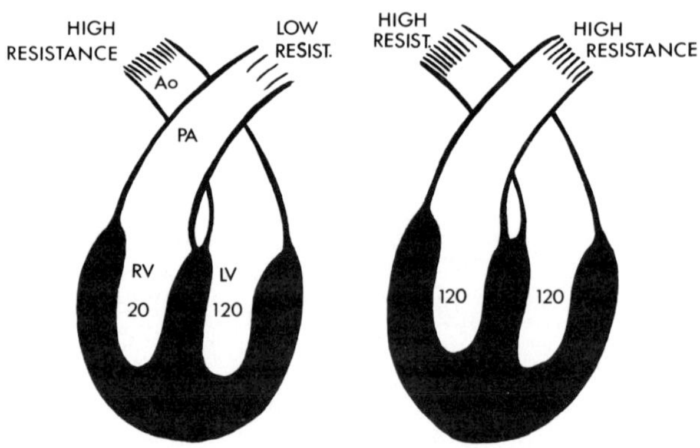

Fig. 2.9. Where the resistance offered by the lung vessels approaches that of the peripheral vessels, the pressure in the right side rises, resulting in pulmonary hypertension. PA, Pulmonary artery; Ao, Aorta.

Most cases of 'surgical' pulmonary hypertension, however, are 'secondary' in the sense that there is some underlying cardiac malformation or disease.

Passive Pulmonary Hypertension. This is not difficult to understand; it is the result of obstruction to forward flow in the left side of the heart. The right ventricle continues to pump blood into the lungs under increased pressure in an attempt to overcome the obstruction in the left heart. As a result, the pressure rises in the pulmonary veins, capillaries and arteries. In general, the closer the obstructive lesion is to the lungs, the sooner the patient will experience pulmonary congestion and the less obvious will be signs of cardiac disease. Thus, pulmonary hypertension is an early and, often, silent finding in pulmonary vein stenosis or cor triatriatum (where there is a membrane across the left atrium), whereas it occurs somewhat later in mitral valve stenosis. It is a very late

A second important consideration when an elevated resistance is found in the lungs is whether this is 'fixed' or 'reversible'. Some indication of reversibility can be obtained by administration of pulmonary vasodilator drugs or 100% oxygen during cardiac catheterisation, but, in a few cases, lung biopsy at operation may be necessary to assess the severity of pulmonary vascular disease. When the changes in the small, muscular arterioles become widespread and far advanced, the pulmonary resistance may increase to the point where pressures on the right side of the heart are equal to or higher than those on the left side. Under these circumstances, desaturated ('blue') blood flows into the left side producing central cyanosis, this being the cause of cyanosis in Eisenmenger's syndrome. At this point, the septal defect or ductus acts as a safety valve to decompress the high pressure on the right side of the heart, and closure is contraindicated.

The mechanism by which changes come about in pulmonary vascular disease is not completely understood. Prior to birth, the structure of the pulmonary and systemic arteries is very similar, reflecting the high resistance in the airless, fetal lung. Normally, expansion of the lungs at birth is followed by a reduction in pulmonary arterial resistance and, over a period of several weeks, a corresponding decrease in the muscle within the walls of the pulmonary vessels converts them to thin-walled, elastic arteries. In a few patients whose pulmonary arterial pressure remains at systemic level, for example due to a large ventricular septal defect, this regression of muscle does not occur and a high resistance is still found in the first months of life. Paradoxically, if there is no fall in pulmonary resistance and the pulmonary pressure equals the aortic pressure, little shunting occurs across the septal defect. Such patients have few symptoms or signs of a ventricular septal defect and tend to develop severe pulmonary vascular disease without evidence of cardiac failure.

More commonly, when a child is born with a large ventricular septal defect, the initial fall in pulmonary resistance continues after the child breathes and expands the lungs, and subsequent changes in the muscular arteries lead to progressive reduction in the obstruction to blood flow through the lungs. The left ventricle discharges progressively more of its contents via the ventricular septal defect into the pulmonary circulation, which comes to represent the path of

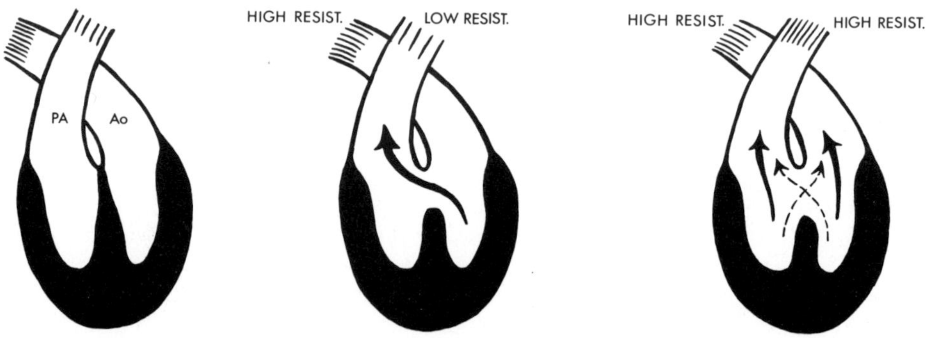

Fig. 2.11. The effect of the pulmonary resistance on the blood flow across a ventricular septal defect. With a low resistance, the shunt is predominantly left-to-right, and with a high resistance it is balanced.

lesser resistance. As more blood is shunted across the ventricular septal defect, the full clinical picture of a large left-to-right shunt emerges, with congested lungs, enlargement of the heart, and failure to thrive. At some point, the fall in pulmonary resistance must be opposed. Otherwise, the entire cardiac output would be discharged into the lungs and no blood would pass into the aorta, a situation incompatible with life. When the ventricular septal defect remains large, a secondary increase in pulmonary resistance results from redevelopment of muscle within the pulmonary arteries and serves to limit blood flow to the lungs. This, then, is the usual haemodynamic picture in cases of large ventricular septal defect surviving the first month of life: there is an elevation of pulmonary artery pressure, partly from increased flow and partly from increased vascular resistance.

It is interesting to contrast the haemodynamics of a large ventricular septal defect with those of an atrial septal defect, for raised pulmonary resistance and even increased pulmonary arterial pressure are uncommon or late complications of the latter. An explanation for this observation was offered by Wood in 1958. Since the right and left ventricles are equally hypertrophied at birth, there is probably no left-to-right shunt across an atrial septal defect initially. Only after the pulmonary arterial resistance has fallen to normal is there an accompanying resolution of right ventricular muscle mass. As the right ventricle becomes thin-walled and compliant, right atrial pressure falls below that in the left atrium, and blood flows towards the more distensible, low-pressure right ventricle through the atrial septal defect and tricuspid valve. By this time, the pulmonary vessels are themselves thin-walled and distensible and tend to accommodate the increased flow at a low pressure for a considerable period of time.

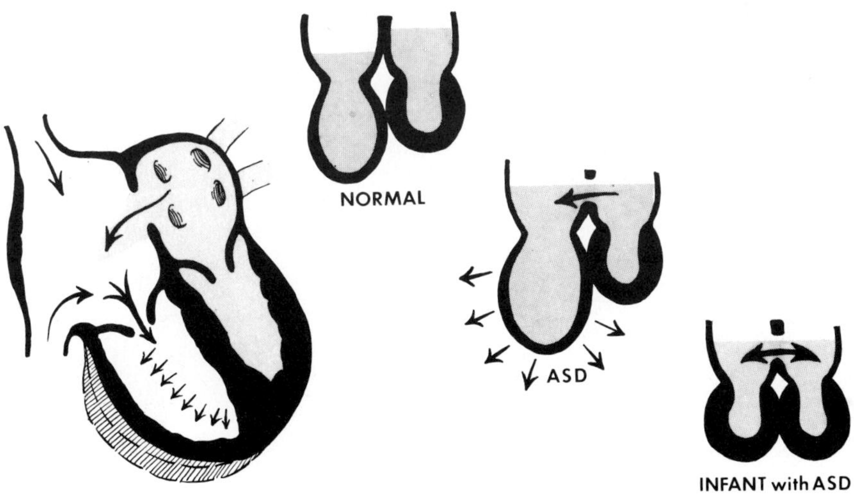

Fig. 2.12. Blood from both atria tends to flow into the right ventricle, which is more easily distended. ASD, Atrial septal defect.

Pressure Relationships in the Cardiovascular System

Aortic and pulmonary artery pressures are normally in the ratio of about six to one as the result of the unequal resistances in the pulmonary and systemic vascular beds. If the cardiovascular system is considered as a tubular pump (as it developed embryologically), the circulation can be represented quite simply. The pressure in the right ventricle varies between 20–30/0–4 mmHg in systole, and that in the left ventricle is about 120/0–8 mmHg. If there is no obstruction at the pulmonary or aortic valves, the systolic pressure will be transmitted unaltered

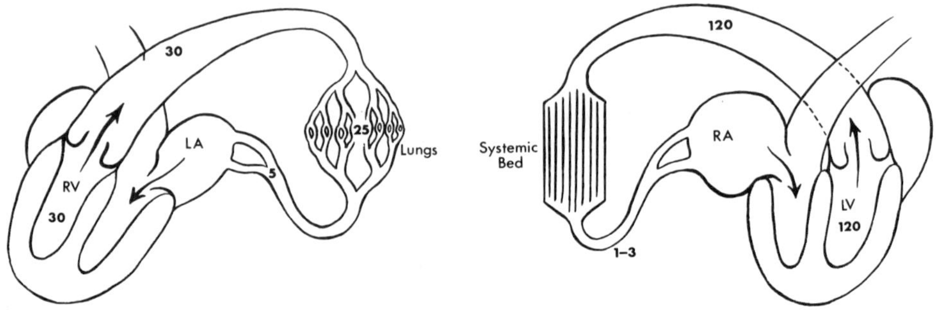

Fig. 2.13. The pressure relationships (mmHg) within the cardiovascular system.

from the ventricles to the main vessels. As the pressure falls towards zero in the ventricles, the pulmonary and aortic valves close. This is the mechanism which maintains the diastolic pressure and a continuous forward flow through the cardiac cycle. Thus, pressure in the pulmonary artery is about 20–30/5–15 mmHg, and, in the aorta, 120/80 mmHg. It follows that the pressure in the ventricle at the end of diastole ('end-diastolic pressure') should be equal to the corresponding atrial pressure, for, at this point in the cardiac cycle, the mitral and tricuspid valves are widely open. Atrial pressure is, in turn, equal to the pressure in the veins which the atrium receives because there are no haemodynamically effective valves between these two structures. Estimation of central venous pressure on the right side or pulmonary venous pressure on the left (usually by wedging a small catheter in a distal branch of the pulmonary arterial tree – the 'pulmonary capillary wedge pressure') gives an indication of both the volume of blood in the circulation and the respective ventricle's ability to pump it.

The Venous Return

Factors responsible for the venous return are:

1. The left ventricle
2. Other contributory factors
    a) Leg muscles plus venous valves
    b) Negative intrathoracic pressure

The continuous flow of blood through the great veins into the right atrium is largely the result of the left ventricular propulsive force. This fact is often obscured if undue attention is paid to the other factors modifying or influencing the venous return. Muscle contractions, particularly in the legs during exercise, are a powerful *aid* to venous return, particularly in the erect position when gravity must be overcome. The valves in the veins ensure a unidirectional flow.

A further factor aiding venous return is the negative pressure within the thoracic cage, which also modifies the pressure in the great veins and right atrium. While negative pressure is not an essential prerequisite for venous return in the normal heart (as demonstrated by the maintenance of cardiac output in a patient under anaesthesia with both pleural spaces open and with intermittent positive pressure respiration supplied by the anaesthetist), it may assume greater importance with some types of congenital heart defects. Following a Fontan operation (see Chap. 6), for example, where the systemic venous return flows directly through the right atrium to the pulmonary arteries, the negative intrathoracic pressure generated by spontaneous respiration may considerably enhance pulmonary blood flow and overall cardiac output.

A minor factor influencing venous return may be the contraction of the great veins which can be observed within the thoracic cage. This cannot contribute greatly in the absence of venous valves near the heart, but the loss of venous 'tone' occasioned by various muscle relaxants and vasodilator drugs may contribute to pooling of blood in the peripheral veins, and so indirectly decrease return to the heart.

Effects of Obstruction and Regurgitation in the Cardiovascular System

Obstruction at the level of the mitral or tricuspid valve tends to be reflected in elevation of the pulmonary or systemic capillary pressure, which results in pulmonary or systemic oedema. This is the picture in *atrial* obstruction.

Where the outflow from the right or left *ventricle* is obstructed, as in pulmonary or aortic stenosis, the ventricle continues to eject blood under a higher head of pressure to maintain the more distal pressure and blood flow as near normal as possible. Thus, the left ventricle may have to generate a pressure of 200–300 mmHg and the right ventricle 100–200 mmHg to maintain the flow and pressure relationships in the aorta and pulmonary artery. Unfortunately, in contrast to atrial obstruction, there is no intervening capillary bed, and the increased burden may be carried for a long period without symptoms. During this asymptomatic period, the muscle of the affected ventricle undergoes generalised, concentric hypertrophy which may become massive. The progressive increase in wall thickness steadily encroaches upon the lumen of the ventricular cavity and may also cause secondary muscular obstruction of the ventricular outflow.

At the same time, the hypertrophied muscle mass needs more blood to meet its metabolic requirements. Coronary blood flow is probably reduced, however, because of the prolonged systolic ejection phase during which coronary flow is suboptimal. In addition, the diminished cavity of the ventricle can accommodate less filling during diastole, and, consequently, less volume of blood is ejected

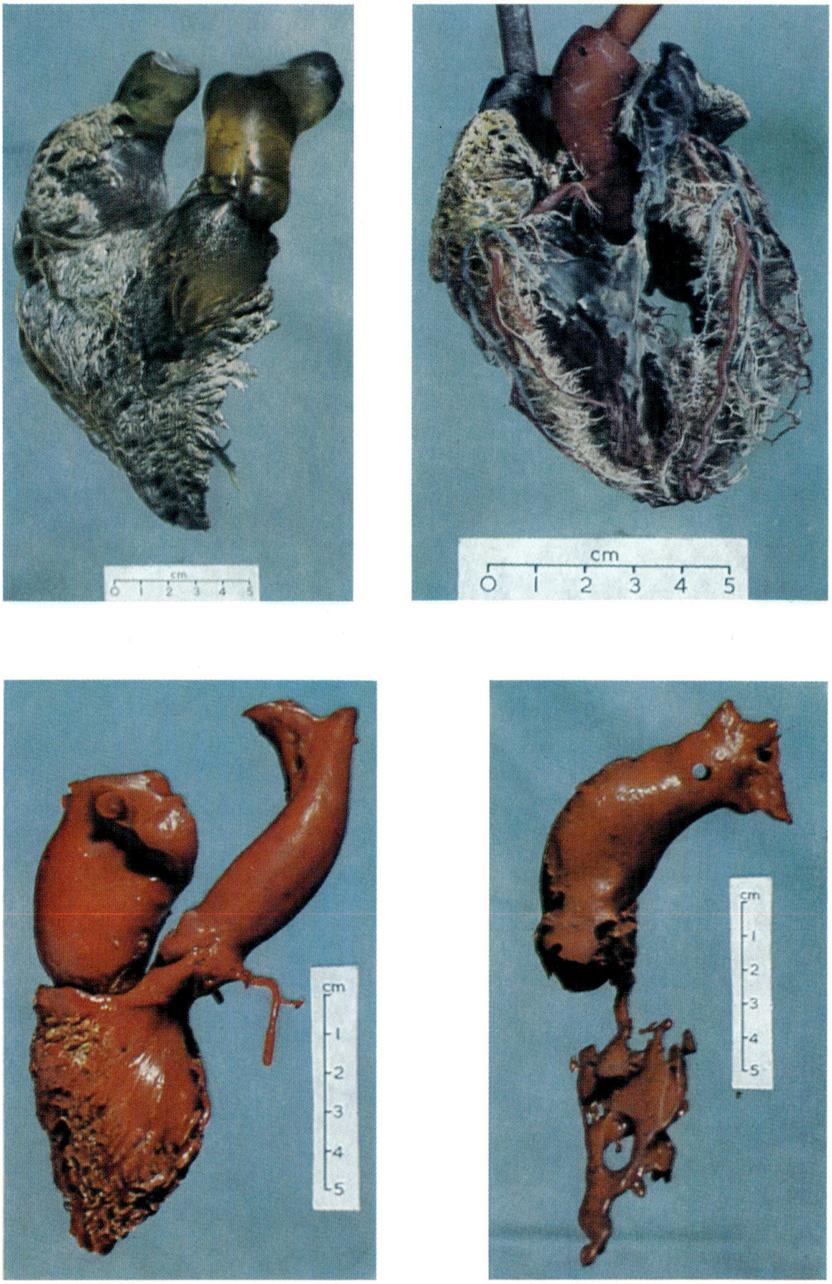

Fig. 2.14. Coloured plastic cases of the right and left ventricular outflow tracts. *Upper*: a normal right atrium, ventricle and pulmonary artery and a cast from a case of severe right ventricular obstruction showing the slit—like cavity and outflow tract. *Lower*: a normal left ventricular outflow and the result of severe aortic stenosis. A flattened left ventricular cavity leads to a huge aorta via a thread—like outflow tract.

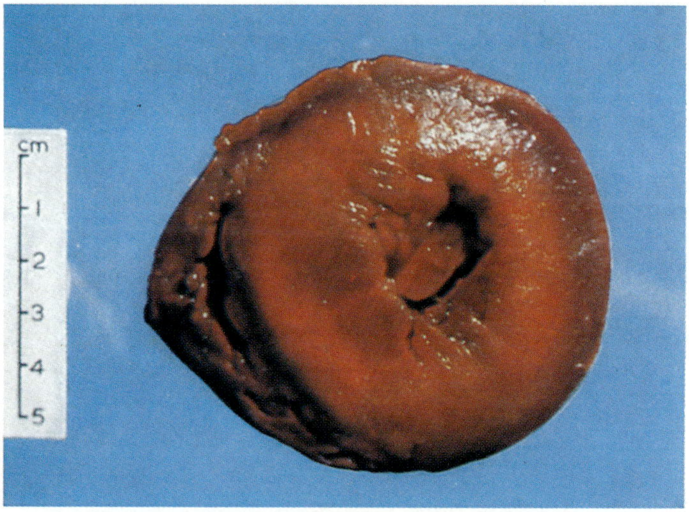

Fig. 2.15. A cross section through a muscle-bound left ventricle associated with aortic stenosis causing sudden death in a girl of 13 years. The right ventricle is flattened.

with each systole. As the heart has only two mechanisms by which to increase or maintain its output, stroke volume and heart rate, it can only compensate for a decreased stroke volume by beating faster. This is again at the expense of the diastolic filling phase. Thus there emerges a vicious circle of an increasing burden with a progressively less adequate supply of blood to the cardiac muscle, sometimes manifest by anginal symptoms.

Failure of the doubly obstructed, hypertrophied and blood-starved ventricle is usually sudden and devastating, a clinical phenomenon occasionally seen in cases of untreated aortic stenosis. It can be readily appreciated that the consequences of unrelieved obstruction to a ventricle emphasise the need for

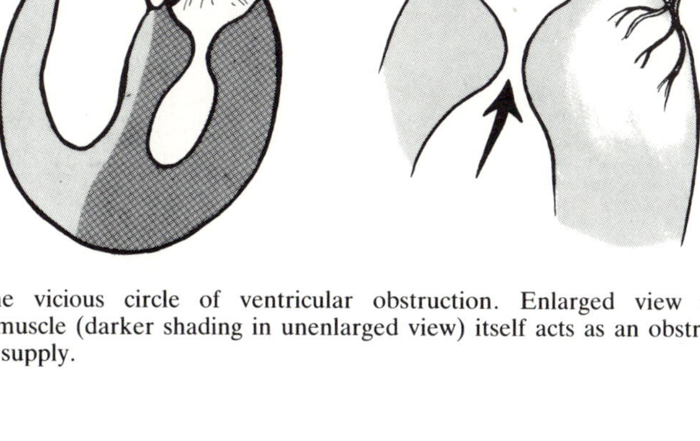

Fig. 2.16. The vicious circle of ventricular obstruction. Enlarged view shows how the hypertrophied muscle (darker shading in unenlarged view) itself acts as an obstruction and has a deficient blood supply.

early relief of obstruction before this cycle is established, and often before symptoms develop.

Where there is regurgitation of blood through a valve, the heart is generally better able to adapt itself to the strain of a volume overload, at least in the initial stages. The cavity of the atrium or ventricle enlarges, and the ventricular stroke volume increases to maintain adequate forward flow. When the ventricle fails in this situation, the progression of events tends to be more gradual, though no less serious in its consequences.

Further Reading

Anderson RH. Cardiac morphology. In: Julian DG, Camm AJ, Fox KM, Hall RJC, Poole-Wilson PA (eds) Diseases of the heart. Baillière Tindall, London, 1989, pp 1–23

Caro CG, Pedley TJ, Schroter RC, Seed WA. The mechanics of the circulation. Oxford University Press, Oxford, 1978

McAlpine WA. Heart and coronary arteries. An anatomical atlas for clinical diagnosis, radiological investigation, and surgical treatment. Springer-Verlag, Berlin, 1975

Poole-Wilson PA. A brief account of the physiology of the heart and circulation. In: Julian DG, Camm AJ, Fox KM, Hall RJC, Poole-Wilson PA (eds) Diseases of the heart. Baillière Tindall, London, 1989, pp 24–36

Walmsley R. Anatomy of left ventricular outflow tract. Br Heart J 1979; 41: 263–267

Walmsley R, Watson H. Clinical anatomy of the heart. Churchill Livingstone, Edinburgh, 1978

Wilcox BR, Anderson RH. Surgical anatomy of the heart. Gower Medical Publishing, London, 1985

Chapter 3

Clinical Aspects of Cardiac Diagnosis

Few undertakings in medicine will reward the physician with greater satisfaction than the clinical examination of the cardiovascular system. A carefully elicited history combined with skilful observation of physical signs will often provide sufficient information to make a diagnosis, while the expeditious use of complementary invasive and non-invasive investigations provides for immediate confirmation or revision of this impression. Because effective medical or surgical treatment is available for most cardiac conditions, accurate diagnosis readily benefits the patient with appropriate therapy, and the physician can observe the results of treatment in a comparatively short period of time. In addition, there has been a recent trend to recommend surgery for many operable lesions without cardiac catheterisation. This again places great responsibility upon the surgeon to satisfy himself that the preoperative clinical diagnosis is both accurate and complete.

Classification of Surgical Heart Disease

A simple but complete classification of heart disease is an essential aid to differential diagnosis. By attention to special clinical points, the diagnostic possibilities are narrowed down further. Special investigations may be used to confirm or further elucidate the nature of the lesion from anatomical and physiological points of view.

A broad distinction between congenital and acquired heart disease in adults is generally easy to make. For example, with an uncomplicated atrial septal defect, the lesion has obviously been present from birth: the bulging ribs over the precordium serve as evidence of an enlarged, overactive heart from an early age, before the final moulding and adult structure of the rib cage has taken place. In contrast, conditions such as isolated aortic valve stenosis continue to be a source of controversy when discovered in middle life. In some cases, the calcified valve is evidence of atherosclerotic sclerosis, which would normally occur later in life, or of previous rheumatic infection. In others, it can be explained as a congenital deformity, asymptomatic during early life but later, due to calcification of the deformed leaflets, constituting a significant and rigid obstruction. The distinction is mainly academic, for the important point is to establish a diagnosis of obstruction at the aortic valve. In contrast, mitral valve disease and aortic stenosis, when they coexist, almost certainly establishes the latter condition as one of acquired rheumatic heart disease.

The vast majority of heart defects encountered in infants and children will, of course, be congenital lesions. But it should not be forgotten that infection and metabolic disorders also may produce acquired cardiac disease early in life.

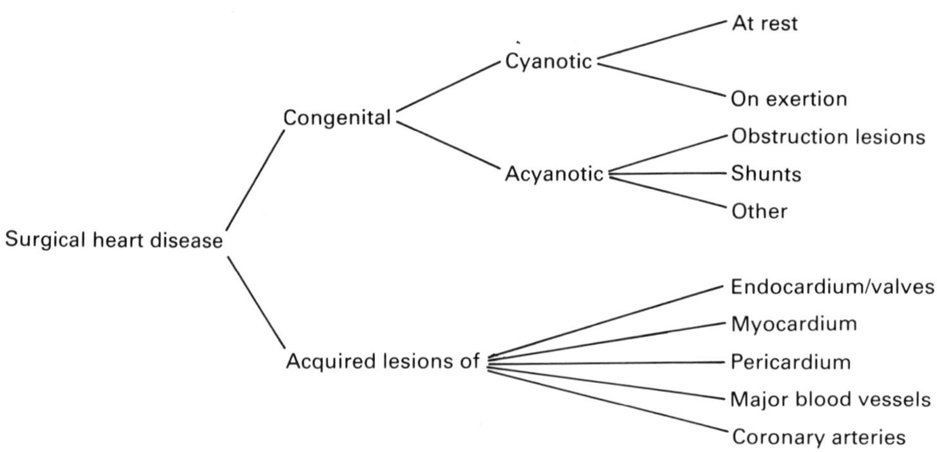

Fig. 3.1. Classification of surgical heart disease.

History

While the standard schemes of history-taking are likely to give all the required information, they may include a good deal of irrelevant detail, and a direct approach with some leading questions is often more productive. One's scheme of questioning will depend, to some extent, on whether the case is one of suspected congenital or acquired heart disease. Information should be deliberately sought on the following points:

1. Breathlessness
2. Chest pain
3. Syncope
4. Palpitation
5. Oedema
6. Haemoptysis

7. Cyanosis
8. Fatigue
9. Claudication
10. Emboli

Breathlessness or Dyspnoea. In its simplest form this represents an awareness of breathing; it is frequently a prominent symptom. It may be central in origin from abnormal drive to the respiratory centre, which gives a pattern of periodic breathing in congestive heart failure (Cheyne–Stokes respiration). But, more commonly in heart disease, its cause lies in loss of elasticity in the lungs. Passive congestion resulting from left heart failure or valvular obstruction, or active congestion from increased pulmonary blood flow with a left-to-right shunt causes the lungs to become turgid and more difficult to inflate. Related manifestations of dyspnoea arising from pulmonary congestion include cough, chestiness, wheezing and recurrent bronchitis. In patients with cyanotic congenital heart defects, breathlessness results from increasing hypoxia and may be accompanied by increased cyanosis or loss of consciousness.

It is useful to fix in some simple manner the point at which dyspnoea appears; for example, the distance that can be walked on the flat or, more usefully, the number of stairs or the distance uphill that a patient can climb at a normal rate without having to rest. If a note is made of this information, it is a good guide by which to judge subsequent improvement or deterioration.

Dyspnoea occurring in the recumbent position is called orthopnea and probably results from increased venous return to the right heart and lungs which cannot be dispatched by a failing or obstructed left ventricle. A similar mechanism may explain paroxysmal nocturnal dyspnoea, in which the patient is awakened by breathlessness and must sit up to obtain relief.

Chest Pain. Chest pain occurs in many forms of surgical heart disease. Excruciating pain in the anterior chest and radiating to the back is characteristic of acute dissection of the aorta, while pleuritic pain in the side of the chest often signifies infarction of the underlying lung consequent to pulmonary thrombosis or embolism. Angina, or cardiac pain occurs when there is a discrepancy between the amount of blood available to and required by the myocardium. This may be due to an increase in the cardiac muscle mass, as results, for example, from systemic hypertension or aortic stenosis. In such cases, angina may occur even though there is a normal coronary arterial tree. In contrast, the coronaries may be narrowed so that they do not deliver enough blood to the muscle. Alternatively, the cardiac output may be insufficient to meet the heart's requirements, in spite of good muscle and coronary arteries. Several of these factors, for example hypertrophy, low cardiac output and coronary disease, may coexist.

If angina is regarded only as substernal pain brought on by exercise and restricted to the classical paths of radiation to the arm, neck, jaw and epigastrum, many cases will be overlooked. It may be only a disagreeable sensation of pressure or tightness, and occasionally is experienced more consciously at other points than the left precordium. While, typically, the pain is precipitated by exertion and relieved by rest, it may occur during cold weather or after eating, or even wake the patient from sleep. An episode not precipitated by activity and lasting longer than a few minutes suggests myocardial infarction.

Ischaemic pain of cardiac origin, then, may be expected with any severe stenotic lesion, and the symptom can often be elicited in cases of pulmonary stenosis or severe mitral stenosis, as well as aortic valve obstruction and coronary artery disease. Less frequently, obstruction of a coronary ostia by tumour or clot, or by dissection of the aorta, also will cause pain from myocardial ischaemia. The pain experienced during a 'spell' in cyanotic heart disease probably originates from the hypoxic myocardium.

Syncope. Fainting or syncope, of cardiac origin, occurs classically in aortic stenosis and its cause on effort is not known with certainty. It may be related reflexly to the very high pressure generated in the left ventricle (in some cases over 400 mmHg has been recorded) or to a decrease in cerebral blood flow as peripheral resistance falls secondary to exercise.

Syncope is, however, by no means exclusively related to severe aortic stenosis. Pulmonary valve stenosis and mitral stenosis with pulmonary hypertension may give rise to a history of syncope on exertion. These latter conditions are generally associated with a fixed low cardiac output that cannot increase with exercise. A less common cause of paroxysmal fainting is a ball-valve thrombus or myxoma of the left atrium intermittently impacting in the mitral orifice.

Palpitation. This is the patient's awareness of his heartbeat. It may be because of increased force of contraction, as occurs with aortic regurgitation, or due to extra or irregular heartbeats. A typical example of the latter is atrial fibrillation, which often supervenes during the course of mitral valve disease.

Oedema. In many forms of heart disease oedema is a late occurrence, and the patient who gives a history of swollen legs, enlarging girth and weight gain will generally be found to have severe congestive heart failure. Characteristically, fluid accumulates in dependent areas, such that an ambulatory patient suffers oedema of the legs while a bedridden one will have sacral oedema. Oedema due to fluid retention in heart failure is often preceded by a history of dyspnoea and, typically, 'pits' on pressure.

Haemoptysis. Any of a number of different underlying pathological processes may be indicated by haemoptysis. Mitral stenosis is a common cause of this symptom. This may be due to bleeding from the congested bronchial mucosa, or from rupture of small congested capillaries. The pink blood-stained frothy sputum of pulmonary oedema is of different and more sinister significance. Patients with this symptom are in a precarious condition, and relief of their obstruction is a matter of urgency.

A more alarming but probably less dangerous form of haemoptysis is the sudden coughing, with little effort, of a large volume of bright red blood – so-called 'pulmonary apoplexy'. This generally occurs in cases with pulmonary venous hypertension, and the sudden loss of bright red pulmonary venous blood may give temporary relief, acting as a physiological venesection.

Another cause of haemoptysis, often with pleuritic pain, is pulmonary infarction. This may result from pulmonary embolism complicating peripheral venous thrombosis in the bedridden patient. Haemoptysis may also arise in cases of pulmonary arterial or venous thrombosis, where there has been a long-standing left-to-right shunt associated with pulmonary atheroma or increasing pulmonary hypertension. Pulmonary arterial thrombosis with massive infarction and haemoptysis is a classical terminal event in patients with Eisenmenger's syndrome.

The causes of haemoptysis can be summarised as:

Bronchitis
Pulmonary congestion (mitral stenosis)
Pulmonary oedema
Pulmonary 'apoplexy'
Pulmonary embolism
Pulmonary artery thrombosis

Cyanosis. The blue discolouration that results from excess reduced haemoglobin in the circulation can be appreciated by most observers at a level of 5 g/100 ml and thus will be influenced by anaemia as well as oxygen saturation. In patients with cyanosis, it is important to establish whether this is central or peripheral, and whether it has been present from birth (although it is quite frequently missed by parents in the early weeks of life) or came on at a later age. Where there is a history of cyanosis, one should enquire whether the child squats or has suffered 'spells' with loss of consciousness, since the combination of cyanosis with squatting or spells is characteristic of Fallot's tetralogy.

Severe cyanosis, squatting and cyanotic attacks with syncope are features suggestive of pulmonary atresia or tricuspid atresia in older childen. Nevertheless, where the degree of cyanosis is disproportionately great even though the child is surprisingly active and not greatly incapacitated, one should suspect the possibility of complex transposition of the great vessels.

Cyanosis developing later in life or coming on only with exertion is likely to be due to the late reversal of a previous left-to-right shunt. An exception to this is the condition of ventricular septal defect with infundibular pulmonary stenosis ('acyanotic' Fallot) where variable obstruction by the infundibular muscle may modify the right-to-left shunt.

Fatigue and Weakness. These are such widespread symptoms and result from such a variety of conditions that their usefulness as an indicator of heart disease is limited. None the less, a patient with inadequate cardiac output may well experience exhaustion or tiredness.

Claudication. This is the peripheral counterpart of angina and signifies an inadequate blood supply to skeletal muscle groups. While the usual cause is peripheral vascular disease, emboli from the heart may be responsible for arterial insufficiency. A history of atheroclerosis in peripheral vessels, conversely, should alert one to the likelihood of coronary atherosclerosis. When claudication is severe, the patient may be so limited in his capacity to exercise that he does not provoke angina, despite the presence of narrowed coronary vessels.

Emboli. Release of clot from the left atrium into the circulation is not uncommon in patients with established atrial fibrillation, and a past history of strokes or vascular insufficiency in the limbs should be sought in such cases. Rarely, emboli may occur in the presence of sinus rhythm, and this should arouse suspicion of bacterial endocarditis or a friable left atrial myxoma. Either may shed particles into the systemic circulation. The presence of a septal defect allows the potential for emboli from the left side of the heart to enter the pulmonary circulation, or emboli from the venous side to pass into the systemic circulation.

Functional Capacity

It may be useful to summarise the degree of disability experienced by a patient with cardiac disease in terms of the amount of activity required to bring on symptoms. The classification adopted by the New York Heart Association (Table 3.1) has been used widely for both this purpose and in relation to the results of surgical treatment.

Table 3.1. New York Heart Association classification of functional class

Class I	No limitation of physical activity
Class II	Slight limitation; symptoms brought on by more than ordinary physical activity
Class III	Marked limitation; symptoms on less than ordinary activity
Class IV	Symptoms present even at rest and without any physical activity

Family and Past History

The metabolic disorders underlying some types of coronary atherosclerosis may be genetically transmitted and reflected in a family history of myocardial infarction at an early age. Enquiry may reveal a past history of rheumatic fever, chorea, scarlet fever or severe tonsillitis, though this is by no means invariable in cases of rheumatic heart disease. Maternal rubella in early pregnancy can result in congenital heart disease, while a family history of heart disease may be relevant in other congenital lesions.

Physical Examination

General

The paramount importance of a thorough examination at the bedside cannot be over-emphasised. In general, a careful physical examination will yield more information than long detailed histories and elaborate investigations.

The patient should be at ease on a firm couch or high hospital bed, with the head and shoulders raised at an angle of about 30°. If the patient is on a low bed,

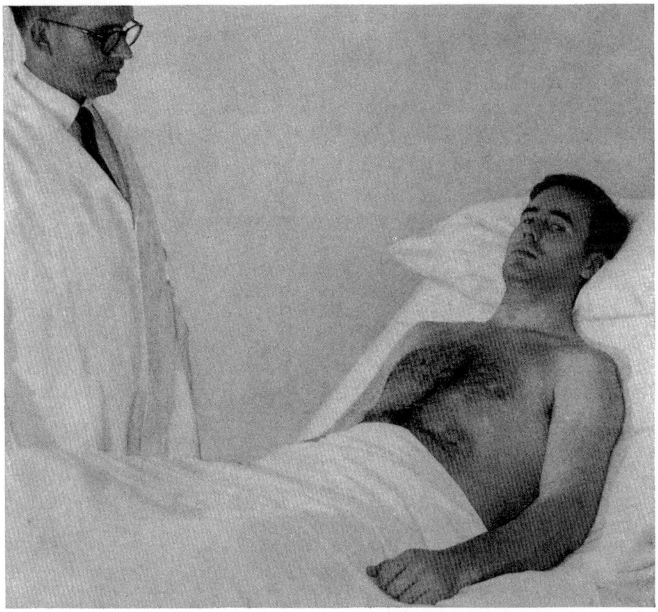

Fig. 3.2. Patient in position for examination at an angle of about 30°, relaxed and in a good light.

the doctor should sit on a chair at the patient's side. The room should be warm and quiet if one is to assess degrees of cyanosis, the state of the peripheral circulation, the pulses and heart murmurs. The legs and toes must be accessible for inspection and palpation.

Little of definite value can be learned from the general physical build, but bulging and deformity of the chest in the region of the precordium may provide a clue to the presence of a congenital heart lesion with long-standing cardiac enlargement. Quite frequently, older patients with ventricular septal defect have a prominent sternum. Skeletal stigmata of the Marfan's syndrome should alert one to the possibility of aortic dissection or valvar regurgitation, while underdevelopment of the lower extremities, suggests coarctation of the aorta. Patients with severe mitral disease are often thin and have a purple malar flush; with associated tricuspid disease there may be, in addition, brown pigmentation of the skin.

A number of chromosomal abnormalities that produce recognisable syndromes are associated frequently with characteristic heart lesions. Most common are Down's syndrome (persistent ductus arteriosus and septal defects), Turner's syndrome (coarctation of the aorta), William's syndrome (supravalvar stenosis), DiGeorge syndrome (aortic arch anomalies), and Noonan's syndrome (valvar pulmonary stenosis).

Cyanosis

A patient may be obviously cyanosed, doubtfully cyanosed, or of a normal colour. Central cyanosis suggests the presence of a right-to-left intracardiac shunt or less commonly, a pulmonary arteriovenous fistula. Red cheeks and bright lips may conversely indicate a left-to-right shunt. Cyanosis is caused by the presence of reduced haemoglobin in the visible vessels of the skin and mucous membranes. It may be peripheral or central in distribution. The former is present in a number of conditions with inadequate peripheral circulation and also may be a sign of severe low cardiac output. Central cyanosis is best detected in the 'warm' areas, that is, lips, conjunctivae and tongue.

In general, the presence of central cyanosis indicates the mixing of venous and arterial blood within the heart or major arteries, but one should keep in mind the possibility of cyanosis due to other conditions, such as lung disease, pulmonary arteriovenous fistula, methaemoglobinaemia and blue dyes.

It is convenient to record the degree of cyanosis observed according to a simple grading. This enables one to judge deterioration or improvement, particularly in the Fallot type of conditions. Four grades of severity can be distinguished.

Grade I. This is cyanosis on exertion only, as might be seen in a patient with a ventricular septal defect and mild pulmonary stenosis. Here, right-to-left shunting would not occur until exercise caused a fall in systemic resistance. In the absence of pulmonary stenosis, cyanosis on exercise in lesions with a predominantly left-to-right shunt is, however, more ominous. Here it may indicate increasing pulmonary vascular resistance.

Grade II. This is cyanosis of a mild degree at rest which is, as a rule, detectable only to a trained observer. A corresponding arterial oxygen saturation would be about 85%. Interestingly, this is in theory the approximate value that would result from complete mixing of systemic and venous blood inside the heart. Such patients are often not regarded as being abnormally coloured by the casual observer.

Grade III. This degree of cyanosis is obvious to the lay observer and includes most cases of recognisable cyanotic heart disease. Arterial oxygen saturation is usually less than 75%.

Grade IV. This is cyanosis or blueness of an extreme degree, commonly seen in severely disabled cases of Fallot's tetralogy, pulmonary and tricuspid atresia, transposition of the great vessels and the terminal phases of reversed shunts.

Differential Cyanosis. An interesting subgroup of Grade I cyanosis is differential cyanosis, or cyanosis of the lower extremities with a normal pink colour of the arms and face. It is rarely seen at rest, and is more likely to be brought on by exertion. Generally, this indicates a reversal of blood flow through a persistent ductus arteriosus either as a result of pulmonary hypertension or consequent to obstruction of the aorta more proximally. Poorly oxygenated pulmonary arterial blood then mixes with that of the descending aorta supplying the lower limbs. With a hypertensive ductus arteriosus, pulmonary arterial blood may eventually flow proximally into the aortic arch, giving a variety of bizarre colour combinations. For example, one could have cyanosis of the feet and left hand together with the left half of the face as well. Such advanced pathology is now rarely encountered.

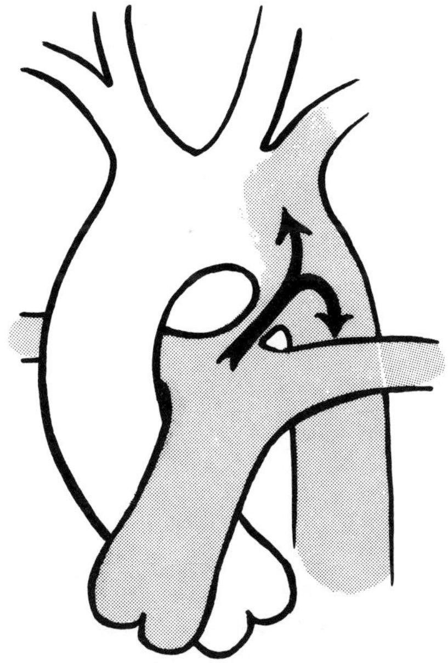

Fig. 3.3. With the reversal of blood flow through a ductus, desaturated blood (*shaded*) is directed to the lower half of the body and possibly the distal aortic arch.

Clubbing

An examination of the fingers should be part of the routine inspection of the hands preliminary to feeling the pulses. The hands are felt, to gain some estimate of the peripheral systemic blood flow: in conditions with low cardiac output they will be cold and the patient may complain of cold hands and feet. Attention should next be directed to the toes to assess the degree of clubbing and the peripheral circulation there. As with differential cyanosis, there may be differential clubbing of the toes in cases of persistent ductus arteriosus with reversed shunt.

The mechanism producing clubbing remains obscure. Clubbing is common in a large number of non-cardiac conditions, particularly suppurative lung disease and bronchial carcinoma. It may occur as part of the condition of pulmonary hypertrophic osteoarthropathy or hepatic failure. It may be mediated through circulation of a vasodilating factor, either arising as a secretion in the lungs or from failure of the lungs to 'remove' such a substance produced elsewhere. This would explain its occurrence in lung disease and also in conditions of right-to-left shunts, where a portion of the blood flow bypasses the lungs.

It is convenient also to grade the degree of clubbing noted.

Grade I. There is a filling in or loss of the angle between the nail and the nail bed. The latter is shiny and prominent. Clubbing appears first in the thumb and great toe, later progressing toward the smaller digits. It will be apparent in patients with even mild or doubtful cyanosis when this has been present for more than 3 months.

Grade II. In addition to the above features, there is a 'watch-glass' contour of the nails, with convexity in two planes, longitudinal as well as lateral.

Grade III. There is an increase in the volume of the soft tissue digital pulp, in addition to the above features.

Grade IV. This is an exaggerated stage of the above, with swelling of the tissues on each side of the nail bed.

Grade V. This is revealed as gross 'drum-stick' formation of the ends of the digits and may be associated with clubbing of the nose.

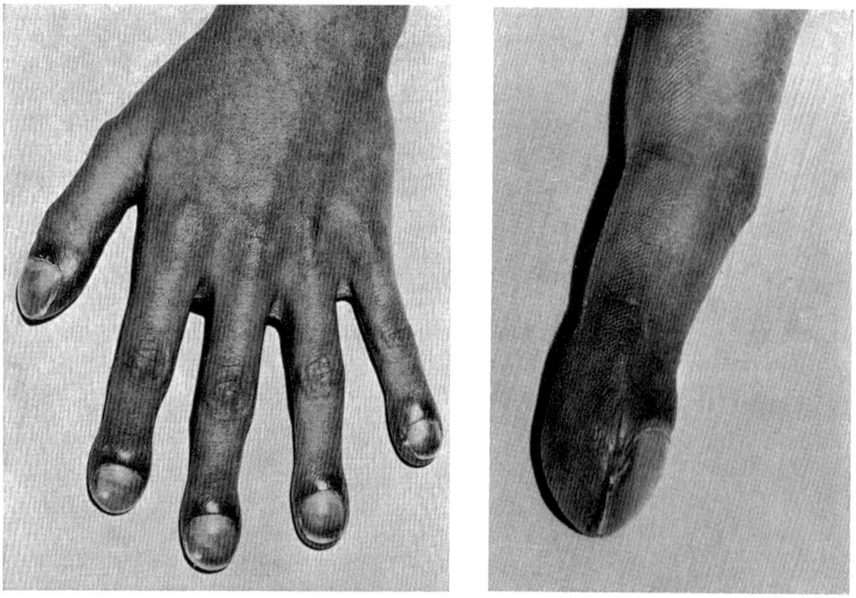

Fig. 3.4. Severe grade V clubbing demonstrating all the above features.

Oedema

During the general inspection and assessment of the patient, before examining the cardiovascular system more specifically, it is convenient to feel for pitting oedema of the ankles as a sign of raised systemic venous pressure or right heart decompensation. Firm pressure, maintained for 15–30 s, is necessary to detect minor pitting, and pressure should be against a firm background, for example the subcutaneous border of the tibia.

The fact that ankle oedema is unlikely in patients confined to bed should be kept in mind. In these cases, it is the sacral area which must be inspected, and digital pressure here will often reveal a considerable sacral pad of oedema. Where there is evidence of much fluid retention, signs of ascites and an enlarged liver should be sought.

Anaemia

Severe anaemia may mask the presence of cyanosis or, by increasing cardiac output, exacerbate symptoms of angina and congestive heart failure. Its presence should alert one to the possibility of endocarditis or haemolysis resulting from prosthetic valve dysfunction. Also, a history of bleeding in the context of anticoagulation for previous emboli, or prosthetic heart valves should be considered. Anaemia can often be detected by comparing the patient's palm with that of the examiner.

Jaundice

Jaundice occurring as the result of cardiac disease is usually of poor prognosis. While haemolysis from a prosthetic heart valve or a high-pressure jet of blood against a prosthetic patch may reach proportions sufficient to cause jaundice, it is more commonly a sign of hepatic dysfunction as the result of severe long-standing congestion or profound low cardiac output. Again, the hand may manifest palmar erythema.

The Cardiovascular System

In examining the heart itself one is evaluating the efficiency of two pumps working side by side. Consequently, we examine the output of the pumps (arterial pulses) and their ability to cope with their input of blood (venous pressure and pulse) and to feel for evidence of over-activity of one or other 'pump'. In addition, turbulence, as blood passes through narrow or irregular channels (thrills), may be detected.

Having made an assessment of the nature of the disorder and its most likely site, it is then useful to listen to the working of the pump in different areas, in order to gain more precise information. The sequence of a cardiovascular examination, then, is *inspection* followed by *palpation* and *cerebration*, and concluding with *auscultation*. Of these, cerebration is by far the most important.

Inspection of the Precordium

Note should be made of the shape and the movement of the precordium.

Shape. Bulging of the chest wall suggests the possibility of an enlarged and perhaps overactive heart from an early age – before firm moulding and ossification of the ribs took place. This would likely be due to a congenital heart lesion. Cases of isolated ventricular septal defect with raised pulmonary flow and resistance are said to commonly have a prominent narrow sternum (pigeon chest), but this finding is not invariable.

Movements. In thin-chested individuals, it is often possible to see areas of pulsation. Over-activity of the left ventricle is confined to the apex, while over-activity of the right ventricle and its outflow tract may be observed along the left sternal border. Again, an active hyperdynamic precordial impulse is suggestive of a volume-overloaded ventricle, while obstructive lesions of the heart are more often associated with a slower, more sustained type of pulsation. These features may be more apparent on palpation of the heart. The possibility of pulsation on the right side in dextrocardia should not be overlooked.

The Pulses

The arterial pulse provides information about the rate and regularity of the heart's action and, more important, gives some indication of the output of the

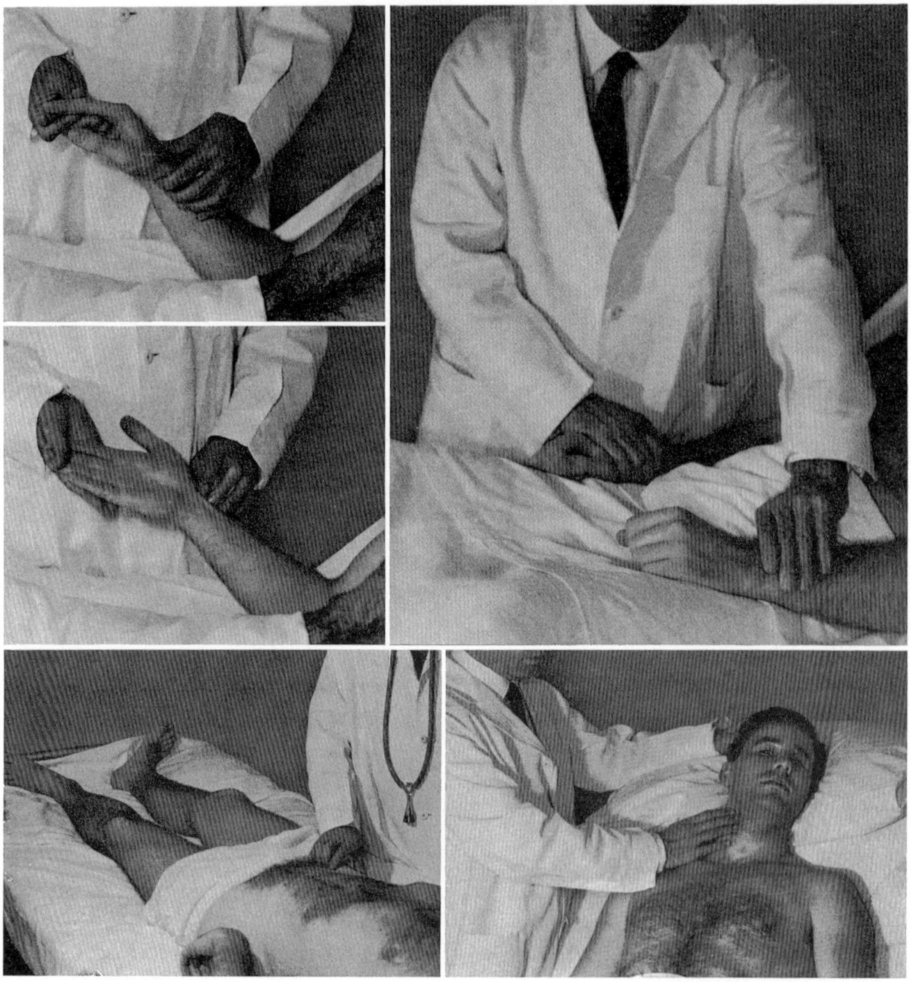

Fig. 3.5. The arterial pulse. *Upper left*: While feeling the radial pulse the fingers are inspected; they give an indication of the peripheral circulation and the nails are examined for clubbing. *Centre left*: While examining the pulse, the palm is inspected for the diffuse redness associated with hepatic dysfunction. *Upper right*: Both radial pulses should be felt and compared synchronously. *Lower left*: In feeling for the femoral pulses the feet should be in external rotation. *Lower right*: The carotid pulse may give valuable information with regard to the pulse contour and associated thrills may be felt.

left ventricle. Additional information can be inferred from the form of the pulse wave.

In examining the pulses it is important to take stock of as many as possible, certainly the carotids, both radials and both femorals. Peripheral transmission of the pulse changes its contour so that the ascending portion and systolic pressure become enhanced and the diastolic pressure becomes lower. Thus, the carotid pulse will represent events near the heart, while overall variations in the amplitude or contour of the pulse may be appreciated more easily in peripheral vessels. When the radial pulse is small and difficult to evaluate, the brachial or axillary pulse may be more helpful. The carotid pulse is often visible in the neck and its palpation will help to distinguish venous pulsation as well as to feel any thrill transmitted to the neck vessels from the aortic arch.

Absence of a pulse (with possible exception of the dorsalis pedis, which is congenitally absent in about one-tenth of the population) is always significant. A diagnosis of coarctation of the aorta can be made immediately; in mitral stenosis with atrial fibrillation, it may provide the only evidence of systemic embolism. In a man with absent femoral pulses, the aortic pulse in the epigastrium should be sought next: if it is present and the femorals are absent, the diagnosis is likely to be aortic thrombosis (Leriche syndrome) and not coarctation.

The normal pulse has a moderately rapid upstroke coinciding with ventricular ejection. As the left ventricular pressure falls, the aortic and ventricular pressures then fall to their different diastolic levels, that in the ventricle being normally close to zero.

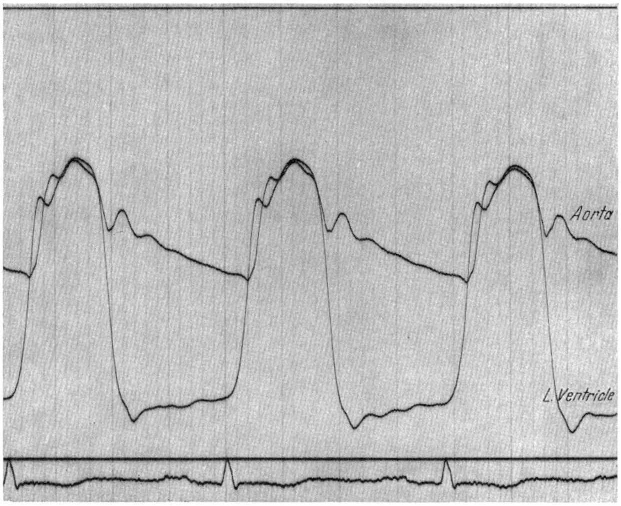

Fig. 3.6. This record shows synchronous pressure tracings from the left ventricle and aorta.

The contour of the pulse changes in severe aortic stenosis because the ejection phase of the left ventricle is prolonged. This produces a flattened type of pulse wave – the so-called slow rising or 'plateau' pulse. A bounding pulse easily visible in the neck and clearly perceptible on palpation should raise the possibilities of persistent ductus arteriosus, aortic incompetence, or an arteriovenous fistula. Where the aortic valve is incompetent, or where there is some other type of rapid run-off from the systemic circulation in diastole, there will be an abrupt fall in pressure during diastole to an abnormally low level. This is the 'collapsing' or 'Corrigan's' pulse. There results also an increased left ventricular stroke volume, producing a rapid upstroke in the arterial wave form. With the patient's wrist elevated, it is often possible to feel such a radial pulse as a slapping impulse against the flat of the hand, reminiscent of the movement of a 'water hammer'. Other features of this haemodynamic state are marked arterial pulsation in the neck, sometimes with movement of the ear lobes, capillary pulsation (best seen in the nail beds and lips) and audible pulse sounds when listening over the brachial or femoral arteries.

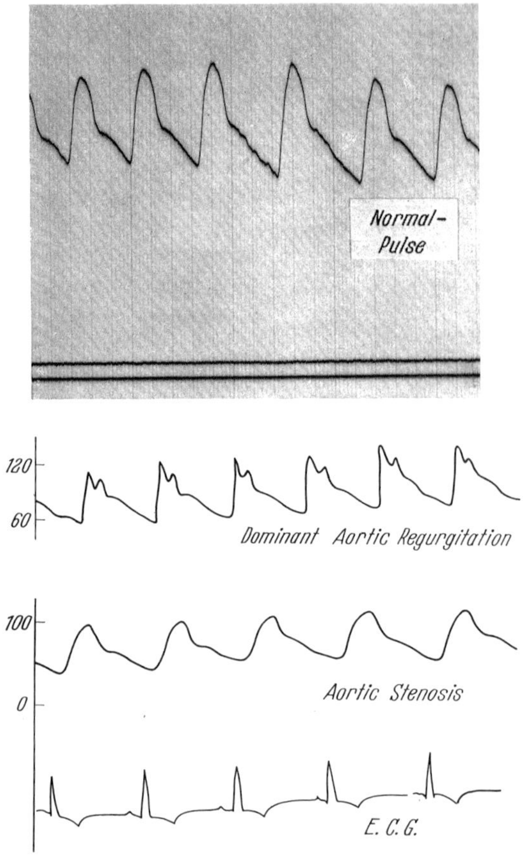

Fig. 3.7. Pulse curves in a normal subject and in cases of aortic regurgitation and aortic stenosis.

Disturbances of rhythm such as atrial fibrillation can also be detected and a number of other characteristic pulse irregularities have been described and are commonly encountered in surgical practice.

Pulsus Bigeminus. This is a disturbance of rhythm where the impulses are coupled, giving alternating strong and weak beats. The first of the coupled beats

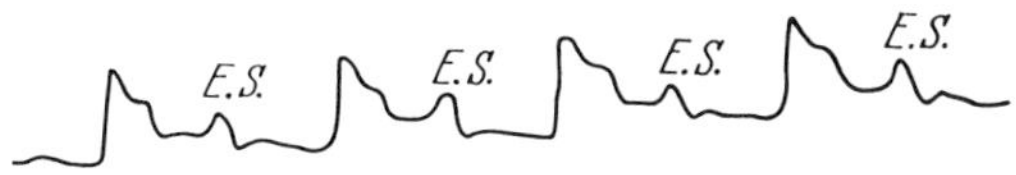

Fig. 3.8. Pulse tracing showing pulsus bigeminus. Each normal beat is followed by an extrasystole (E.S.) and a compensatory pause.

is a larger than normal pulsation due to the compensatory pause following the extrasystole. Pulsus bigeminus may be a sign of digitalis intoxication.

Pulsus Alternans. This is a disturbance of force. Here, beats are regular (i.e. there is no compensatory pause) but each alternate beat is of reduced form or amplitude. It is of grave prognostic significance and generally indicates severe left ventricular failure, resulting from hypertension, coronary artery disease or aortic stenosis.

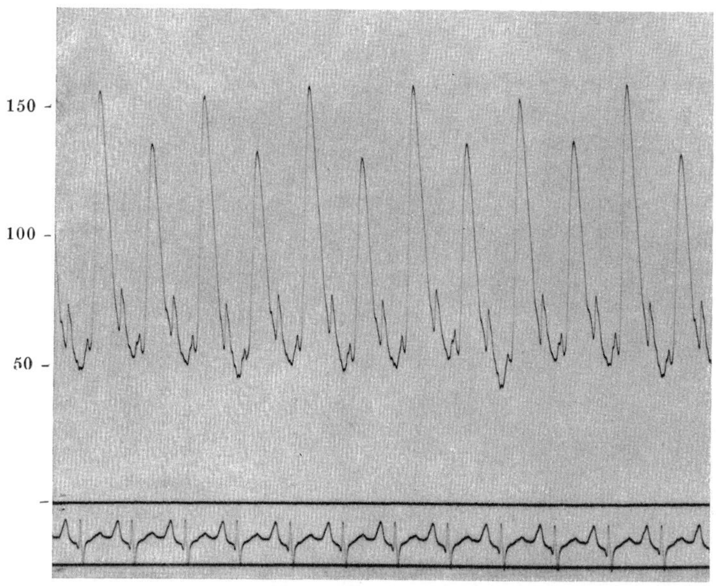

Fig. 3.9. Pulse contour in a case of pulsus alternans. Each successive beat has reduced or increased force.

Pulsus Paradoxus. In normal circumstances, a deep inspiration reduces intrathoracic pressure and causes pooling of blood within the pulmonary circulation and a slight (3–10 mmHg) decrease in systemic blood pressure. When there is limitation of diastolic filling of the heart, for example, by constrictive pericarditis, this decline in blood pressure is more pronounced. Indeed, the peripheral pulse may become impalpable, while paradoxically, the heart sounds are unchanged. A wide variety of conditions may produce pulsus paradoxus, including obstruction of the superior vena cava, pulmonary disease, severe congestive heart failure and pericardial tamponade.

Blood Pressure

The assessment of the blood pressure with a sphygmomanometer is an important part of the examination. In cases of persistent ductus arteriosus and aortic incompetence the systolic blood pressure will be high and the diastolic pressure low. This produces a wide *pulse pressure*. The converse occurs in aortic stenosis or severe low cardiac output, where the systolic pressure is low and there is a small fall in pressure during diastole: this produces a narrow pulse pressure.

When the blood pressure in the arms is unexpectedly high, the possibility of coarctation of the aorta should be considered and blood pressure in the leg measured. On the other hand, where a diagnosis of coarctation has been made and the systemic blood pressure is lower than anticipated, it is well to remember the possibility of coarctation with associated aortic stenosis or an anomalous right subclavian artery arising below the coarctation.

The measurement of blood pressure at frequent intervals is of great value in the postoperative management of cardiac surgical cases, particularly in helping to assess shock and haemorrhage. It can also be of value in the early detection of systemic embolism within the arterial tree. For example, after mitral valvotomy a rise in blood pressure may be the first sign of this complication, preceding evidence of ischaemia or loss of function in the area of occlusion. After closure of a persistent ductus arteriosus, there is usually narrowing of the pulse pressure as a result of obliterating the fistulous leak. In coarctation, the blood pressure may not fall immediately postoperatively and may actually rise, emphasising that mechanical obstruction of the aorta is not the only factor maintaining the high blood pressure. The pressure usually falls slowly over a period of several days or weeks.

The Venous Pulse

This may yield a great deal of information and is best studied on the right side of the neck. The patient should be sitting up at an angle of about 30°, and there should be a good and movable light source for tangential illumination.

The first observation to be made is the level of the venous pressure, by noting the height to which the veins are distended above the level of the right atrium or, conventionally, the sternal angle. The right hand should gently compress the region of the liver or right hypochondrium. This increases the venous pressure and distends the external jugular vein – the so-called hepatojugular reflex. This manoeuvre also helps to emphasise venous pulsation and, at the same time, gives an indication of the size and tenderness of the liver.

The next feature to be examined is the venous pulsation, and to distinguish this from arterial pulsation. Apart from the position of the pulse in the line of the veins, venous pulsation has a rapid flicking quality unlike arterial pulsation. Also, venous waves are more easily seen than felt.

Normally, three waves are detected, *a*, *c* and *v*, and they can be most conveniently timed by listening to the heart sounds while observing the venous pulsation. The *a* wave just precedes the first heart sound and the *v* follows the second sound. The *c* wave, in between, just follows the first heart sound. In addition to the three positive waves, two negative waves or pressure deflections are described – the *x* and *y* descents.

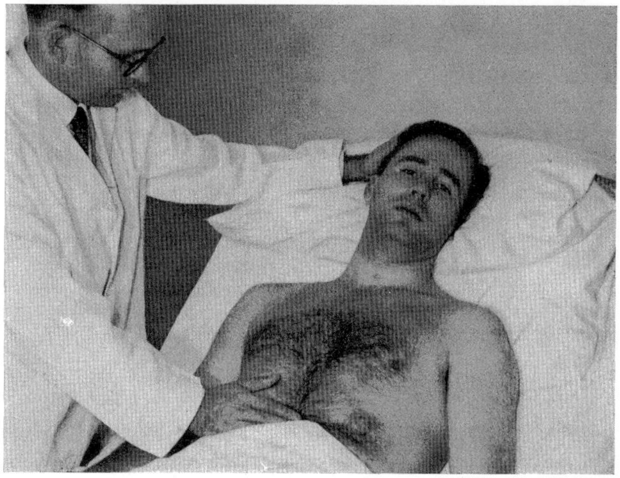

Fig. 3.10. For inspection of the jugular pulse, the neck muscles should be relaxed. Pressure exerted with the right hand over the liver will elicit the hepato-jugular reflex.

The a *Wave*. This is due to atrial contraction, which briefly increases atrial pressure. Usually, it is the largest visible positive wave and may be enhanced by inspiration. It is absent in atrial fibrillation and will coincide with a fourth heart sound when this is present. Accentuation of the *a* wave is suggestive of tricuspid or pulmonary valve stenosis.

The c *Wave*. There has been a good deal of controversy regarding the *c* wave, so-called because it is coincident with the carotid pulse and, therefore, synchronous with ventricular systole. It is not due only to the carotid pulse in the neck, as can be demonstrated by its presence in cardiac catheterisation pressures recorded from the right atrium. One explanation is that it arises from a displacement of the tricuspid valve cusps into the atrium. This is brought about by the rise of ventricular pressure during systole.

The x *Descent*. Following on from the *c* wave there is a decline in venous pressure towards the end of ventricular systole. This is because concentric contraction of the ventricles pulls down the atrioventricular ring, reducing right atrial pressure. Atrial relaxation may also make a contribution.

a

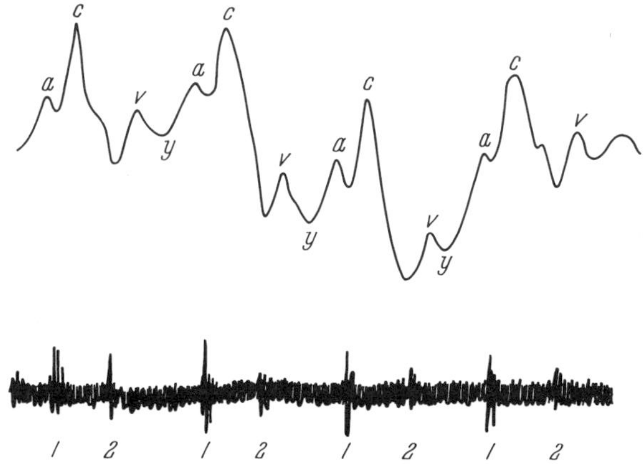

Fig. 3.11. The normal jugular phlebogram shown diagrammatically.

The v *Wave*. With the tricuspid valve firmly closed throughout ventricular systole, blood continues to flow from both vena cava into the right atrium which is, at that time, virtually a closed chamber. There is, consequently, a progressive rise of right atrial pressure producing a positive *v* wave. Regurgitation of blood through an incompetent tricuspid valve will accentuate the *v* wave.

The y *Descent*. With the *y* descent the cardiac cycle is completed. When the ventricle relaxes, the pulmonary valve closes due to the fall in right ventricular pressure. When this falls below the right atrial pressure, the tricuspid valve opens and there follows a rapid decrease in right atrial pressure as blood pours from atrium to ventricle. This fall of pressure is reflected in the venous pulse as the *y* descent.

In the presence of *tricuspid stenosis*, the right atrial pressure will be high and there will be elevation of pressure throughout the venous system. Also, with normal rhythm, there will be increased force of right atrial contraction producing large *a* waves. The rate of the *y* descent will be slow because, during diastole, blood can only escape slowly from the right atrium across the narrow valve orifice into the right ventricle.

Giant a *Waves*. These represent a high pressure in the right atrium and can occur from any cause of obstruction to right atrial emptying. Thus right ventricular hypertrophy, pulmonary hypertension or pulmonary stenosis may be the cause. Resistance to right ventricular filling may also be increased by septal hypertrophy either as an isolated condition or as a part of left ventricular (and septal) hypertrophy – the Bernheim phenomenon.

Giant v *Waves*. In tricuspid rugurgitation, there occurs a reflux of blood into the right atrium during ventricular systole, causing an exaggerated rise of atrial pressure coincident with systolic contraction of the ventricle. These reflux systolic waves are giant *v* waves. Large *v* waves have been described also in atrial septal defect, particularly in children, due to excessive filling of the right atrium against a closed tricuspid valve. In this case, filling is not only from the vena cava but also from the left atrium.

Cannon Waves. Large positive venous waves at the time of atrial contraction occur characteristically in complete heart block. In these circumstances, there is dissociation between atrial and ventricular contractions. When they occur at the same time, the right atrium contracts against a closed and even prolapsed tricuspid valve, producing a steep rise of pressure in the jugular veins.

Left Atrial Pressure Waves. A venous wave pattern identical with that found in the right atrium can be recorded from the left atrium either by direct puncture at operation or trans-septal catheterisation. Left atrial pressure can also be inferred indirectly from the pulmonary capillary venous tracing obtained at cardiac catheterisation or from a Swan–Ganz catheter. A study of such left atrial pressure waves may be helpful in diagnosing and distinguishing mitral stenosis and regurgitation and left ventricular dysfunction, particularly the diastolic function.

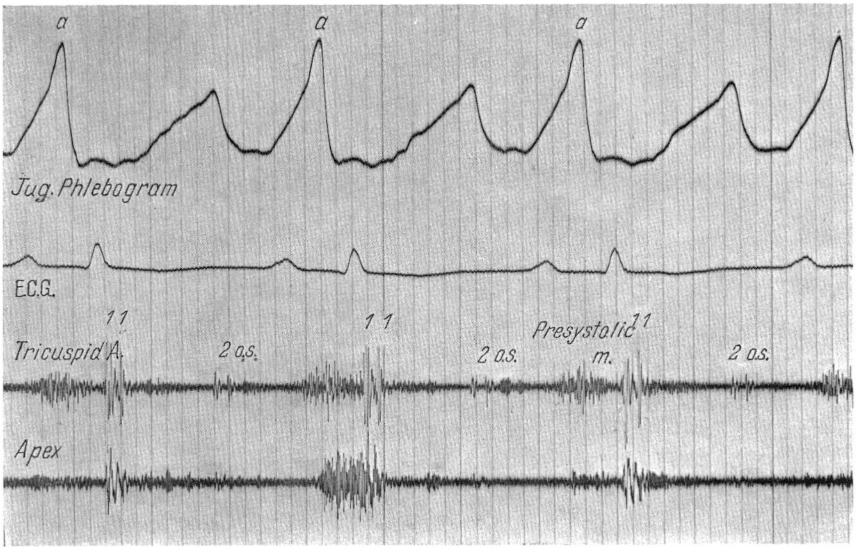

Fig. 3.12. Giant *a* waves in a case of tricuspid stenosis. O.S., Opening snap; m, murmur.

Palpation of the Liver

The liver is felt as part of the examination of the venous pulse when trying to elicit the hepatojugular reflex, as noted previously. Additional information should be obtained with regard to (a) size, (b) tenderness and (c) pulsation.

In right heart failure or right heart obstruction the liver is likely to be enlarged and may be painful or tender as the result of distension of its capsule. When a fluctuating venous pressure is transmitted to it from the heart, the liver will also be pulsatile. Thus, in tricuspid valve stenosis and regurgitation, there may be marked liver pulsation in time with the venous pulse. Occasionally, liver pulsation will be more easily observed than other signs of tricuspid valve disease or right heart failure.

True liver pulsation should be distinguished, by its timing, from systolic pulsations transmitted from the ventricles or aorta through the liver.

Palpation of the Ventricles

This is one of the most important parts of the clinical examination of the heart. By this means, it should be possible to assess which ventricle carries the burden of the cardiac lesion and, also, the nature of this burden. Examination is for evidence of (a) which ventricle is under strain and (b) whether the load is obstructive in nature or is due to an increased stroke volume.

The *left ventricular impulse* is normally felt at the apex of the heart in the region of the left nipple or just below the left breast in a woman. It is the most lateral and lowest point at which a finger is lifted on the precordium. Generally a localised impulse, in standard schemes of cardiological examination, the 'apex beat' is usually noted in relation to the ribs and its distance from the midline or the mid-clavicular line. This position can vary widely however, depending upon underlying lung disease and physical build. In many patients, it can be felt with certainty only by tipping the patient to the left, a manoeuvre which itself displaces the apex beat. Thus, the assessment of the *nature* of the left ventricular impulse is of far greater value than a description of its position.

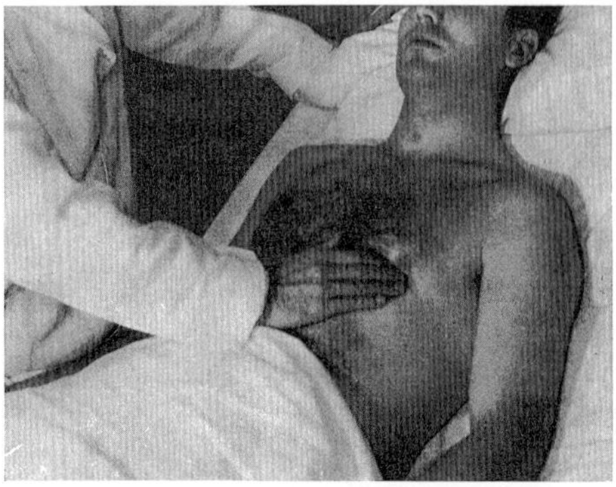

Fig. 3.13. The position of the left ventricular impulse is located.

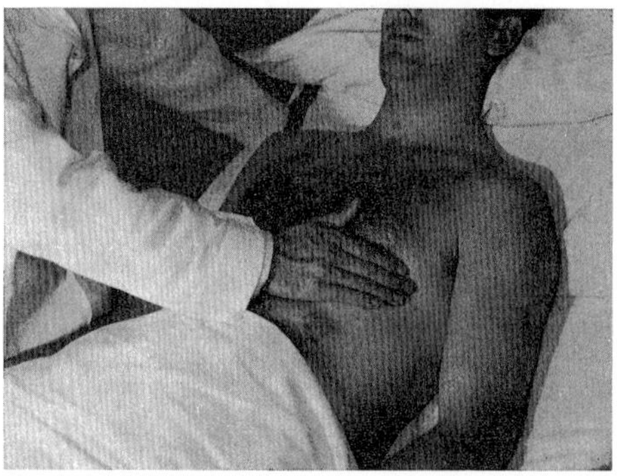

Fig. 3.14. Evaluation of the left ventricular activity – force and character of the impulse.

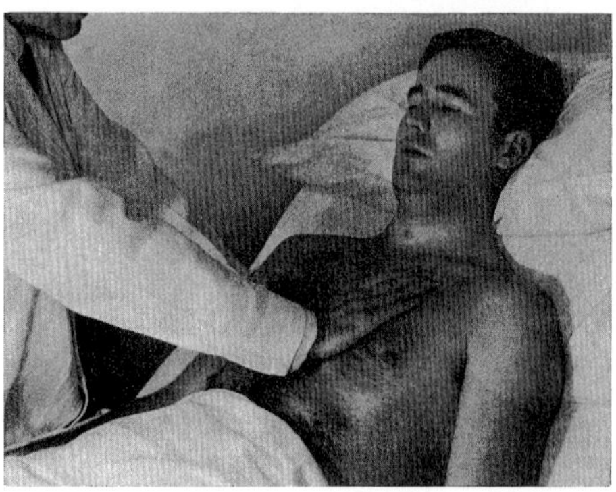

Fig. 3.15. The right ventricular impulse is felt along the left sternal border.

Where the left ventricle is *obstructed*, as in aortic stenosis, it will be hypertrophied and will transmit a localised but powerful heaving and sustained type of impulse to the flat of the hand. Where the left ventricle is pumping *extra volumes* of blood, as in ventricular septal defect, persistent ductus arteriosus or aortic incompetence, the impulse from the now enlarged left ventricle may be diffuse, but its character will be more active, turbulent and hyperdynamic.

Similar observations apply to the right ventricle. The *right ventricular impulse* is palpable to the left of the sternum, normally, in the third and fourth interspaces, and again is felt best with the flat of the hand.

Obstructive lesions of the right ventricle also result in a sustained heave, but over a rather wider area than with the left ventricular impulse. This is best illustrated in pulmonary valve stenosis with intact ventricular septum, but it can be appreciated in most cases where pressure is increased in the right ventricle. When the right ventricle ejects an increased volume of blood, it becomes dilated and over-active such that one feels a diffuse, rocking impulse over the region of the right ventricular outflow. This is best illustrated in cases of atrial septal defect, where, in addition, the dilated and pulsating pulmonary artery may be felt over the second left interspace.

In assessing the work of the right or left ventricle, it is again convenient to grade it according to the degree of over-activity (load or volume work). This can be done on an arbitrary scale of 0 to ++++, the former being normal. An assessment made by the same observer on each examination can then be used to judge clinical improvement or deterioration.

Thrills and Palpable Sounds

The passage of blood through narrow segments or, alternatively, the passage of large volumes of blood through normal-sized channels, is liable to give rise to turbulent blood flow. This turbulence can be appreciated as a palpable vibration or, if less intense, as an audible murmur heard only with the stethoscope.

Murmurs may be audible over a confusingly wide area of the precordium and the site of maximal loudness may not be easy to determine. The palpable thrill, on the other hand, is less diffuse and consequently of greater value in localising the probable site of the lesion giving rise to the turbulence.

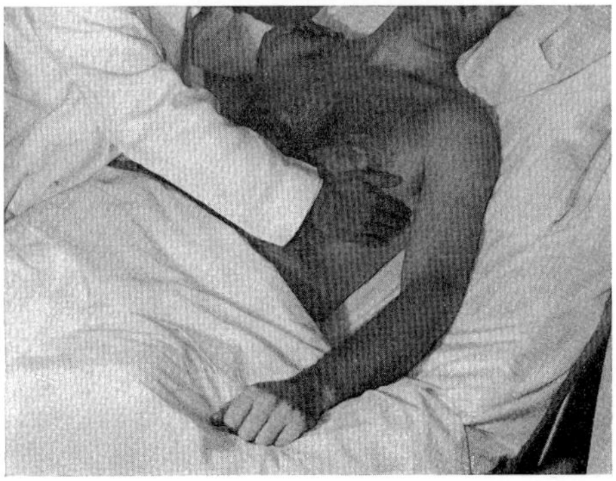

Fig. 3.16. In feeling for the mitral thrills the patient should be rolled slightly over towards the left.

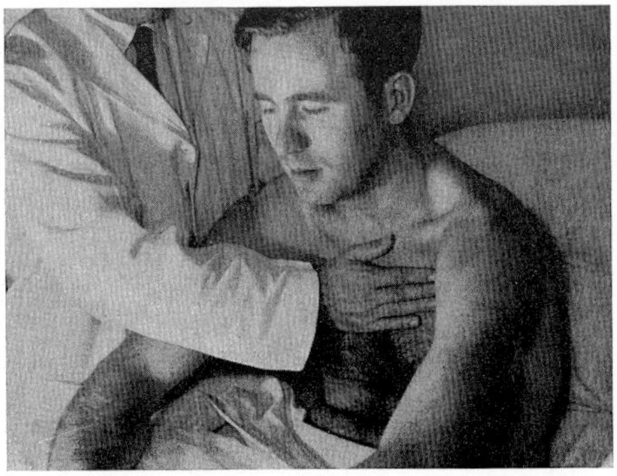

Fig. 3.17. Thrills emanating from the aortic and pulmonary valves are best felt with the patient sitting up and with the breath held in expiration.

In this way, obstructions at the aortic, mitral or pulmonary valves are often localised with accuracy by palpating a thrill at the appropriate area, while murmurs from these lesions (particularly in aortic stenosis) are likely to be widely conducted throughout the precordium.

The diastolic thrill of mitral stenosis is best felt with the patient rolled slightly over to the left. Thrills emanating from the base of the heart (aortic and pulmonary valves) are best felt with the patient sitting forward and with the breath held in expiration. The thrills of infundibular stenosis and of ventricular septal defect are generally felt in the third and fourth left interspaces respectively, and a muscular ventricular septal defect felt somewhat lower on the precordium.

Closure of the cardiac valves gives rise to the heart sounds but the shock waves they produce are not generally palpable. On the other hand, where valve closure is forceful and under increased pressure, the vibrations of the 'closing sound' can often be detected by the examining hand. Thus, in mitral stenosis the loud first sound and occasionally the 'opening snap' of the mitral valve may be felt at the patient's apex, and, in conditions with severe pulmonary hypertension, the forceful closure of the pulmonary valve can sometimes be felt over the base of the heart.

Summary Illustrating Some of the Foregoing Points in Clinical Diagnosis

Suppose that a young female patient presents with a history of breathlessness on exertion. Her pulses are small in volume and possibily reveal atrial fibrillation, her extremities are cold, suggesting a reduced cardiac output and there may be increased jugular venous pulsation.

Inspection of the precordium reveals a slight heave to the left of the sternum. On palpation, this is of a sustained nature in the distribution of the right ventricle and with the severity of + to ++. At the same time, a palpable second 'sound' over the base of the heart can be appreciated, suggesting, with the right ventricular heave, that the pulmonary artery pressure is raised. On palpation at the apex no left ventricular thrust or over-activity can be felt, but the slapping first 'sound' may be palpable and a thrill can be felt as the cardiac impulse recedes from the hand in diastole.

These findings can be summarised thus:

Small volume, irregular pulse
Cold periphery
RV++ LV0*
M_1 and P_2 palpable*
Diastolic thrill at apex

Thus, before recourse to the stethoscope, it is clear that this woman probably has mitral stenosis with some increase of her pulmonary artery pressure (pulmonary hypertension) as revealed by the over-active right ventricle, *a* wave and palpable pulmonary valve closure. The stethoscope can now be used as it

*RV++ = right ventricle, ++; LV0 = left ventricle, 0; M_1 = mitral component of first heart sound; P_2 = palmonary component of second heart sound.

should be used – in order to validate the previous findings and to assess them with more accuracy. In this case, it is not really being used to make the diagnosis.

In other words, what to listen *for* should be known on the basis of information available from inspection and palpation. Listening first is not the surest way to diagnosis, since the sensitive ear will give too much auditory information, confusing the clinical picture. With the clinical information already available, listening can be selective and give the maximum useful information.

In the present case, a loud mitral first sound is expected because it was palpable, and we know we shall hear a rumbling diastolic murmur as revealed by the thrill. Once observed these features can be noted quickly. Then listening can be more selective and careful, for an opening snap of the mitral valve, suggesting its pliability, and for the blowing systolic murmur which may suggest associated mitral or tricuspid regurgitation. Likewise, at the base, a loud second sound due to pulmonary hypertension is expected, possibly a basal diastolic murmur of, say, pulmonary regurgitation (the turbulence of which is not generally palpable).

Auscultation: Heart Sounds

As suggested above, the stethoscope can be most usefully employed in listening for specific features, with guidance from the history and other physical signs, and should not be regarded as the primary tool for making a diagnosis. However, accurate auscultation can elicit a great deal of information once the mechanism underlying the sounds and murmurs is understood. Consequently, the emphasis here is on an explanation of the 'mechanics' or underlying haemodynamics of the auditory phenomena. Thereafter, facility and skill in the use of the stethoscope will follow with diligence, practice and an intelligent application of the ear. The

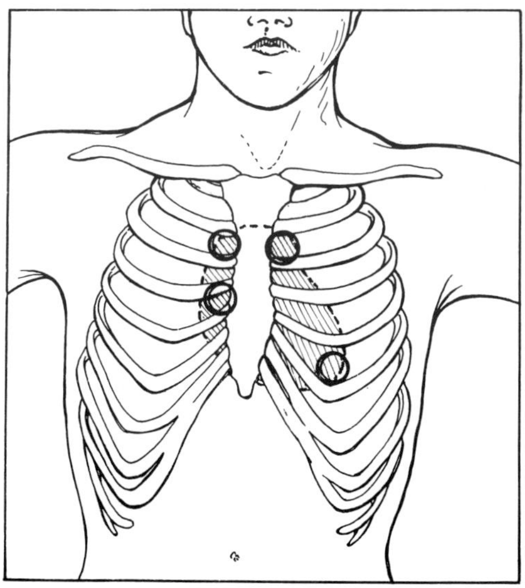

Fig. 3.18. Auscultatory areas of the precordium.

attitude of 'listening hopefully' for a diagnosis to present itself is unproductive and is to be avoided.

Two clearly defined sounds can be distinguished in each cardiac cycle and are readily heard over the whole precordium. The gap between the first and second sound represents the systolic phase of the cardiac cycle, and the rather longer gap before the next first sound represents the diastolic. Third and fourth heart sounds can be heard in certain circumstances by the trained observer, while a number of additional sounds can sometimes be perceived.

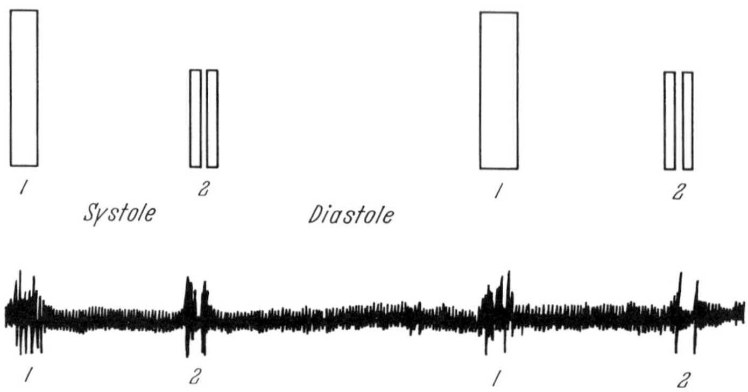

Fig. 3.19. Diagrammatic representation of the first and second heart sounds.

The First Heart Sound. This is probably caused almost wholly by closure of the mitral and tricuspid valves. Since it is the rule for electrical and mechanical events on the left side of the heart to slightly precede those on the right, the valves close asynchronously. Thus, under normal conditions, mitral valve closure precedes tricuspid valve closure, causing the first heart sound to be split into two components. The first component relates to closure of the mitral valve, and the second is due to closure of the tricuspid valve. This split of the first heart sound is not always clearly heard with the stethoscope, but it is a normal phenomenon and can be distinguished on the phonocardiogram. The first sound is heard most clearly when listening over the mitral and tricuspid areas of the heart. It is rather lower in pitch compared with the second sound, a factor which is said to be due to the muscular component of the sound.

The intensity of the first heart sound reflects both the mobility of atrioventricular valve leaflets (particularly the mitral valve) and their position at the time ventricular systole causes them to close. Rapid approximation of leaflets which were widely open, for example in tachycardia, produces a loud first heart sound. Delayed valve closure as the result of elevated left atrial pressure also accentuates the first heart sound, classically a sign of mitral stenosis with mobile valve cusps. Calcification of the mitral valve results in a soft first heart sound, as does poor left ventricular function, while a first heart sound of varying intensity suggests heart block with disassociated atrial and ventricular contractions.

The Second Heart Sound. This is most clearly heard over the base of the heart and is due to the closure of the aortic and pulmonary valves. As with the first heart sound, left heart events precede those of the right so that the second sound also is normally split, the aortic component (A_2) preceding that of the pulmonary (P_2). This splitting of the second sound at the base is easily heard in most normal people and is particularly conspicuous in children.

A characteristic feature of the second sound is the variation in splitting of the components with respiration. Normally, with inspiration there is increased filling of the right heart with blood so that the ejection phase of the right ventricle is prolonged. As a result, pulmonary valve closure is further delayed, and splitting of the second sound is therefore widened. On expiration the splitting again narrows. This is called 'physiological' splitting.

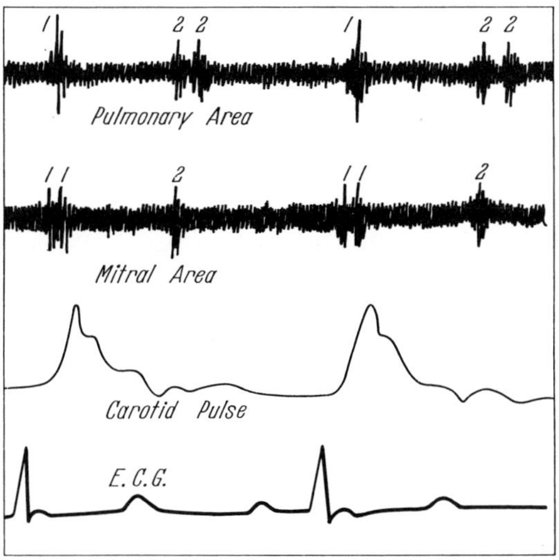

Fig. 3.20. Idealised figure representing the split of the first sound at the mitral area and the split second sound at the pulmonary area.

In general, the two components of the second heart sound are best heard at the base with the patient sitting up. In order to elicit this variation of splitting with respiration, the patient should then be instructed to breathe rhythmically and quietly through the open mouth.

In listening critically to the second heart sound, the following information should be noted:

1. Whether two distinct components are present
2. The width and respiratory variation of the interval between the components
3. The loudness of each separate component of the sound

The *presence of two distinct components* suggests that both the aortic and pulmonary valves are present and functioning. As a rule, the aortic (first) component of the second sound is best heard to the right of the sternum in the second interspace (aortic area). The pulmonary (second) component of the second sound (P_2) is most clearly heard in the corresponding left interspace or a

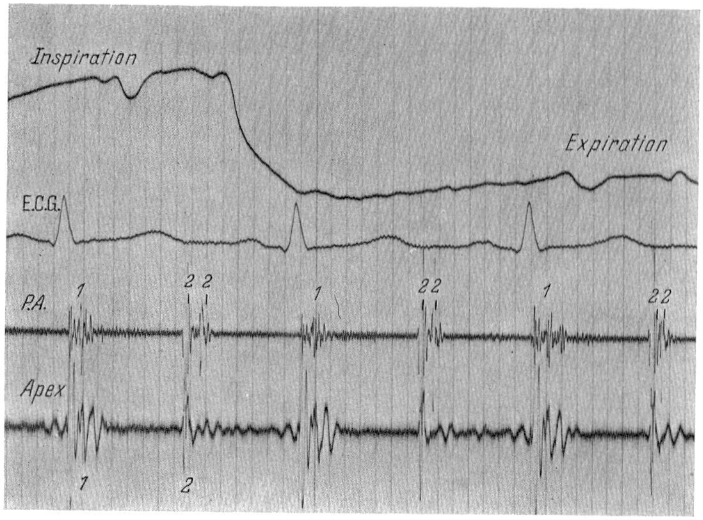

Fig. 3.21. Phonocardiographic tracing showing (a) the composite nature of the first sound at the apex, (b) the splitting of the second sound at the pulmonary area, and (c) the respiratory variation of the second sound.

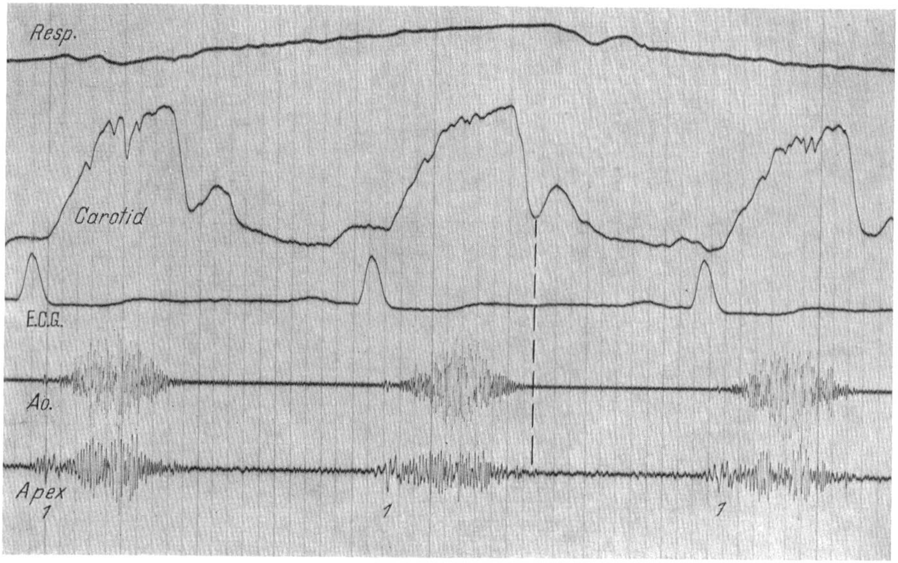

Fig. 3.22. Phonocardiogram from a case of aortic stenosis showing an 'absence' of the second sound which should occur with the notch of the carotid trace.

little lower. Where one or other valve is diseased, as in aortic or pulmonary stenosis, its closing sound may be inaudible. A rigid, distorted or calcified valve may be totally immobile and unable to close or to make a sound on closing. Thus, in severe calcific aortic stenosis, the aortic component of the second sound is generally absent and, since the aortic valve closure is the louder of the two components, there is an apparent 'absence' of the sound at the base.

A single second heart sound, both components being present but heard at the same time, occurs when both ventricles and great arteries are at the same pressures. This situation is found in a large ventricular septal defect with pulmonary hypertension. The second heart sound also will be single when there is atresia of one or the other outlet valves.

The *varying interval between the components* is also called the 'width' of splitting. The normal respiratory variation in the time interval between the two components of the first heart sound may be altered by several mechanisms.

In cases of atrial septal defect, the splitting of the second sound is wide, easily audible and does not vary appreciably with respiration. In other words, there is 'fixed' splitting of the second sound. Two mechanisms are contributory. The flow of blood from the left atrium across the atrial septal defect occurs independent of respiration and is of such magnitude as to obscure the small inspiratory increase of venous return to the right atrium. This factor is abolished by closure of the interatrial defect. Conduction delay in the right bundle as a result of the right heart volume overload also causes delayed closure of the pulmonic valve in atrial septal defect, and this tends to persist after intracardiac repair.

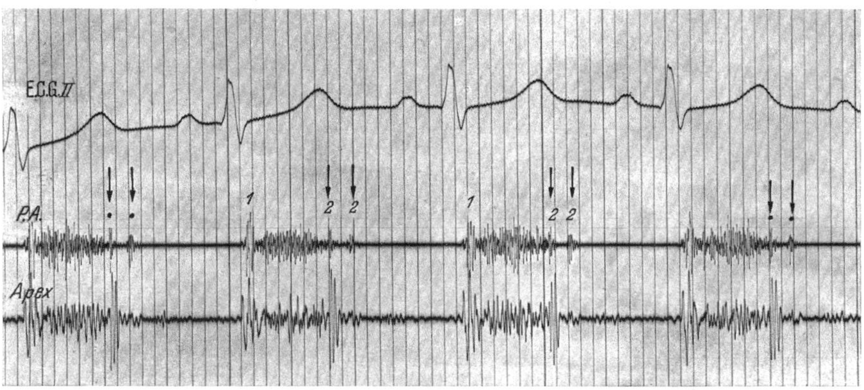

Fig. 3.23. In this case of atrial septal defect the two components of the second sound are widely spaced and 'fixed', i.e. they do not vary with respiration.

When there is impairment of the left branch of the conducting bundle, there is delayed activation of the left ventricle, so that in certain circumstances, aortic valve closure may actually come after pulmonary valve closure. As the pulmonary component still has its normal respiratory variation, there can in these circumstances be narrowing of the distance between the two components with inspiration and widening with expiration, as the pulmonary component approaches and recedes from the markedly delayed aortic valve closure. Such a state of affairs is known as 'paradoxical' or 'reversed' splitting of the second sound. This phenomenon will occur in other conditions that prolong left ventricular ejection also, including systemic hypertension and aortic stenosis.

The *loudness of the two components of the second sound*. The splitting of the second heart sound into two components indicates the presence of two functional valve units. But the loudness or intensity with which they close is an indication of the diastolic pressure in the vessel which causes the valve leaflets to approximate. Thus, in systemic hypertension with an aortic diastolic pressure of, say, 140 mmHg, there is a loud ringing closure of the aortic valve, best heard to the right of the sternum. In the evaluation of cardiac cases for surgery, one is concerned with the presence of pulmonary hypertension, and the loudness of the pulmonary valve closure is listened to critically. This is best heard to the left of the sternum in the pulmonary valve area. Where there is significant elevation of pulmonary artery pressure, the pulmonary component of the second sound is loud and ringing, a sign which usually confirms collateral clinical evidence of pulmonary hypertension. If this is severe, the shock of the pulmonary valve closure may be so marked as to be felt, with the flat of the hand held over the pulmonary area, as an appreciable impulse.

The Third Heart Sound. This is of low-pitched intensity and usually best heard at the apex of the heart. A ventricular filling sound heard during the rapid portion of ventricular filling, it is caused by the in-rush of blood in early diastole and thus closely follows the aortic second sound. It is more easily appreciated in children and young adults, where a third heart sound is a normal physical finding. Pathological processes giving rise to a third heart sound, usually later in life, include a large dilated left ventricle (as occurs in left ventricular failure), anterior myocardial infarction, and mitral or aortic regurgitation.

The Fourth Heart Sound. Also due to ventricular filling, the fourth heart sound results from atrial contraction and therefore immediately precedes the first heart sound and ventricular systole. It is caused by blood being pumped into a non-compliant ventricle and thus is indicative of hypertrophy or fibrosis, as seen commonly with systemic hypertension or coronary artery disease. Its occurrence is hardly ever a normal physical finding and it should alert one to underlying myocardial pathology.

Auscultation: Additional Sounds

In addition to the heart sounds already described, a number of extra sounds may be audible in systole or diastole. The best known of these are the ‘opening snap’ of the mitral valve and the pulmonary and aortic ‘ejection clicks’.

The *opening snap* of the mitral valve strongly suggests that the valve is abnormal. This sharp, snapping sound is best heard to the left of the sternum and just medial to the apex beat. Being related to mitral valve opening, it is heard just after the normal second heart sound, i.e. in early diastole and immediately before the rumbling diastolic murmur caused by the flow of blood through the valve. It indicates a thickened, stenotic mitral valve but one with pliable leaflets which, from a surgical point of view, is favourable for valvotomy. A heavily calcified valve rarely gives rise to an opening sound or, if it does, the sound is indistinct. An opening sound is less common in mitral regurgitation but may be present with mobile leaflets.

The high-pitched opening snap may be confused with the pulmonary component of the second heart sound unless one remembers that pulmonary valve closure is heard most clearly in the pulmonary area, and the mitral valve opening sound at the apex.

A mid- to late-systolic click is characteristic of mitral valve prolapse, in which movement of the billowing leaflet is suddenly arrested at the full length of its elongated chordae.

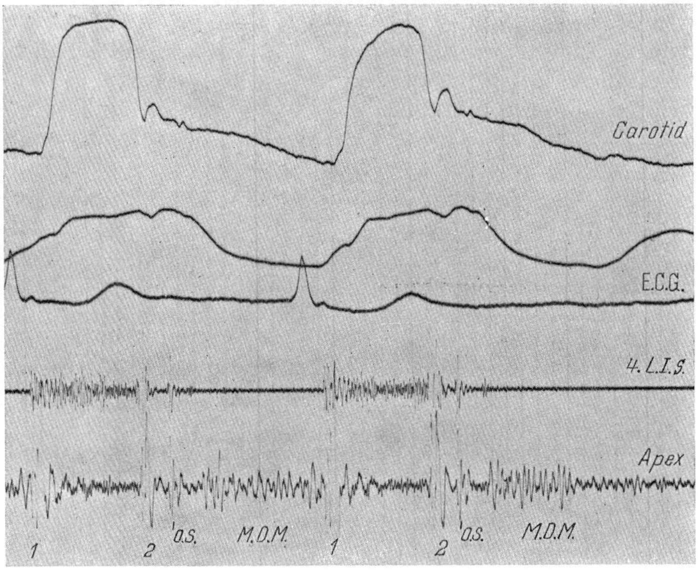

Fig. 3.24. The opening snap (o.s.) is most clearly audible medial to the apex. It follows the second sound and immediately precedes the mitral diastolic murmur (M.D.M.). L.I.S., Left intercostal space.

Aortic and pulmonary *ejection clicks* are high-pitched sounds produced by the sudden arrest of upward movement in mobile but restricted valve cusps. They are heard just after the first heart sound and coincide with the start of the systolic

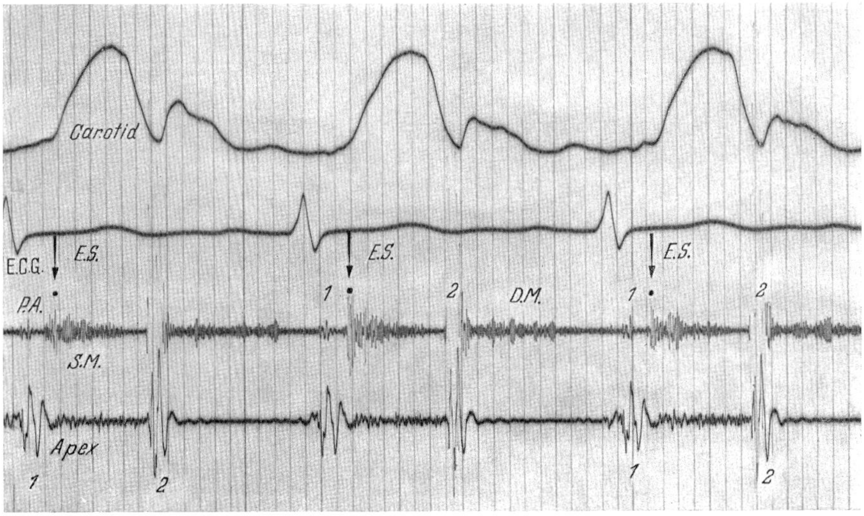

Fig. 3.25. In this case of persistent ductus arteriosus with pulmonary hypertension, an ejection sound (E.S.) can be distinguished coincident with the start of the systolic murmur (S.M.) at the pulmonary area. There is also a loud second sound and a diastolic murmur (D.M.) of pulmonary regurgitation.

murmur caused by blood flow through a narrow or deformed aortic or pulmonary valve. Heard best in the fourth interspace to the left of the sternum or at the apex, the aortic ejection click may be transmitted up towards the root of the neck. Just as the mitral opening snap may be mistaken for a widely split second sound, so aortic and pulmonary ejection sounds may resemble a split first sound.

Auscultation: Murmurs

These represent turbulence of blood flow at a frequency sufficient to give rise to audible vibrations. The loudness of a murmur is generally proportional to the pressure gradient along which the blood passes but not necessarily an indication of the severity of the lesion. Similarly, the length of the murmur is an indication of the time during which there is a pressure difference between two cavities or structures. A small flow of blood through a severe obstruction is likely to give rise to a loud murmur, whereas a very large flow across a mild obstruction may produce minimal turbulence. Alternatively, if a stenosis amounts to almost complete obstruction, the flow of blood will be so slight as to cause no murmur at all. Thus, more significance can be attached to the length of a murmur, its character or quality and its distribution.

The *length* of the diastolic murmur in mitral stenosis is some indication of the severity of the obstruction, for it indicates prolonged, turbulent flow of blood through the obstructed orifice. Similarly, the late systolic murmur associated with prolapse of the mitral valve denotes a lesser degree of mitral regurgitation than the pansystolic murmur of free mitral valve incompetence. Much the same considerations apply to pulmonary and aortic systolic murmurs.

The *character* of a murmur can be of considerable importance in correctly interpreting its site of origin and significance. A diastolic murmur arising from the mitral and tricuspid valves has a low-pitched rumbling quality, which can hardly be confused with any other murmur. On the other hand, diastolic murmurs from the aortic and pulmonary valves are of a high-frequency, decrescendo quality. Systolic murmurs emanating from the mitral and tricuspid valves have a blowing quality, like the wind, while aortic and pulmonary systolic murmurs are of a harsher spurting nature. When the heart rate is very rapid, it may be easier to infer the site of origin of a murmur by its character than by attempts to time it in relation to the cardiac cycle. Sir Thomas Lewis said 'know your mitral murmurs like you know the bark of your dog!'.

While the *distribution* of murmurs or their area of maximum intensity and direction of radiation can be helpful, better localisation can usually be gained from careful appraisal of associated thrills when present. Murmurs are not necessarily confined to the immediate area of the heart and precordium. For example, the continuous murmur of a persistent ductus arteriosus is heard most clearly below the left clavicle but may be readily heard also over the patient's back. Similarly, the harsh ejection murmur of aortic stenosis is usually transmitted to the carotid arteries and can be heard in the neck. Murmurs of collateral vessels in coarctation of the aorta or bronchial collateral arteries in pulmonary atresia also give rise to systolic or continuous bruits heard over the intercostal spaces posteriorly.

By timing murmurs in relation to the cardiac cycle, and remembering basic haemodynamics, it is not difficult to identify the probable origin of a murmur. During systole, blood will flow (1) forward across the aortic and pulmonary valves, (2) backward through incompetent mitral and tricuspid valves, (3) across a defect between the ventricular chambers, or (4) through a communication between systemic and pulmonary circulations distal to the aortic and pulmonary valves.

Because ventricular pressure increases to initiate flow across the semilunar valves, the murmur begins after the first heart sound, becomes loudest in the middle of systole, and declines as flow diminishes at the end of ventricular contraction. Thus, the typical aortic or pulmonary systolic murmur is 'ejection' or 'diamond' in its configuration, whether caused by stenosis of the outflow tract or increased flow across a normal valve (see Figs. 3.20, 3.22).

Murmurs that begin with the first heart sound indicate blood flow to a lower pressure chamber at the very beginning of ventricular systole. This is possible across an incompetent atrioventricular valve or through a ventricular septal defect. The murmur usually lasts into the second sound and thus is pansystolic. Associated findings, such as the character and radiation of the murmur and signs of ventricular overload, must be taken into consideration to complete the diagnosis.

Diastolic flow in the cardiac cycle occurs normally from the atria to the ventricles, across the mitral and tricuspid valves. Stenosis or increased flow across these valves would be expected to result in a late or mid-diastolic murmur when atrial contraction propels the largest portion of blood into the ventricles. There is thus 'presystolic accentuation' of the murmur. A leaking aortic or pulmonary valve, in contrast, allows regurgitation of blood into the ventricle as soon as ventricular pressure falls below that in the great vessel. These murmurs are, consequently, 'immediate' or 'early' diastolic murmurs.

Whenever there is a communication between a high-pressure and a low-pressure structure without an intervening one-way valve, the potential exists for turbulent blood flow throughout the cardiac cycle and, hence, a continuous

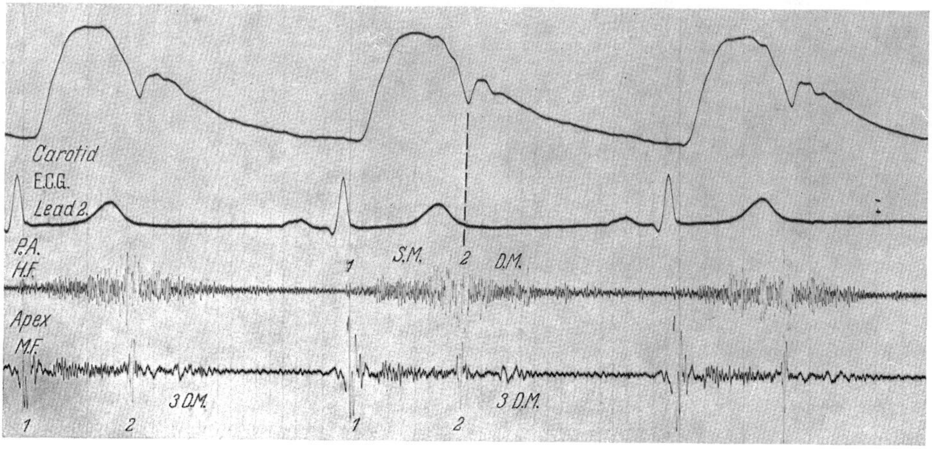

Fig. 3.26. The characteristic murmur of persistent ductus arteriosus which waxes in systole and wanes in diastole.

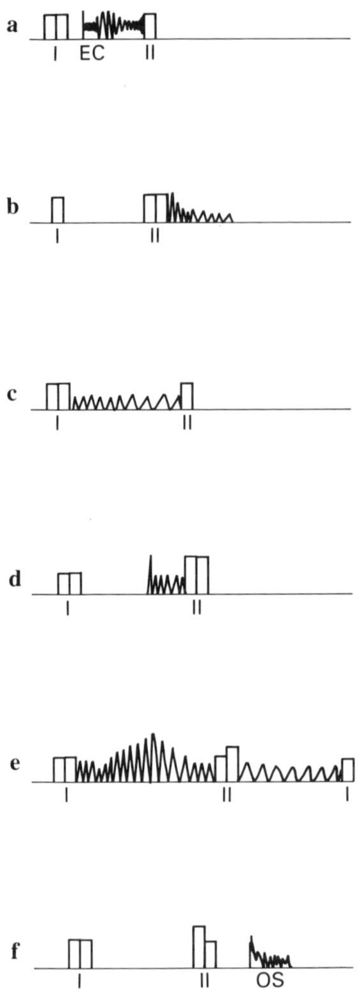

Fig. 3.27. Diagrammatic representation of cardiac sounds and murmurs. **a** Systolic ejection murmur (aortic stenosis) **b** Immediate diastolic murmur (aortic regurgitation). **c** Pansystolic murmur (VSD). **d** Late systolic murmur and click (mitral prolapse). **e** Continuous murmur (PDA). **f** Opening snap/diastolic murmur (mitral stenosis). OS, opening snap.

murmur. The most common cause is a persistent ductus arteriosus, but continuous murmurs occur also with an arteriovenous fistula, a coronary artery fistula, a ruptured sinus of Valsalva aneurysm, an aortopulmonary window, aortopulmonary collateral vessels and surgically-created systemic pulmonary shunts. In these situation, the length of the murmur may be an especially good guide to the pressure difference between the two structures. For example, a persistent ductus arteriosus where the murmur ends early in diastole suggests equilization of aortic and pulmonary arterial pressure and hence pulmonary hypertension.

Special Considerations in Infants and Young Children

The examination of the cardiovascular system in a small infant with tachycardia and respiratory distress or in the toddler who screams at anything clad in white may, on first attempt, appear to be a complete impossibility. However, with attention to proper technique, it is soon appreciated that this group of patients are almost 'transparent' as regards physical signs of cardiovascular disease.

In contrast with adults, the history is usually obtained from the patient's parents. When there are older children in the family, useful comparison can often be made with them, to elucidate a history of difficult breathing, poor feeding, slow weight gain, abnormal colour or limitation of activity. In this respect, it should be remembered that the infant's 'stress test' is feeding, particularly when there is increased pulmonary blood flow. Some symptoms, such as breathlessness and cyanosis, may become apparent only when the child begins to walk or otherwise increase his physical activity.

Physical examination of a young infant may be helped by ensuring that it is warm, dry and fed. Care should be taken to prevent exposure to both infection and cold during the examination. Young children usually prefer the security of a parent's lap and will respond to a few minutes spent gaining their confidence. In the occasional patient who cries throughout the examination, one must concentrate upon auscultatory findings during inspiration, when there is usually a brief period in which heart sounds can be heard.

In recording blood pressure, it is important to use a cuff which is appropriate for the size of patient, as too small an apparatus will give falsely elevated values. Often, the diastolic pressure cannot be determined accurately in children and just the systolic pressure, frequently obtained better by palpation, is recorded.

Because of the short length of the neck, elevation of the jugular venous pressure is less readily appreciated. However, the liver is quite distensible and its enlargement is an equally reliable sign of heart failure, particularly in infants.

The thinness of the chest wall permits most heart sounds and many murmurs to be appreciated by palpation in children, and both left and right ventricular impulses can be easily seen if there is cardiac enlargement. Indeed, murmurs tend to radiate widely, and a thrill is thus particularly useful in locating their origin. Unlike adults, in children murmurs are not invariably associated with cardiac pathology, and one must be alert for the venous hum of blood in the thoracic veins and the so-called innocent murmur that results from turbulent blood flow in a normal pulmonary artery. Both of these will vary with posture and exercise.

Further Reading

Leatham A. An introduction to the examination of the cardiovascular system, 2nd edn. Oxford Medical Publications, Oxford University Press, Oxford, 1979

Physiologic principles of heart sounds and murmurs. American Heart Association monograph no. 46. American Heart Association, New York, 1975

Wood P. Diseases of the heart and circulation, 3rd edn. Eyre & Spottiswoode, London, 1968, pp 1–84

Chapter 4

Special Investigations

In the routine investigation of a cardiological problem, information is needed on the red and white cell counts, the haemoglobin content of the blood, and the presence of abnormal constituents in the urine. In addition, a standard posteroanterior and left lateral X-ray view of the chest should be available, together with an electrocardiogram (ECG). These commonplace investigations can scarcely be classified as having a special nature, but they should precede other more sophisticated diagnostic procedures.

An estimation of the haemoglobin content of the blood, as a general index of the patient's state of health, is valuable for all patients. A falling haemoglobin may suggest the onset of bacterial endocarditis, haemolysis or haemorrhage related to anticoagulation. In cyanotic congenital heart disease, the haemoglobin content and degree of polycythaemia provide an index of the severity of the lesion. A rising haemoglobin is evidence of deterioration, particularly in Fallot's tetralogy, while, conversely, a postoperative decline in the red cell count can be a valuable guide to the adequacy of surgical palliation.

The urine will be examined as a routine procedure in all cases of heart disease. Apart from abnormal constituents, a measure of the daily volume serves as an indication of the response to treatment, particularly in cases of myocardial failure. The presence of microscopic haematuria may raise a suspicion of bacterial endocarditis.

Chest Radiography

This is an essential part of the examination and can almost be regarded as part of the 'inspection' of the heart. In addition to supplying objective information, a permanent record of the shape and size of the heart and the degree of vascularity of the lung fields is made for comparison at subsequent examinations. On studying the chest film, particular attention should be directed to (a) the bony cage, (b) the cardiac outline (silhouette), (c) the lung fields and (d) areas of calcification.

The Bony Cage

It is worth remembering that congenital anomalies frequently coexist, so that it is not unusual to discover anomalies of the ribs or vertebral column in association with congenital heart disease. Hemivertebrae, with resulting scoliosis, may occur, and supernumerary or bifid ribs are occasionally present. In patients who have undergone a thoracotomy early in life, periostial changes and fusion of ribs may occur, while absence of a rib generally indicates that it has been removed for surgical access.

One feature to look for carefully is rib notching. After about 5 years of age, it is invariably present and bilateral in classical coarctation of the aorta. Unilateral rib notching is sometimes seen after the Blalock–Taussig shunt operation, due to the development of a rich collateral arterial network supplying the arm on the side of the divided subclavian artery. Rib notching has also been observed in severe cyanotic heart disease, such as pulmonary atresia, where large collateral vessels supply the lungs. Erosion of the ribs may be seen occasionally in a long-standing aneurysm.

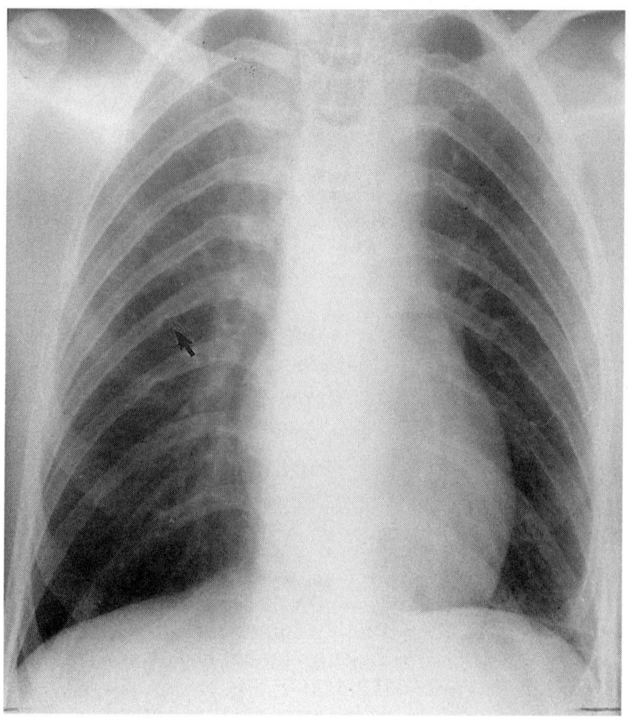

Fig. 4.1. A case of coarctation of the aorta showing notching of the ribs (*arrow*).

The Cardiac Outline

It is possible to gain an impression of an increase in the bulk of the cardiac shadow from casual inspection, but, in obstructive lesions, muscular hypertrophy is initially concentric, with little increase in the size of the heart. A large heart suggests conditions associated with a large stroke volume, such as aortic regurgitation, mitral regurgitation or a septal defect. When cardiac enlargement develops rapidly in the presence of a stenotic lesion, it signifies myocardial failure and dilatation. A postoperative increase in the size of the heart shadow may be due to a number of these factors, but it is equally likely to be the result of accumulation of pericardial fluid. The size of the heart is conveniently measured and compared with the diameter of the chest, the *cardiothoracic ratio*, normal measurement being under 50%. The ratio should be entered in the patient's notes at each examination.

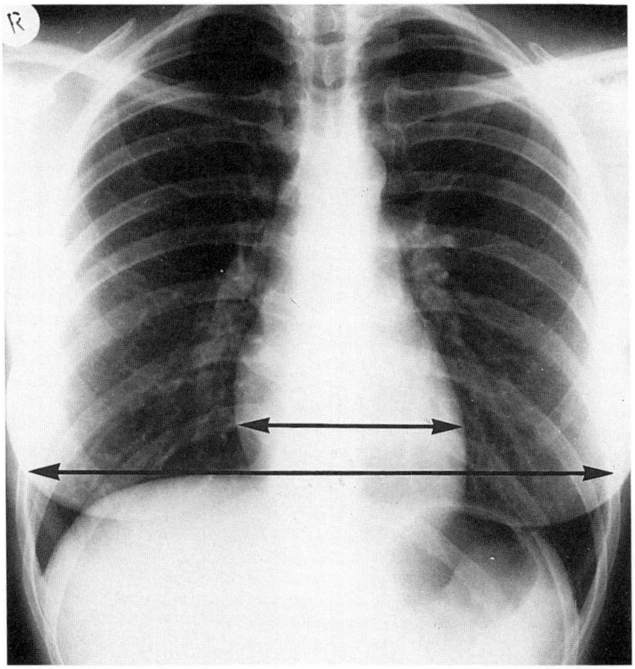

Fig. 4.2. The cardiothoracic ratio is a measure of the transverse diameter of the heart and the greatest width of the chest between the inner boarders of the ribs.

Localised areas of enlargement on the cardiac silhouette can be of great value in diagnosing hypertrophy or dilatation, so that it is essential to have a clear image of what constitutes the normal outline of the heart viewed in the posteroanterior projection. This is indicated in the accompanying drawings. These contours will not invariably be visible on all chest X-rays, but when a localised projection is observed, its underlying cause can often be inferred from a mind's-eye anatomical concept of the outline of the heart within the chest.

The *superior caval* shadow, forming the most superior part of the right cardiac border, is not of great diagnostic value. But occasionally, a corresponding

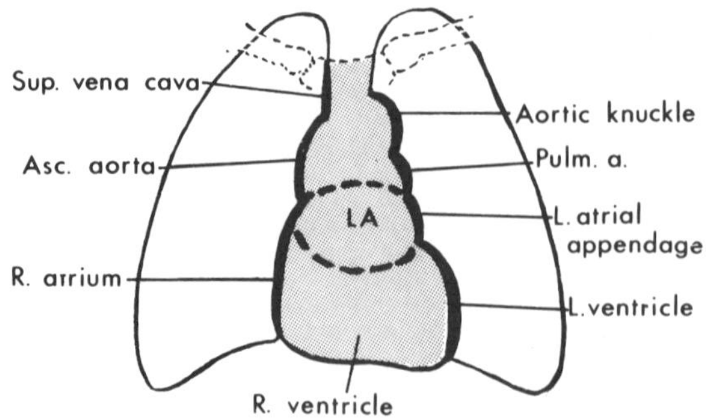

Fig. 4.3. An interpretation of the bulges on the cardiac shadow as seen in the standard posteroanterior chest radiograph.

shadow may be appreciated on the left side and indicates the presence of a left superior vena cava. When the arch of the aorta lies on the right side, it may cause the normal superior caval shadow to appear unduly prominent.

The *thoracic aorta* is visible in two areas on the posteroanterior projection: the ascending part above the valve may contribute to the right border of the heart, while the distal arch forms the 'aortic knuckle' on the left border.

A prominent ascending aorta is the rule in significant aortic valve stenosis and represents one example of post-stenotic dilatation. It should be looked for in every case of aortic stenosis, and its absence should make one reconsider the diagnosis or suspect the possibility of a sub-valvar obstruction. In atherosclerotic unfolding of the aorta, syphilitic aortic regurgitation or the dilated aorta of

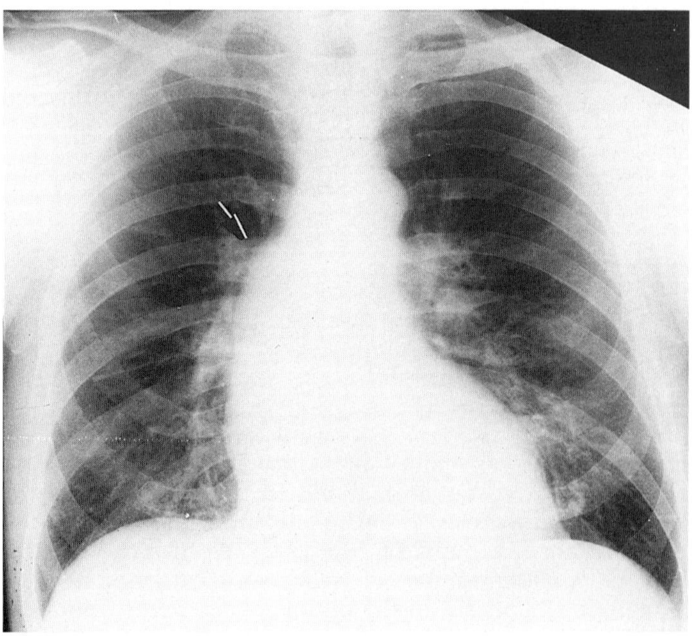

Fig. 4.4. The post-stenotic bulge (*arrow*) of the ascending aorta is well seen in aortic valve stenosis.

a

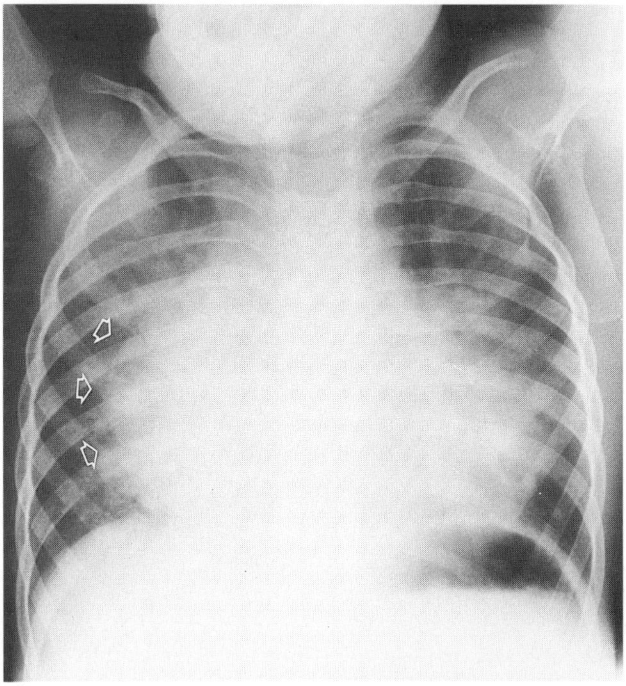

b

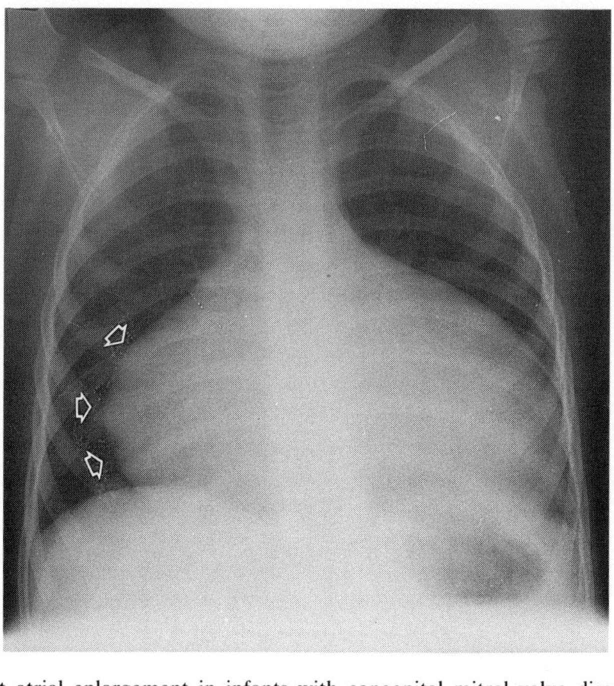

Fig. 4.5. Right atrial enlargement in infants with congenital mitral valve disease, left superior vena cava and complete absence of the interatrial septum (**a**) and Ebstein's anomaly of the tricuspid valve (**b**).

essential hypertension, the ascending aorta will again be prominent, but the rest of the aorta, including the 'knuckle', should be equally conspicuous.

The size of the aortic knuckle is a good indication of the size of the aorta. Its position also discloses the side of the aortic arch, that is the side of the trachea on which the aorta passes from anterior to posterior mediastinum. Normally, this is on the left, but about one-quarter of patients with Fallot's tetralogy have a right aortic arch. In the presence of a left-to-right shunt, a small aortic knuckle favours a diagnosis of atrial or ventricular septal defect, while a large knuckle argues for a persistent ductus arteriosus. This can be a useful differential feature. In general terms, a small aorta, in cases with an obstructive intracardiac lesion, is consistent with a small cardiac output; while a normal-sized aorta suggests mild or moderate obstruction and normal cardiac output.

In coarctation of the aorta, the aortic knuckle may appear to be absent, with a prominent left subclavian artery: alternatively, one may see a 'double aortic knuckle' caused by overlapping shadows of the left subclavian artery and the post-stenotic dilatation of the descending aorta below the coarctation.

The *right atrium* occupies the lower portion of the right heart border and its enlargement shows as a ballooning in this area, extending down to the diaphragm and blunting the right cardiophrenic angle. This may indicate stenosis or regurgitation at the tricuspid valve.

In contrast, *left atrial* enlargement is seen as a globular shadow of increased density within the cardiac silhouette, as this chamber does not contribute normally to either the left or right heart border. This usually produces a double

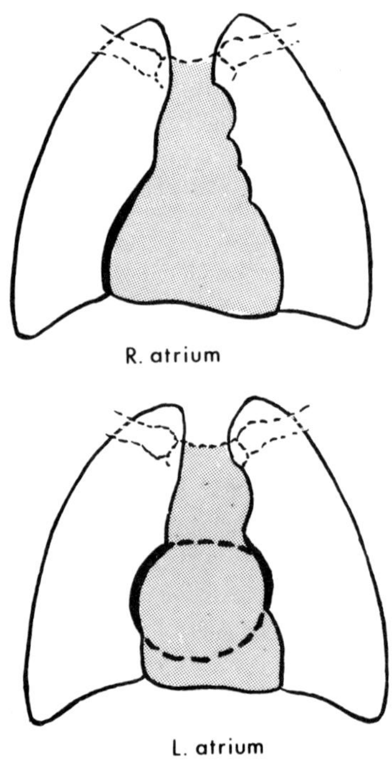

Fig. 4.6. The features of right and left atrial enlargement as seen in the chest radiograph.

density behind the right atrial shadow and widening of the tracheobronchial angle by elevation of the left main bronchus. In the lateral view, posterior displacement of the oesophagus by an enlarged left atrium may be appreciated also.

Very considerable enlargement – sometimes called aneurysmal dilatation of the left atrium or 'giant left atrium' – protrudes beyond both cardiac borders and may be confused with right atrial enlargement. The lower border adjacent to the right cardiophrenic angle, tends in these cases to swing sharply inwards, forming an acute angle between the heart and diaphragm, in contrast to the blunt angle of right atrial enlargement. In addition, the convexity of the left atrial appendage on the left border of the heart shadow tends to be unduly prominent. Aneurysmal dilatation of the left atrium in the presence of mitral valve disease favours a diagnosis of mitral regurgitation, while either stenosis or regurgitation may produce lesser degrees of enlargement.

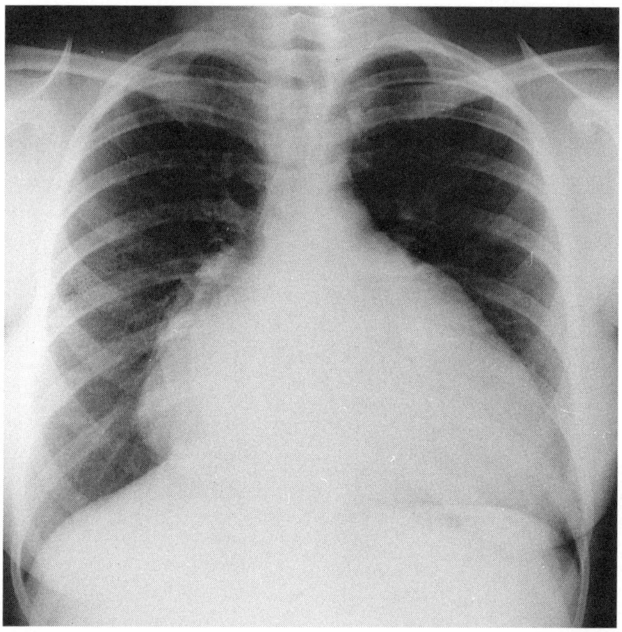

Fig. 4.7. A grossly enlarged left atrium in a case of mitral valve disease. The left atrial shadow projects on the left cardiac border and forms a double density behind the right atrium.

It is worth re-emphasising that there can be considerable concentric hypertrophy of the obstructed right or left ventricle without evidence of enlargement of the *ventricular silhouette*. Where these chambers are grossly hypertrophied or dilated, they have a characteristic contour. The right ventricle lies adjacent to the central tendon of the diaphragm, and enlargement of this chamber tends to elevate the heart and 'round off' the apex. Sometimes this contour is obscured by the diaphragm or can be seen through the stomach gas bubble. On the lateral chest X-ray, an enlarged right ventricle fills in the space between the sternum and the cardiac shadow.

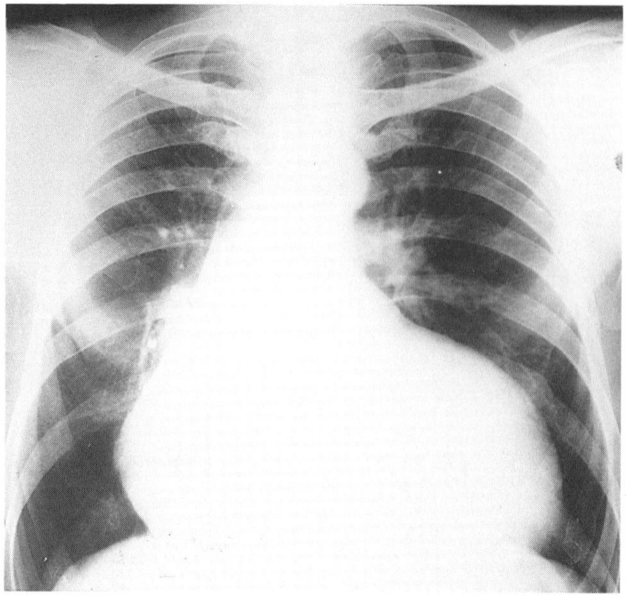

Fig. 4.8. An enlarged left ventricle in a case of aortic regurgitation.

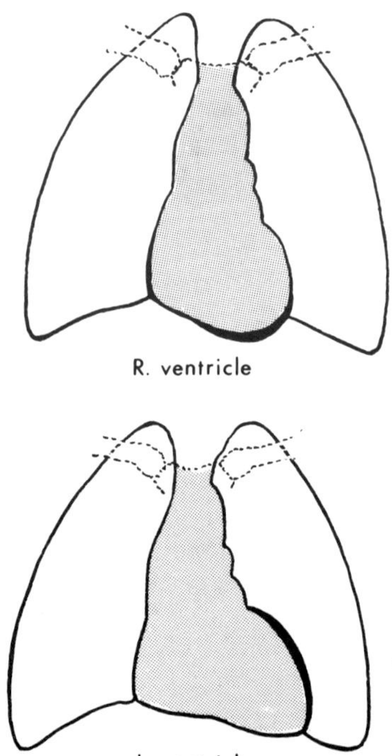

Fig. 4.9. Diagram illustrating the features of right and left ventricular enlargement.

With hypertrophy, the left ventricle, which constitutes the normal left lower border of the cardiac silhouette, enlarges outwards and downwards towards the diaphragm. This produces a 'sharp apex', unlike the elevated, round apex of right ventricular enlargement. A localized bulge on the lateral border of the heart suggests, in contrast, an aneurysm of the left ventricle following myocardial infarction.

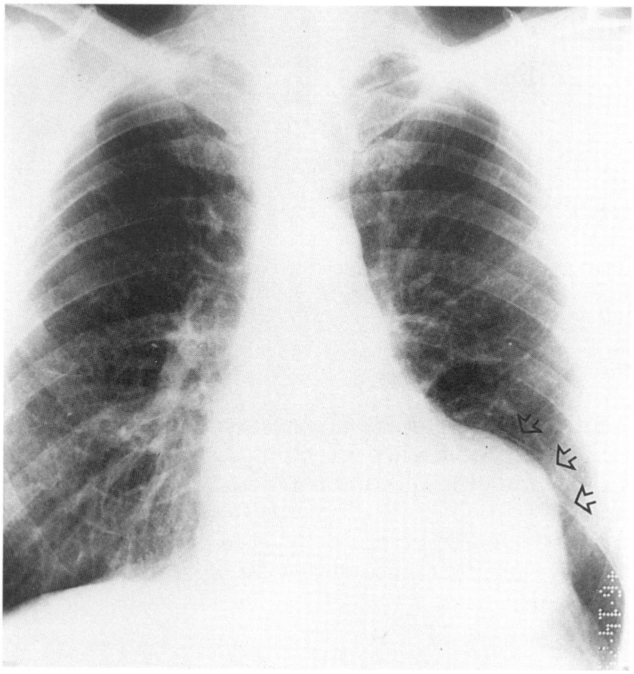

Fig. 4.10. Left ventricular aneurysm.

The Lateral Chest Radiograph

A true lateral picture should always be available, since it is only with the aid of two projections that any doubtful opacity of the lungs or abnormal cardiac shadow can be accurately located within the chest. The interpretation of oblique views of the cardiac contour falls more within the field of the radiologist and physician cardiologist, as do oesophagograms, which give an impression of the vascular and cardiac conformations adjacent to the barium-filled oesophagus. Enlargement of the left atrium displaces the oesophagus backwards in a sickle-shaped curve. Anomalies of the aortic arch and proximal pulmonary arteries produce characteristic indentations which are diagnostic of these malformations.

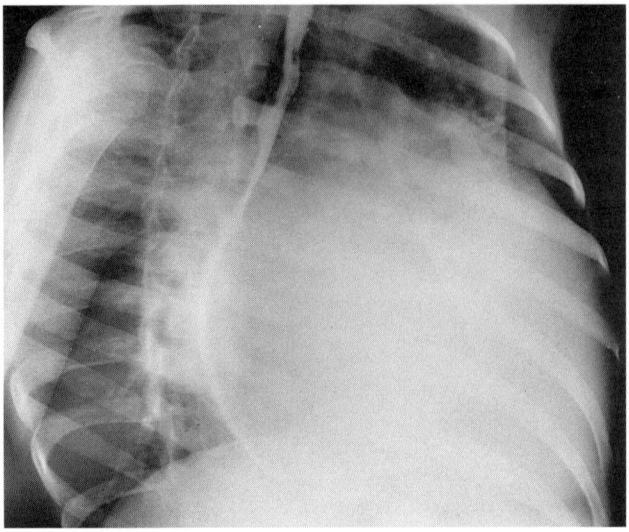

Fig. 4.11. Posterior displacement of the barium-filled oesophagus due to left atrial enlargement, in this case as the result of a large ventricular septal defect.

The Lung Fields

Examination of these is important in any cardiac condition, chiefly for the degree of vascularity or presence of pulmonary venous congestion. Other features, such as pleural effusions and haemosiderosis, should also be noted.

Reduced vascularity, known as *oligaemic* lung fields, occurs in pulmonary atresia or pulmonary stenosis, occasionally as an isolated lesion or, more often, as a part of a complex cardiac malformation. In pulmonary atresia, there may be

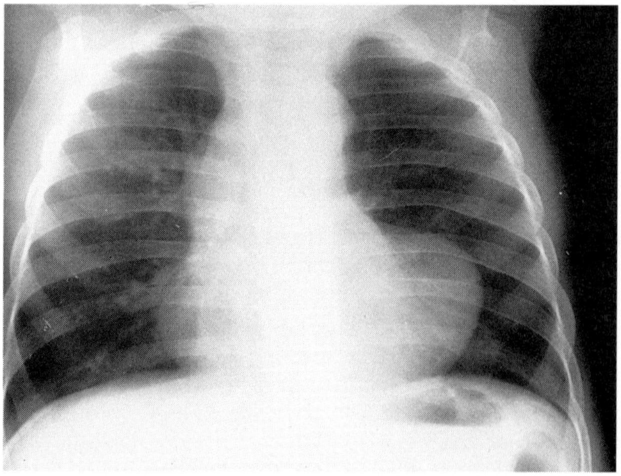

Fig. 4.12. Oligaemic lung fields in pulmonary atresia with ventricular septal defect. Note the concavity in the position of the pulmonary trunk, giving the heart a 'boot-shaped' appearance.

a prominent proximal pulmonary artery as the result of post-stenotic dilatation, but the shadows of the vessels diminish rapidly leaving the periphery of the lung fields 'clear'. This picture should not be confused with that seen in severe pulmonary hypertension. Here, the peripheral subdivisions of the vascular tree become narrowed or occluded, producing clear lung fields in the outer zones, but the hila and middle zones of the lung are occupied by prominent and enlarged pulmonary arteries. In a patient with central cyanosis and a communication between the systemic and pulmonary circulations, such a picture is characteristic of Eisenmenger's syndrome.

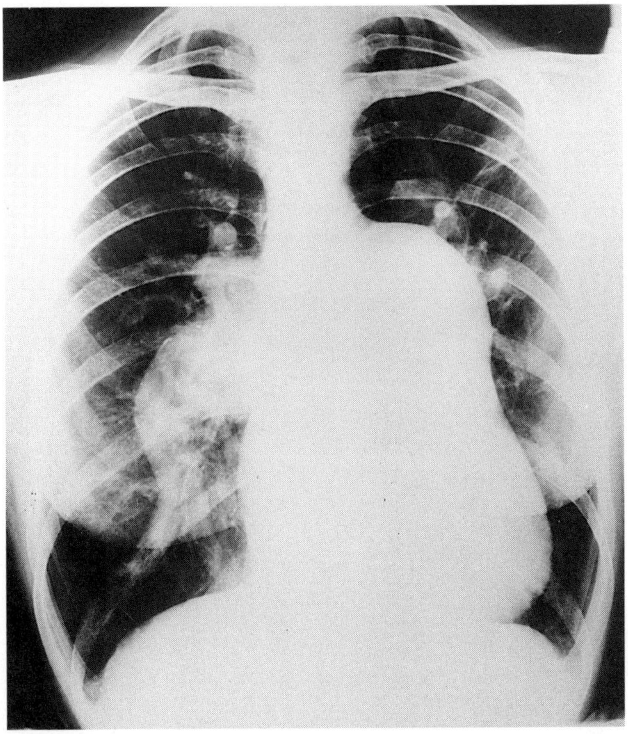

Fig. 4.13. The lung fields in pulmonary hypertension with reversed shunt through an atrial septal defect. The outer one-third of the lung fields is clear.

In some cases of severe pulmonary stenosis or pulmonary atresia, the lung fields are uniformly and diffusely mottled with vascular shadows somewhat reminiscent of miliary tuberculosis. On close inspection, the proximal pulmonary arterial trunks are absent, rudimentary or spidery in pattern. This diffuse, uniform mottling is due to extensive bronchial artery–pulmonary artery anastomoses which support the pulmonary circulation.

Where there is increased vascularity of the lungs, one must differentiate between 'passive congestion' (also called pulmonary venous hypertension) and 'active congestion' as the result of increased pulmonary blood flow. *Passive congestion* may reflect any condition that causes an elevation of left atrial and pulmonary venous pressure, the most common being mitral stenosis and left

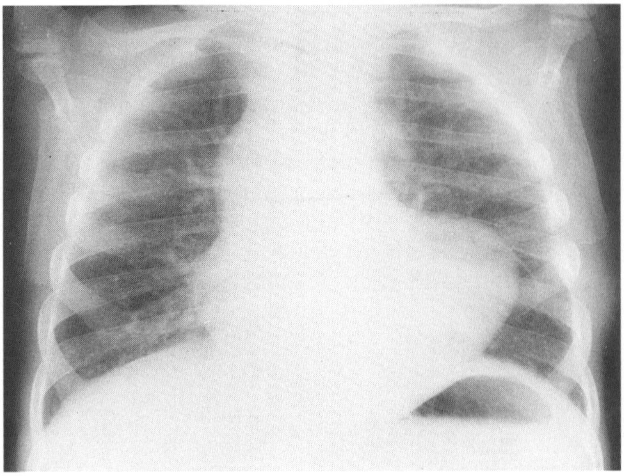

Fig. 4.14. In severe pulmonary stenosis or pulmonary atresia the bronchial vascular pattern predominates as a uniform shadowing from collateral blood flow despite poor development of the main pulmonary vessels.

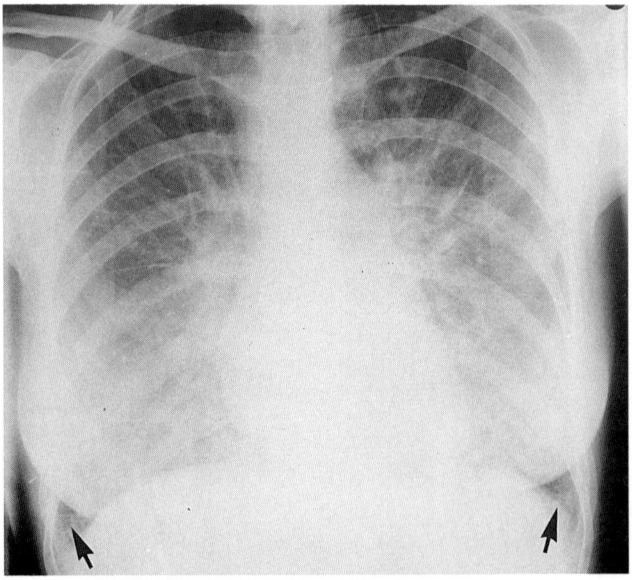

Fig. 4.15. Congestion of the lungs associated with mitral stenosis (passive congestion). Short horizontal basal lines in the costophrenic angle known as Kerley B-lines are seen on both sides. (*arrows*).

ventricular failure. In the early stages of passive congestion, blood flow is diverted to the upper lobes of the lung such that these vessels become equal or greater in size than those in the lower lobes. Interstitial oedema subsequently causes a hazy or congested appearance which is more noticeable in the base and hila. When interlobular septa become prominent from distension of lymphatic channels, short horizontal lines about 1.0–1.5 cm long develop in the costophrenic angles. These are *Kerley B-lines* and generally correspond to a mean pulmonary venous pressure in excess of 20 mmHg. At this time, there are usually symptoms of pulmonary oedema and paroxysmal nocturnal dyspnoea, with associated collections of fluid in the lung fissures or pleural space.

Also known as *pulmonary plethora*, *active congestion* of the lungs is due to a great increase of blood flow through the pulmonary bed which results in uniform increase of vascularity, involving both the arteries and the veins. Plethoric lung fields occur in any condition with a large left-to-right shunt, particularly atrial septal defect, ventricular septal defect and persistent ductus arteriosus.

Asymmetric pulmonary perfusion usually indicates the presence of stenosis in one of the proximal pulmonary arterial branches. This may occur naturally (not infrequently at the site of the ligamentum, causing obstruction to the left pulmonary artery) or following a systemic pulmonary anastomosis.

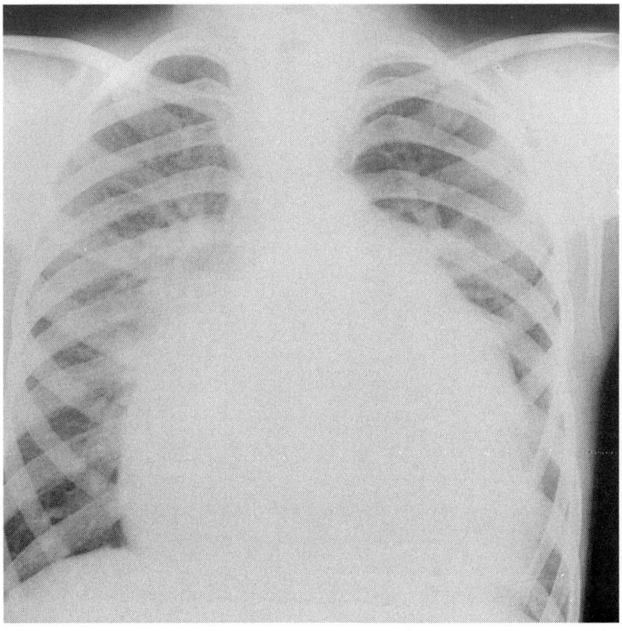

Fig. 4.16. Hyperaemic lung fields indicating a large left-to-right shunt in a ventricular septal defect. Note the pulmonary artery and overall cardiac enlargement.

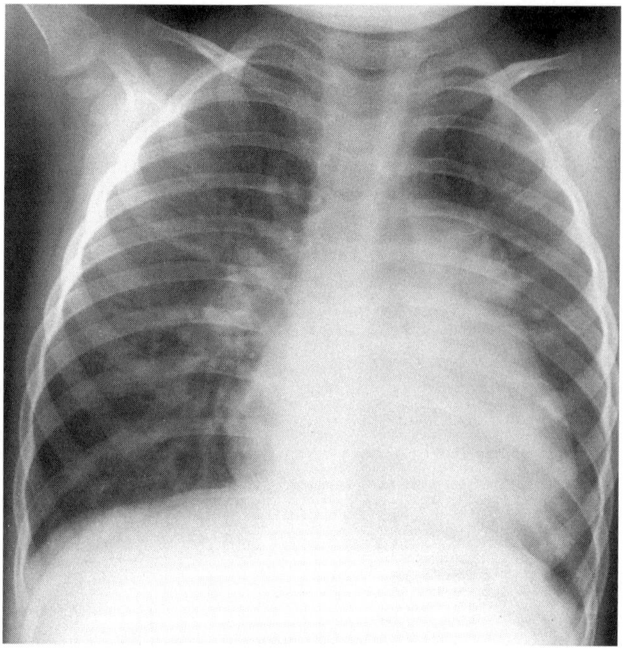

Fig. 4.17. Pulmonary plethora due to a pesistent ductus arteriosus. The main pulmonary arteries and aortic knuckle are enlarged.

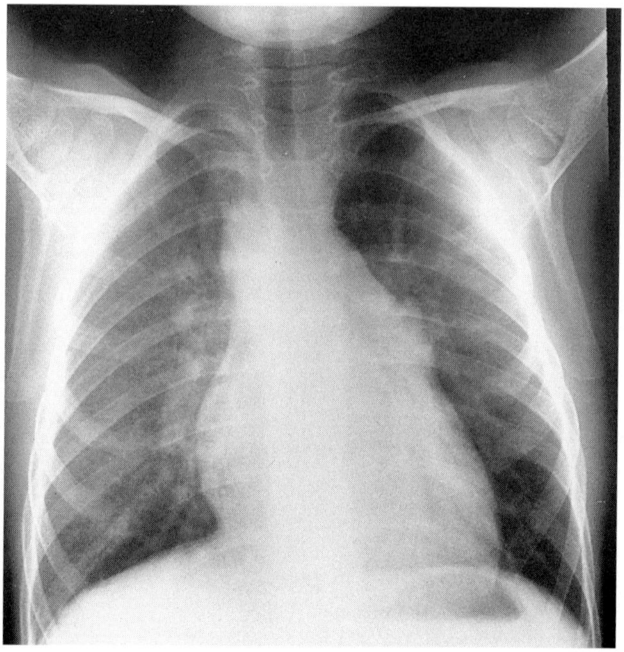

Fig. 4.18. Unequal lung perfusion in a patient with pulmonary atresia and ventricular septal defect. A right aortic arch is present.

Areas of Calcification

These may be observed in the lung fields, the pericardium or the heart and great vessels. A number of pulmonary lesions may become calcified and rarely indicate associated cardiac pathology. Calcification of the pericardium, however, occurs with inflammation resulting from tuberculosis, and may or may not be associated with haemodynamically important constriction.

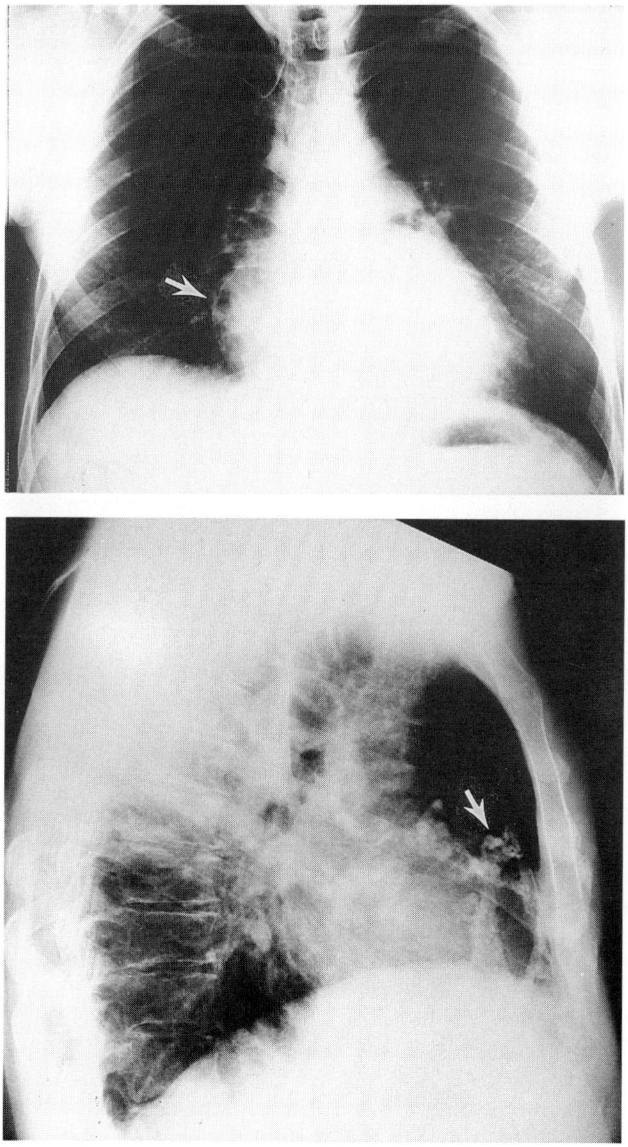

Fig. 4.19. Pericardial calcification (*arrows*) in the posteroanterior and lateral views of the plain chest X-ray.

Within the arch and descending thoracic aorta, calcification occurs commonly with advanced age and also may be seen in the wall of an aneurysm or healed dissection. In the ascending aorta, it suggests a diagnosis of syphilitic aortitis.

In the heart itself, deposits of calcium are not infrequently seen in the aortic and mitral valves in conjuction with obstructive pathology. Whilst biological tissue implants may calcify in any position, such calcification is not invariably accompanied by loss of function. Calcification of the mitral annulus in elderly subjects is not generally associated with valvular obstruction. Similarly, coronary arterial calcification in the elderly does not have the same implication of obstructive disease as it does in younger patients. Areas of calcification within the myocardium usually indicate a healed myocardial infarction, often with the formation of an aneurysm containing laminated blood clot.

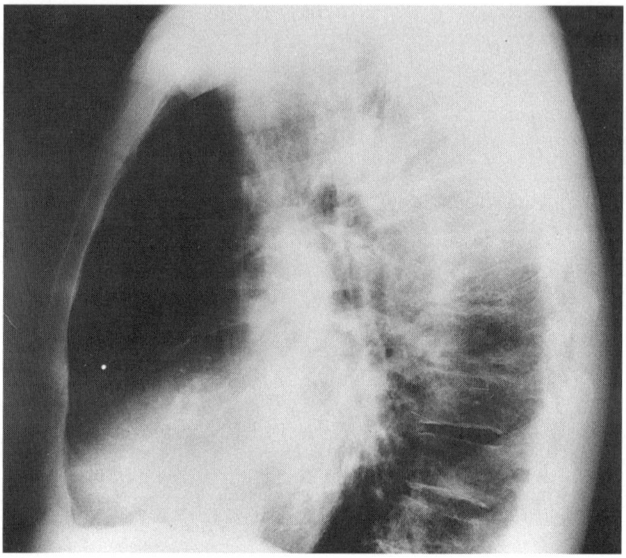

Fig. 4.20. Calcified aortic valve.

Electrocardiography

The interpretation of the electrocardiogram (ECG) in heart disease has become a complex and sophisticated study, and, for the the finer shades of interpretation, one's cardiological colleague should be consulted. It is important, however, for the cardiac surgeon to have some rudimentary concept of the electrocardiographic pattern in order to be able to add to or confirm his clinical impression.

It should be emphasised that the ECG in no way represents the cardiac impulse or the pressure changes within the ventricles. It is simply a recording of the electrical activity or impulses which pass through and are generated by the myocardial cells. These electrical events precede the actual mechanical events of the cardiac cycle.

By convention, it is customary to have recordings of the three standard limb leads (I, II and III), three unipolar limb leads (AVR, AVL and AVF) and six unipolar precordial leads (V_1 to V_6). The wave pattern produced is basically similar in all leads, the various components being identified by the letters P, Q, S and T.

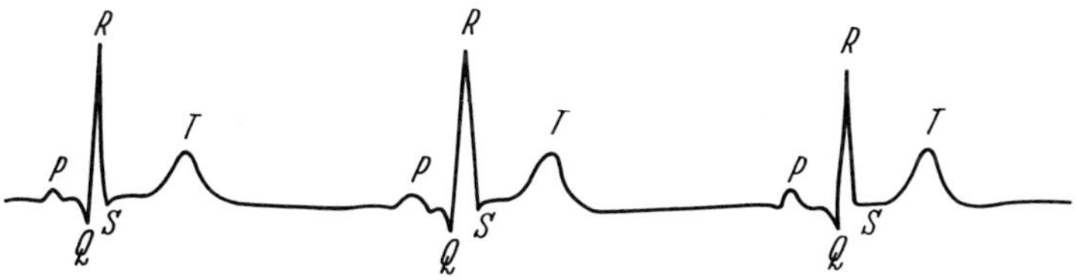

Fig. 4.21. Diagram of the normally seen electrical deflections of the ECG.

The P wave represents the passage of electrical activation through the atria. This normally proceeds in a leftward and downward direction from the sinus node to the atrioventricular node, producing a positive wave in leads on the left side of the body and a negative deflection on the right side. The time interval between the P wave and the beginning of QRS complex is the PR interval, which corresponds to both atrial activation and passage of the electrical impulse through the atrioventricular node, the bundle of His and its branches of Purkinje's tissue. Activation of the latter structures does not cause a wave on the usual ECG but can be detected with an intracardiac electrode during special electrophysiological investigations. The normal PR interval in an adult ranges from 0.12 to 0.20 s; in general, it is shorter at younger ages and faster heart rates.

Activation of the ventricular muscle mass produces the QRS complex, again with positive deflections indicating that the activation is moving toward the electrode, negative deflections away from it. The normal duration of the QRS complex is less than 0.08 s, regardless of age or heart rate. The T wave represents repolarization or re-establishment of the membrane potential in the ventricles and is generally of the same direction as the dominant wave in the QRS complex. Between the QRS complex and T wave, the period without electrical activity is called the ST segment or interval. Occasionally, an additional positive deflection may be observed between the T wave and P wave on the precordial leads, the so-called U wave. Although the aetiology of the U wave is controversial, it appears to be influenced by metabolic factors.

The ECG can be of help to the cardiac surgeon in identifying some congenital malformations, in confirming or interpreting disturbances of rhythm, in estimating hypertrophy of one or more chambers of the heart, and in documenting myocardial ischaemia or infarction.

Disturbance of Rhythm

Probably the most common arrythmia encountered in surgical practice is *atrial fibrillation*. It is usual in cases of rheumatic mitral stenosis and not infrequently occurs postoperatively if not present before operation. Less often, it complicates other lesions in conditions in which the atrium is enlarged, such as atrial septal defect or mitral regurgitation. The presence of atrial fibrillation in association with aortic stenosis should prompt one to consider a rheumatic aetiology for this condition and the possibility of coincident involvement of the mitral valve.

Clinically, there is total irregularity of the volume and rate of the pulse. The atria contract ineffectually, in a completely disorganised fashion, usually at a rate in excess of 400/minute. The pulse, which indicates the ventricular response to this barrage of electrical activity, will be determined by the number of impulses conducted through the atrioventricular node. The ECG is diagnostic, with absence of P waves and a variable interval between the ventricular complexes.

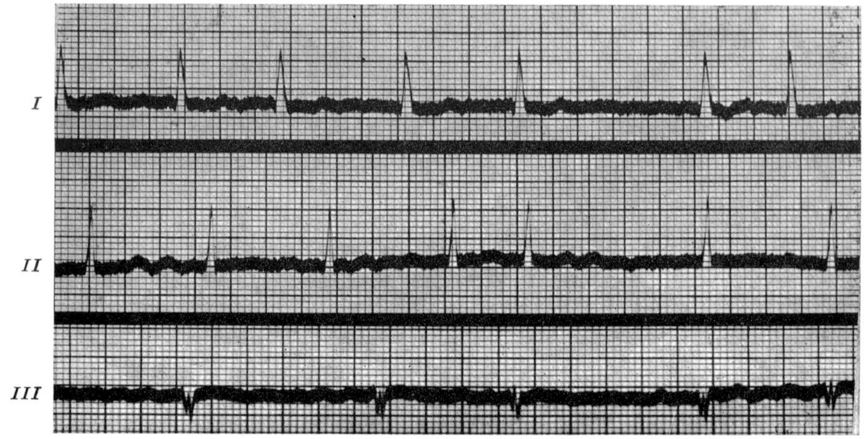

Fig. 4.22. Atrial fibrillation. The P waves are absent and the QRS complexes are irregularly spaced.

Other types of supraventricular tachycardia – that is, abnormally fast heart rhythms originating above the intraventricular conduction system – usually produce a regular pulse. In *atrial flutter*, contractions of the atria are regular at a rate of 300/minute, which may be conducted one-to-one into the ventricles, giving a pulse of the same rate. More commonly, every second or third beat is conducted, such that the ventricular response is 150 or 100/minute. The sinus node, atria and atrioventricular junction also may be the source of rapid, regular heart rhythm. In general, the ECG will show a narrow QRS complex, which is useful in differentiating these from the more sinister ventricular arrythmias. Their treatment depends upon the origin of the abnormal rhythm and the extent to which it embarrasses the cardiac output. Most are responsive to electrical cardioversion or pharmacological control.

Extra heart beats coming from the ventricles are, unfortunately, quite common during cardiac surgery, particularly when dealing with diseased ventricles (for example, due to severe aortic stenosis or coronary artery disease). Occasional, isolated ventricular ectopic beats generally are of little consequence apart from causing a pause in the pulse. When they occur frequently or there are several in a row, they are more foreboding, as the ectopic focus may subsequently dominate the cardiac rhythm and result in *ventricular tachycardia* or *ventricular fibrillation*. In ventricular tachycardia, there is an abnormal area of excitability ('ectopic focus') in the ventricle, giving rise to a rapid regular rhythm. Activation usually does not proceed through the conduction system, so the QRS complex is wider than normal and of a different configuration. This

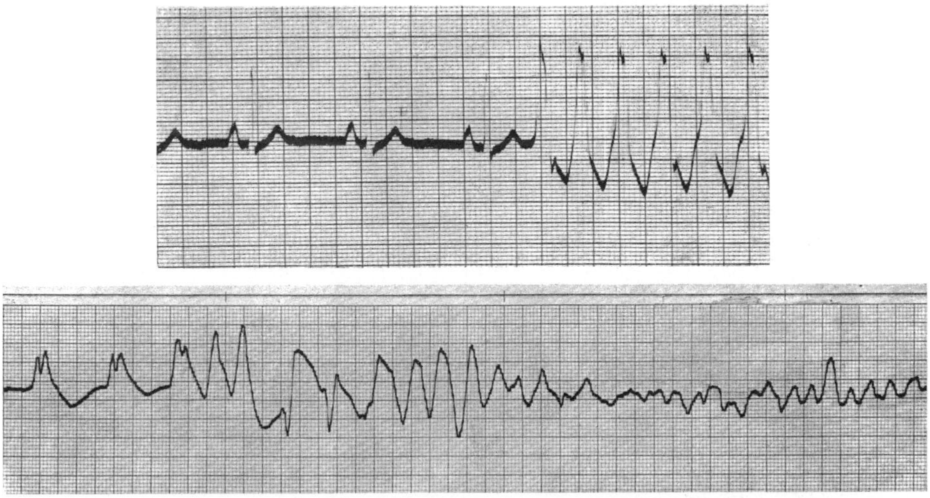

Fig. 4.23. The onset of ventricular tachycardia (*upper*) and decompensation into ventricular fibrillation (*lower*).

electrocardiographic picture should be familiar to all cardiac surgeons, since it is likely to proceed to ventricular fibrillation if the abnormal focus cannot be controlled.

Ventricular fibrillation probably results from a series of ectopic foci within the ventricular muscle mass, with large segments of the ventricle contracting independently. Such a rhythm cannot produce a co-ordinated ventricular contraction and, if untreated, is invariably fatal.

A regularly recurring irregularity, every second beat being premature and followed by a compensatory pause, is known as *pulsus bigeminus*. It may indicate digitalis intoxication. The ECG reveals this as a normal beat followed by a ventricular ectopic beat.

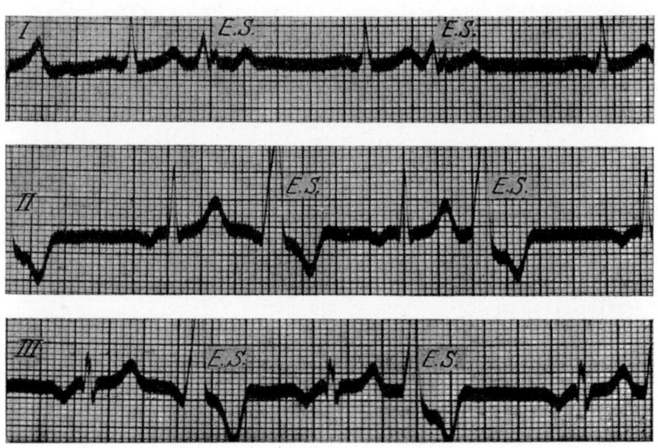

Fig. 4.24. Pulsus bigeminus – each normal complex is followed by an extrasystole (E.S.).

The wide QRS complex of ventricular ectopics must be differentiated from *bundle branch block*. Here, an electrical impulse originating above ventricular level suffers impaired or interrupted conduction through one or the other branch of the bundle. This may be due to a disease process affecting the conduction tissue or due to trauma during surgery. It results in a widening and splintering of the QRS pattern. In general, if the QRS complex has a positive deflection in the left precordial leads (V_5 and V_6), it is the left bundle branch which is affected. Conversely, right bundle branch block causes a positive complex in electrodes on the right side of the heart (V_1 and V_2).

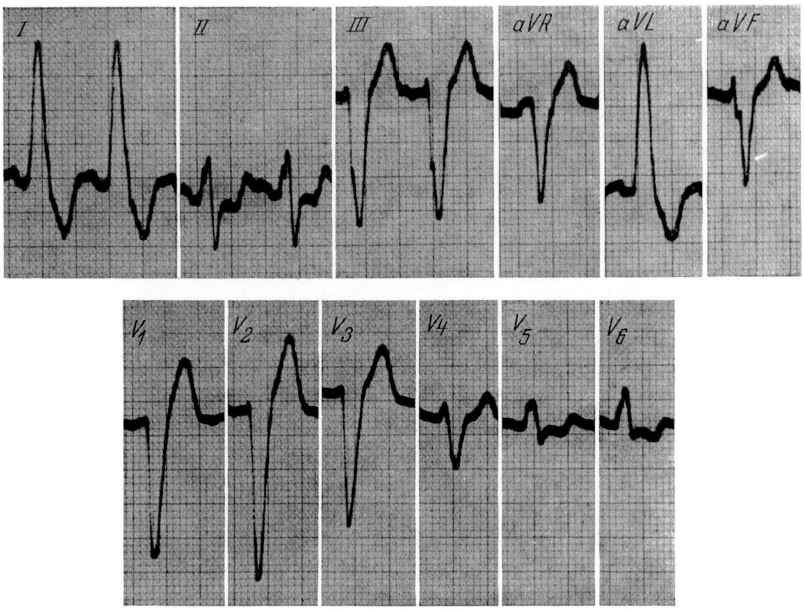

Fig. 4.25. Left bundle branch block. The ventricular complexes are widened and slurred.

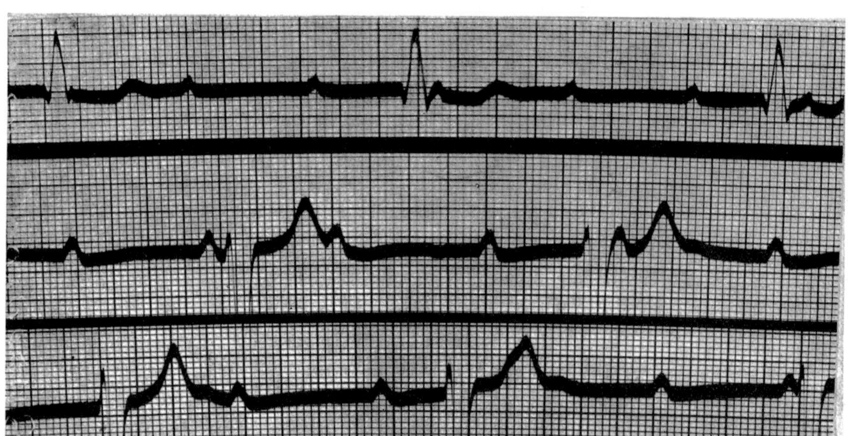

Fig. 4.26. Complete heart block. The P waves are unrelated to the ventricular complexes.

Abnormally slow heart rates (bradycardia) may indicate a condition of *heart block*. Because an impulse that originates in the atria cannot pass into the ventricles, activity of the two structures becomes dissociated, each following its own independent rhythm. The ventricular rate indicated by the QRS complex, is, in the main, much slower than the atrial (P wave) rate. The PR interval is, of course, quite inconstant. This arrythmia can be congenital, but it more commonly occurs as a complication of myocardial infarction or degenerative changes within the heart's conducting tissue. Since the advent of open heart surgery, traumatic heart block also has been recognised as a complication of some operative procedures. Heart block that requires treatment may be amenable to drug therapy, but patients often require implantation of a permanent pacemaker system or treatment by temporary pacing in the early postoperative period.

The cardiac surgeon should be aware of the various types and significance of postoperative rhythm disturbances, for management will depend upon a precise diagnosis.

Cardiac Hypertrophy

Enlargement of the atria may involve the right or left atrium, and the changes are reflected in the P wave. Left atrial hypertrophy, which is characteristic of mitral stenosis, produces a widened, flattened and bifid P wave. This is often best seen in standard limb lead II and is known as the 'P mitrale'. Right atrial hypertrophy is revealed as a tall spiked P wave, sometimes known as the 'P pulmonale'. It may be present in any condition causing increased right atrial pressure, for example pulmonary valve stenosis or pulmonary hypertension.

Hypertrophy or enlargement of the ventricles can be diagnosed most readily from the unipolar precordial or 'V' trace leads. As the left ventricle is normally thicker than the right ventricle, the deflections produced by that structure dominate the normal electrocardiographic picture. In general terms, the normal

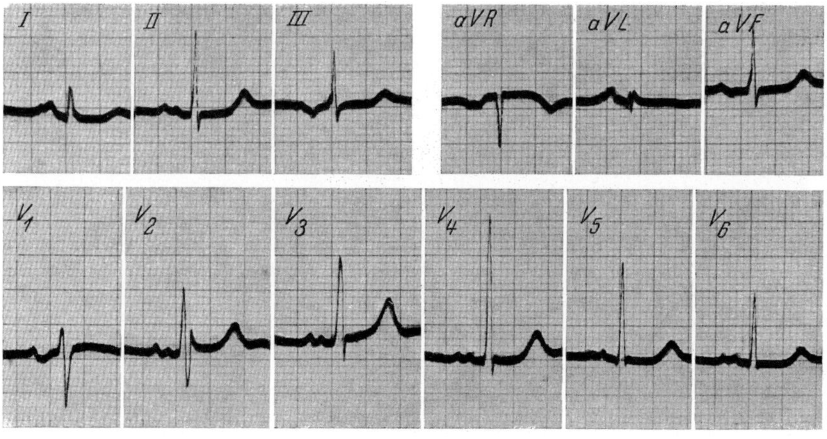

Fig. 4.27. P mitrale. The wave is broad and with a double deflection.

adult pattern obtained is as follows. Over the right ventricle (V_1–V_3), the predominant deflection is an S wave and the R is insignificant. Over the ventricular septum, the R and S waves become roughly equal in size, and over the left ventricle (V_5–V_6), the R wave is dominant while the S recedes in magnitude.

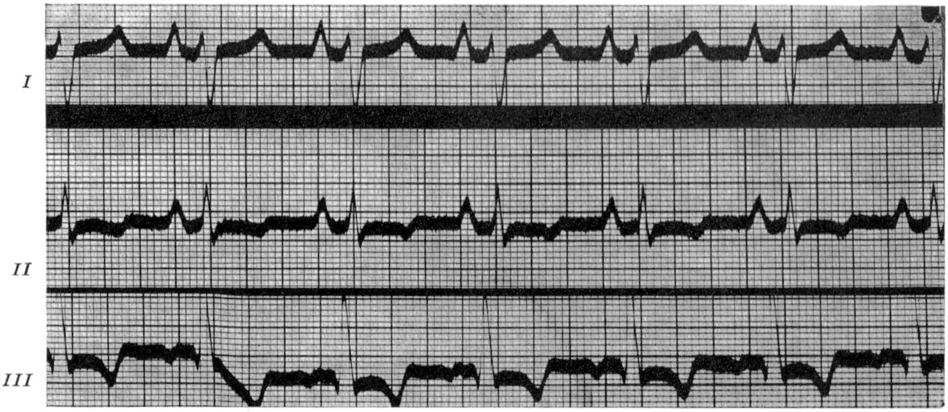

Fig. 4.28. The high spiked P waves of right atrial hypertrophy, shown in the three standard limb leads.

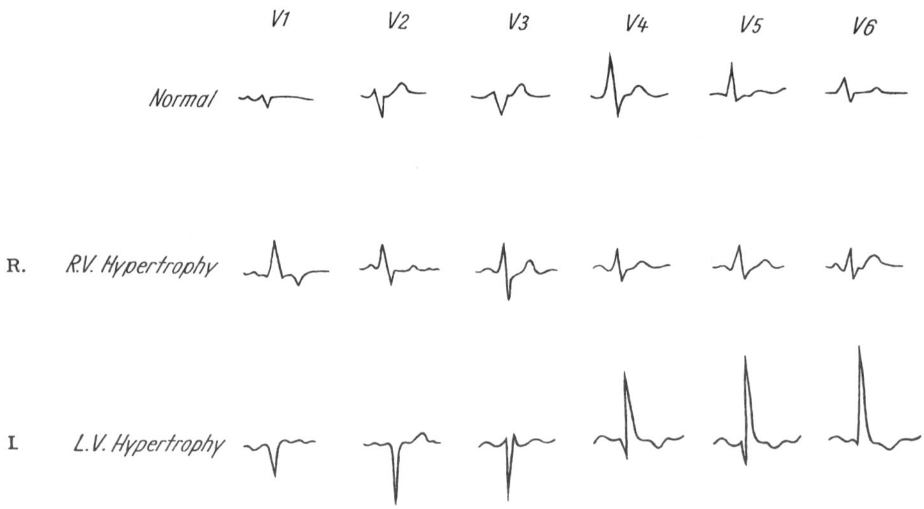

Fig. 4.29. The normal V leads (*upper*) and the characteristic changes of right (*centre*) and left (*lower*) ventricular hypertrophy.

It is convenient, although clearly an oversimplification, to regard the positive deflection (R wave) as representing the activity of the ventricle beneath the exploring electrode. With hypertrophy of this muscle mass or enlargement of the ventricular chamber, there follows an increased amplitude of the positive electrical deflection. Thus, in right ventricular hypertrophy, the positive voltage or R wave should be increased in the leads taken over that ventricle, i.e. larger R waves in, say, V_1, V_2 and V_3. While, in left ventricular hypertrophy, there would be a corresponding increase in the positive electrical deflection (R wave) over the left ventricular leads (V_4–V_6). The magnitude of deflection, which is abnormal and diagnostic of ventricular enlargement, varies with age and should be verified with cardiological tables if necessary.

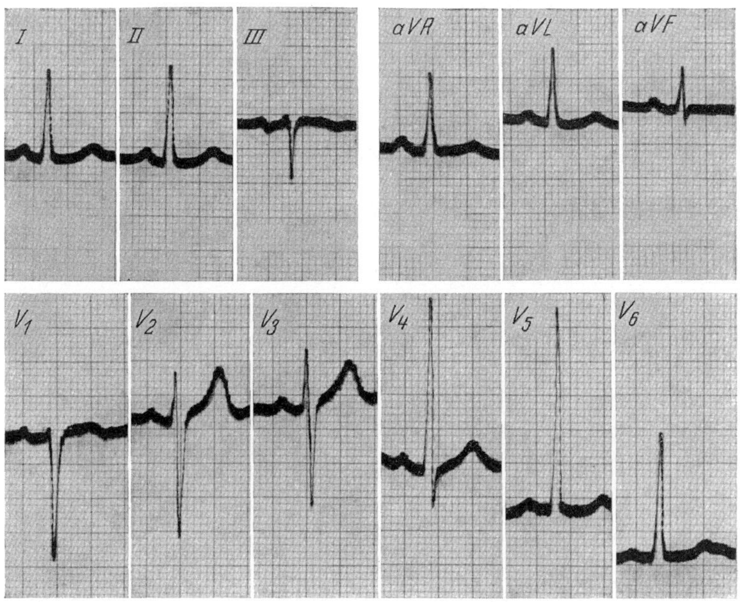

Fig. 4.30. The picture of left ventricular hypertrophy with large positive deflections over V_4–V_6.

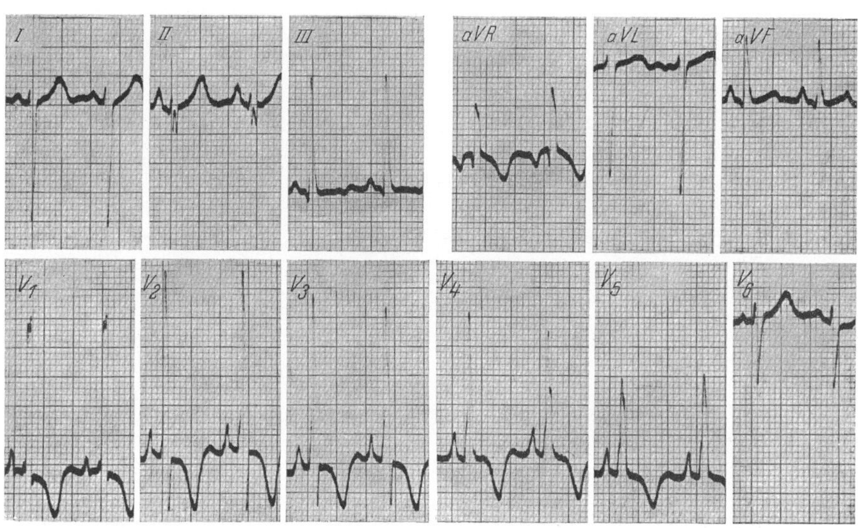

Fig. 4.31. Right ventricular hypertrophy and strain. Note the big positive deflections in V_1–V_4 and the deeply inverted T waves.

In cases of severe ventricular hypertrophy it is usual to see an inversion of the T wave over the distribution of the enlarged chamber, the so-called 'strain pattern'. Where this is marked, the T is not only inverted but the ST segment may also be depressed below the isoelectric point. The cause of these deflections is not known with certainty, but they resemble in some respects the patterns seen in ischaemic heart disease and also correlate with ventricular hypertension. It may be reasonable to assume that the grossly hypertrophied underlying muscle is, in fact, outstripping its blood supply. Certainly in aortic stenosis, the development of a 'strain pattern' with antecedent left ventricular hypertrophy on the ECG indicates a dangerous degree of aortic obstruction.

Two pitfalls should be avoided in interpreting T wave inversion as ventricular 'strain'. First, it is usual for the T wave to be inverted in V_1 and it may be inverted normally in V_2 or even V_3 in young children. Such patients lack other evidence of ventricular hypertrophy on the electrocardiogram. Second, both ST depression and T wave inversion can occur as a result of digitalis.

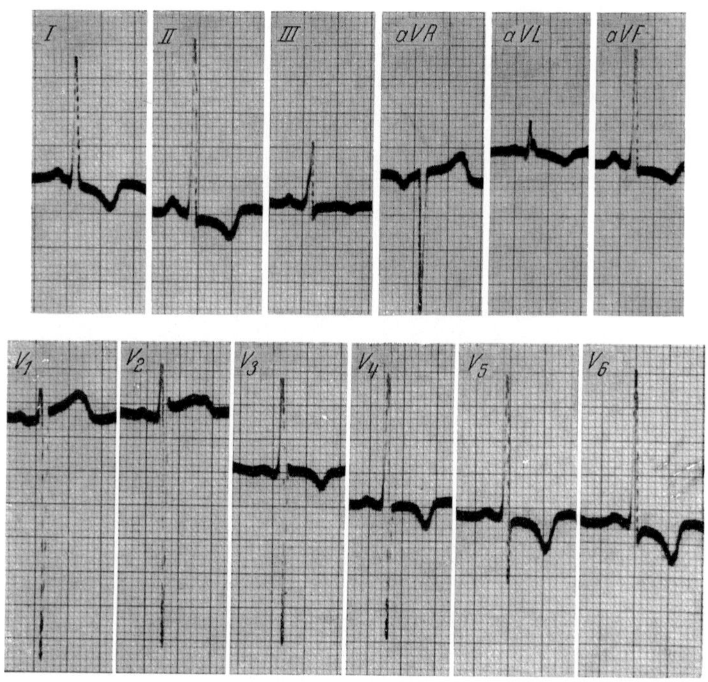

Fig. 4.32. Left ventricular hypertrophy and 'strain'. T wave inversion is seen in V_3–V_6.

Myocardial Ischaemia

Inadequate blood supply to the heart muscle results in ECG changes that indicate which part of the heart is affected and also the duration of the ischaemic episode. These changes may be observed transiently after a deliberate period of aortic occlusion in the operating theatre or as the more permanent outcome of coronary artery disease or injury. In simplified terms, an area of ischaemia causes inversion of the T waves and corresponds to potentially salvageable heart muscle, while elevation of the ST segment is present early in the course of more severe myocardial injury. When the heart muscle dies, the normal R wave is generally lost, and a Q wave takes its place.

Which part of the heart is involved is suggested by the particular combination of electrocardiographic leads that show changes of ischaemia or infarction. Thus, damage to the inferior or diaphragmatic surface will be seen in leads II, III and AVF, while lateral wall infarction is reflected in leads I, AVL and V_6. Persistent elevation of the ST segments for more than a few weeks raises the possibility of a ventricular aneurysm.

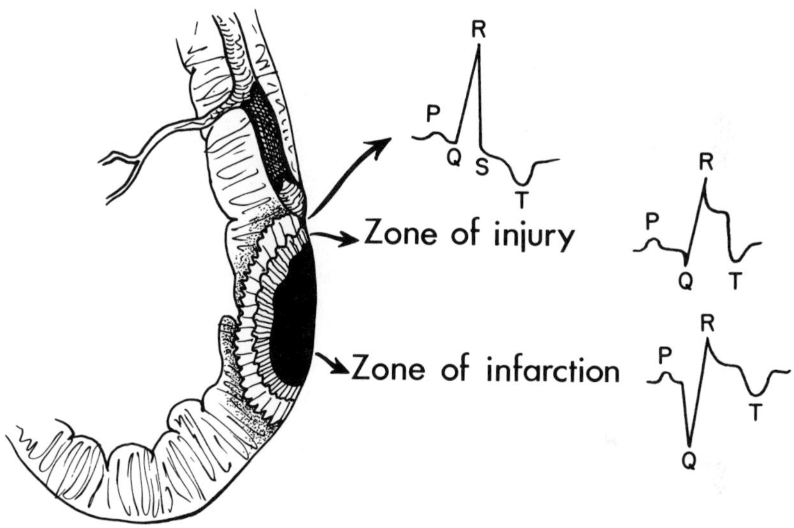

Fig. 4.33. The ECG changes in myocardial infarction.

Morphological Diagnosis

A few malformations alter the disposition of the conduction tissue in a way that is sufficiently constant and characteristic to produce diagnostic changes in the ECG; still other defects are suggested by typical ECG findings. In atrioventricular septal defects or single ventricles, for example, abnormalities of the inlet part of the ventricular septum cause the conduction tissue to lie in a more posterior or anterior position and produce a 'superior' QRS Axis. This information, interpreted in the light of clinical findings and other investigations, often will permit an accurate diagnosis prior to cardiac catheterisation.

Phonocardiography

This is the graphic recording of heart sounds and murmurs. Formerly developed to extend auscultation in the timing of cardiac sounds and identification of their aetiology, phonocardiography has been superseded, for the most part, by other non-invasive methods of cardiac investigation. It is still of value to students of cardiology in educating the ear to appreciate the more subtle variations in heart sounds and murmurs, and to correlate their timing with other events of the cardiac cycle, particularly as demonstrated by echocardiography.

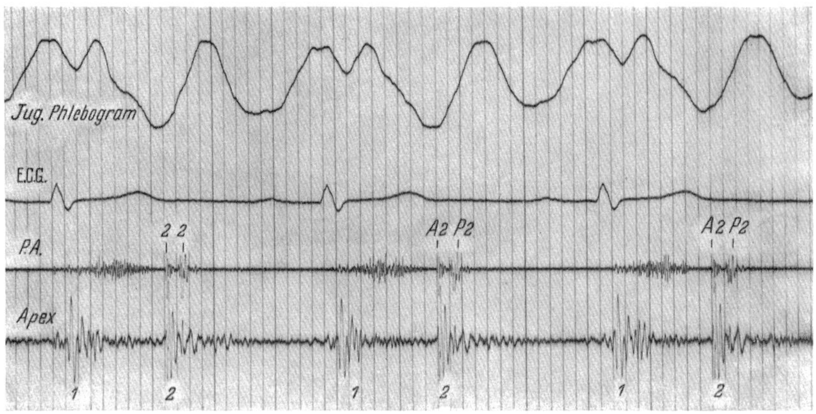

Fig. 4.34. The phonocardiogram relates the heart sounds to other events in the cardiac cycle. In this tracing the two components of the second sound are clearly indicated.

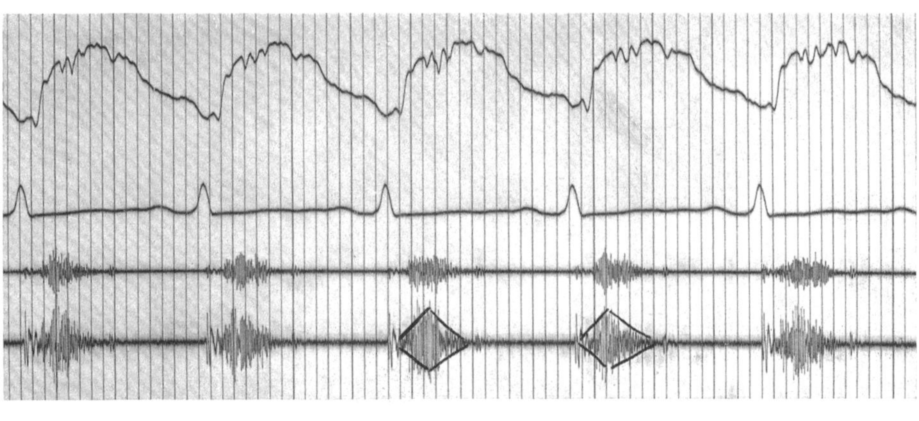

Fig. 4.35. An obstructive systolic murmur from a case of aortic stenosis. The murmur has a diamond shape and follows the first heart sound.

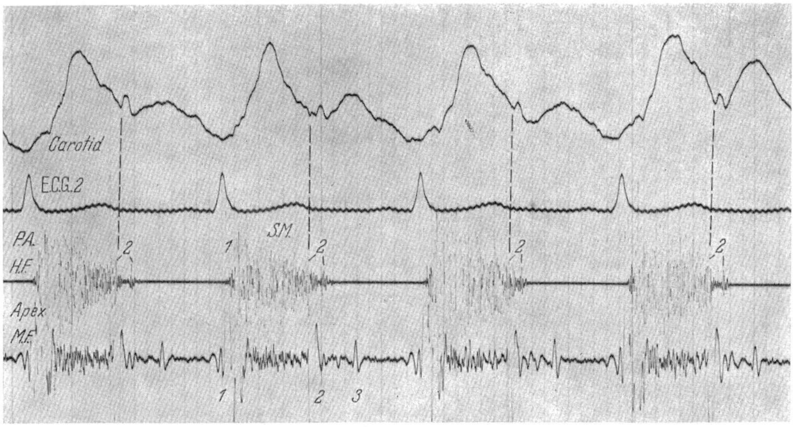

Fig. 4.36. The systolic murmur of ventricular septal defect. The murmur is coincident with the first sound and occupies the whole of systole.

Echocardiography

High-frequency sound waves which are bounced off the heart and great vessels form the basis of several powerful, non-invasive methods used to study cardiac structure and function. Such waves traverse different mediums, like muscle or blood, at different speeds. And, when they pass from one medium to another, part of the sound waves are reflected back toward their origin. The time required for this ‘echo’ to return to the sending device (or ‘transducer’) that emitted the original wave and the amount of energy which is reflected back indicate both the distance between an object and the transducer and the type of tissue which has been penetrated. The resulting echocardiogram will depend upon the frequency of sound waves used, the way in which they were directed toward the heart and the manner in which the returning echoes are electronically processed.

The earliest clinical echocardiograms were produced by directing a single beam of ultrasound (at a frequency of around 2.0–2.5 MHz) through the heart at various positions and recording the echoes as a function of time. Because this conveyed information about the movement of structures within the heart, it was called *M-mode echocardiography*. Such tracings generally are very clear and provide good resolution of structural detail, but they are limited by the smallness of the area that can be visualised at any given time. The images obtained from M-mode studies are well suited to measuring the size of cardiac chambers, showing the direction and extent of movement in the ventricular septum or free wall, and documenting motion of cardiac valves. Because the recordings do not actually portray the heart’s configuration, it requires some expertise to appreciate and interpret the significance of M-mode echocardiograms.

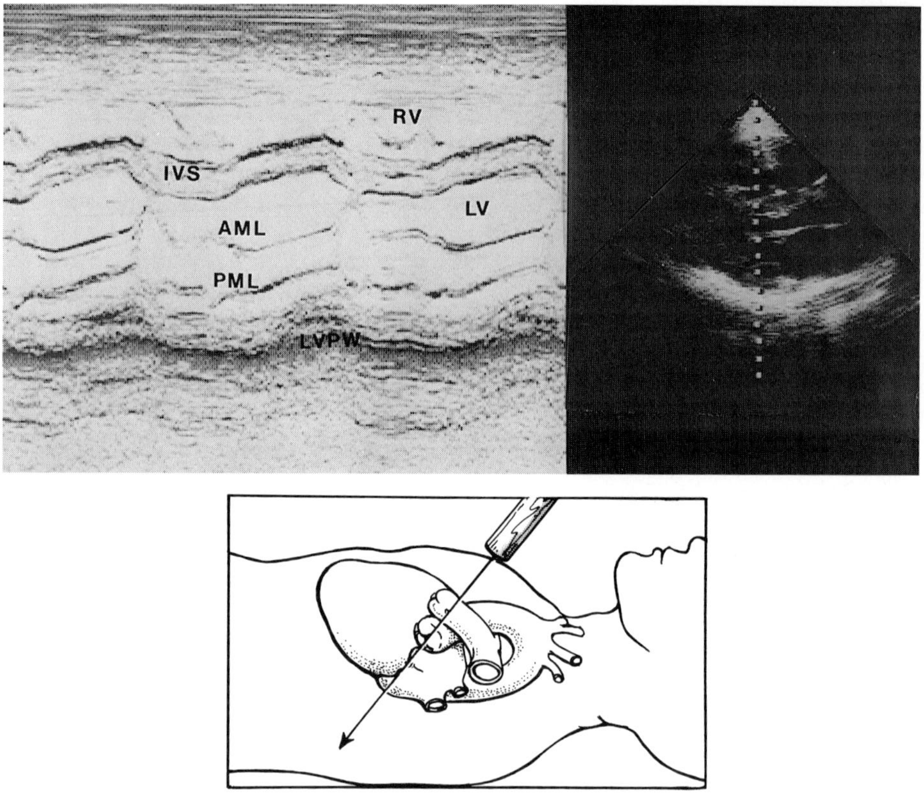

Fig. 4.37. View obtained with M-mode echocardiography. AML, PML, Anterior and posterior mitral leaflets; IVS, interventricular septum; LVPW, left ventricular posterior wall.

By scanning across the heart with multiple beams of ultrasound (which may be accomplished by a variety of mechanical or electronic modifications), it is possible to obtain a moving image that is more easily recognised as an anatomical representation of a slice through the heart. In contrast with the 'core' of information seen on the M-mode echocardiogram, this method visualises a wedge or slice, from which the relationships of various cardiac structures may be appreciated. It has been given several names: *sector scanning, cross-sectional, real-time* and *two-dimensional echocardiography* are among the more common. Several advantages have made real-time echocardiography an integral part of nearly all cardiac investigations. The thin chest wall of infants and children permits good resolution with high frequency ultrasound (3.0–6.5 mHz) and the examination can be carried out (and repeated, if necessary) with minimal disturbance to the patient. It is especially well suited to demonstrating malformations of the atrioventricular valves, septal defects, pericardial fluid and the size of cardiac chambers. One special application is the diagnosis of cardiac defects before birth, which can be done reliably by examination of the fetus *in utero*. When an abnormality is detected, the baby can then be delivered in a centre equipped to deal with heart problems in small infants. Another use is

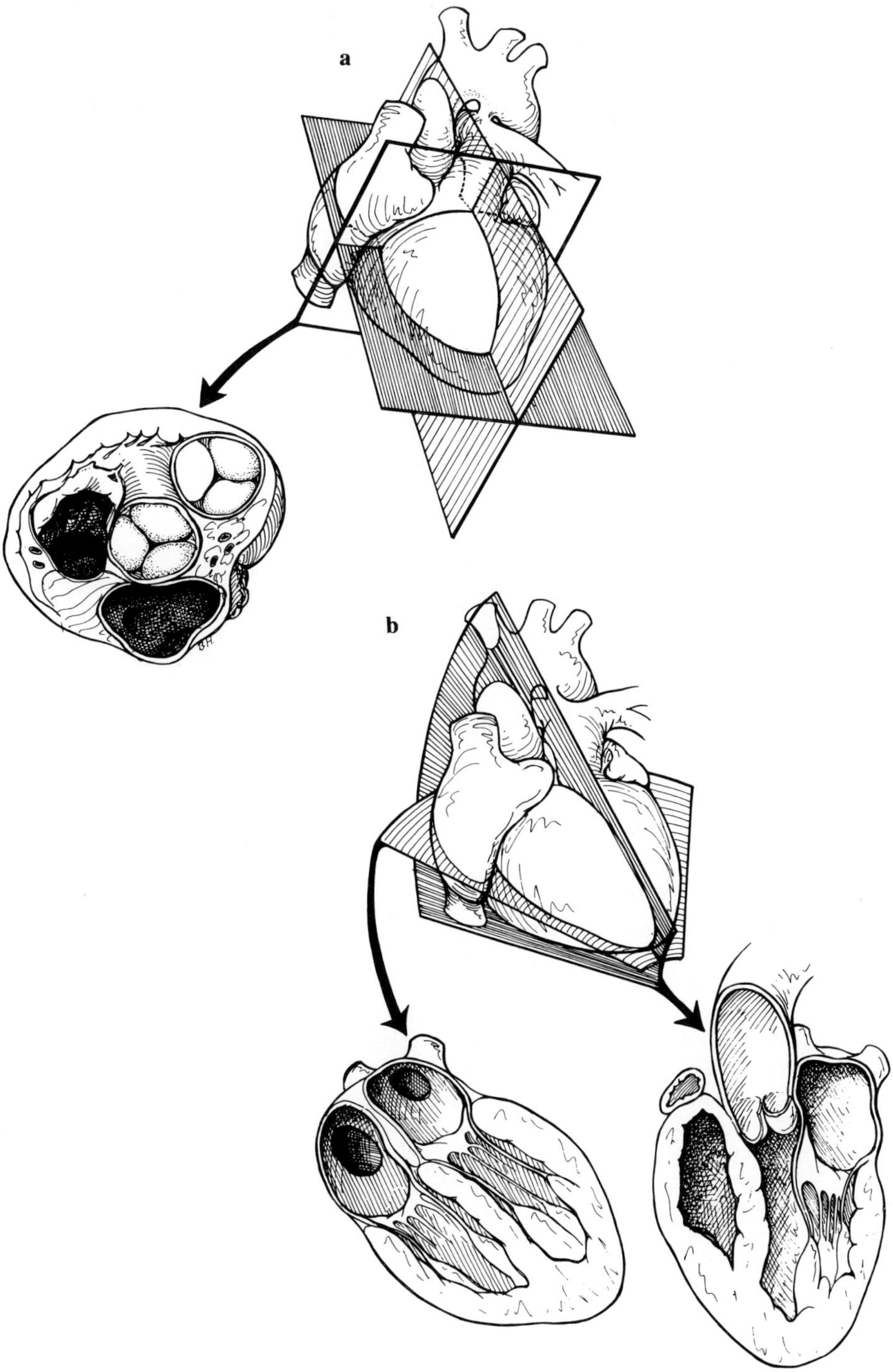

Fig. 4.38. Two dimensional echocardiogram 'cuts' of the heart.

contrast echocardiography. Here, the microbubbles, which normally are present in an injected bolus of saline, are followed through the cardiac chambers. This is a very sensitive and simple way to determine, for example, whether a low systemic arterial saturation early after open heart surgery is due to inadequate ventilation or to a right-to-left intracardiac shunt.

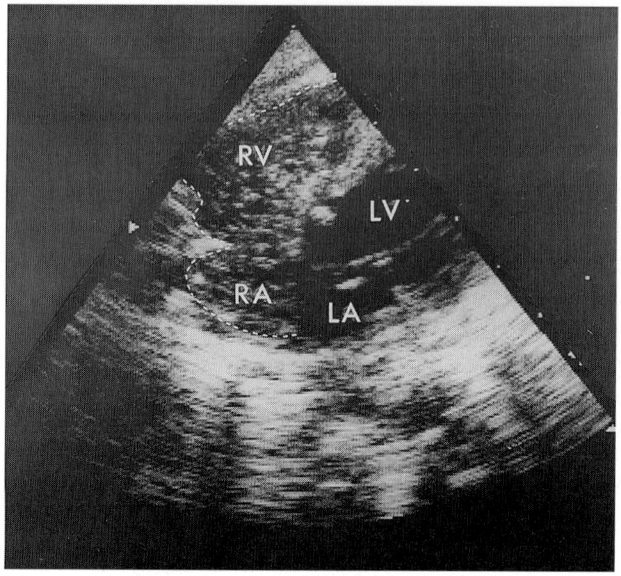

Fig. 4.39. Contrast echocardiogram.

Ultrasound is employed in a rather different way in *Doppler echocardiography*, to obtain knowledge about the velocity and direction of blood flow within the heart and great vessels. The Doppler effect is easily observed in everyday life: sound waves given out by a moving object, such as the whistle of a passing train, change in pitch according to the speed at which the train approaches or leaves the observer. The train whistle moving towards an observer becomes high-pitched as its sound waves are compressed, and it seems lower moving away from the observer because the waves are elongated. (The same is true if the observer moves in relation to a stationary source of sound waves.) It is possible to calculate the speed of a moving object by observing the change in frequency (pitch) of the sound waves.

In clinical echocardiography, the ultrasonic beam is reflected from the red blood cells with a frequency that is proportional to the velocity of the blood-flow and usually within the audible range. By 'sampling' at various places, it is possible to detect a jet of blood passing across a stenotic or leaking valve, across a septal defect or through a persistent ductus arteriosus. When the jet of blood is exactly perpendicular to the sensing transducer, further calculations may be made (from the Bernoulli equation) to predict the pressure difference that generated that particular velocity of blood flow. Thus, it may be possible both to identify a stenotic or obstructed heart valve and to estimate the pressure gradient across it.

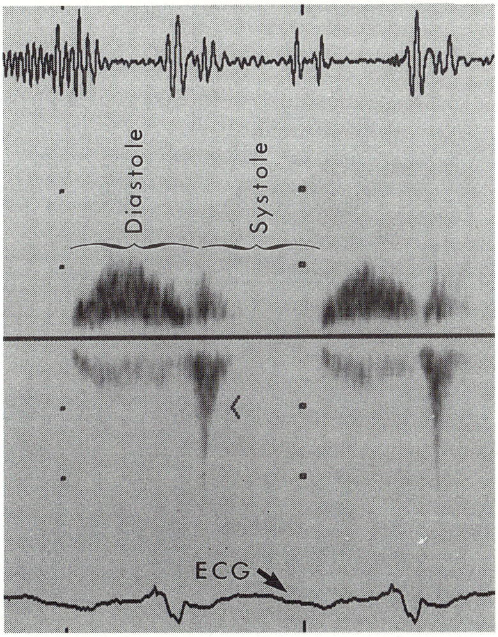

Fig. 4.40. Doppler study showing flow across a heart valve.

An even newer technique, which combines the structural or positional information obtained from real-time echocardiography with the haemodynamic inferences of Doppler examination, is *colour Doppler echocardiography*. Here, the direction of blood flow, determined by Doppler sampling over the entire

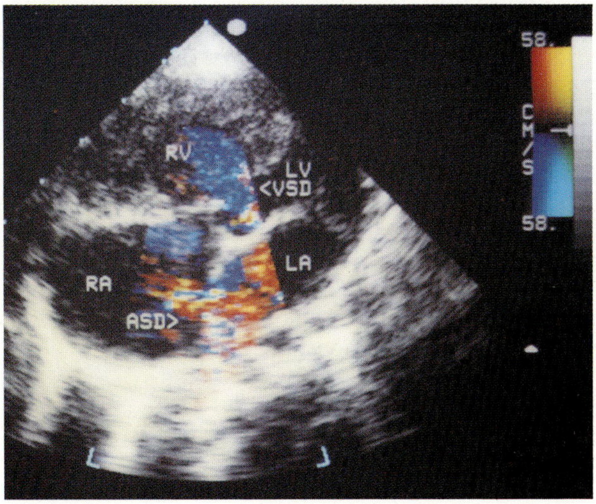

Fig. 4.41. Colour doppler study in a patient with defects in both the atrial septum (ASD) and the ventricular septum (VSD).

area imaged by the sector scan, is coded into colours: red represents flow toward the transducer; blue, flow away from the transducer; and speckled colour, turbulence. These colours are then superimposed on the real-time echocardiogram, such that one can see both the movement of a structure within the heart and, simultaneously, the direction of blood flow through it.

More recent advances in technology have permitted echocardiographic studies to be done from the surface of the heart during surgery and from the transoesophageal route.

Radionuclide Studies

In contrast with other non-invasive techniques for imaging the cardiovascular system, radionuclide studies provide information that relates more to cardiac function than anatomical structure. The general procedure is that an isotope which produces the appropriate radiation is introduced into the circulation through a peripheral vein, and its passage through or concentration within the heart is monitored by use of a gamma camera. The radioactivity 'seen' by the camera is electronically processed and a computer is used to translate the activity measurements into a picture of the heart or time activity curve.

When information about ventricular performance or intracardiac shunts is required, the blood-pool is labelled with a substance that remains in the circulation, commonly technetium-99m on red blood cells. Activity may be recorded just the first time the substance passes through the heart (*first-pass study*), or after it has become dispersed evenly throughout the circulation (*equilibrium study*). From such measurements, it is possible to estimate the ejection fraction of each ventricle, the volume of the ventricular cavity, an impression of ventricular wall movement, and the amount of blood shunted from the systemic to the pulmonary circulation. This type of investigation is called *radionuclide ventriculography*.

Using a radionuclide which is taken up into the myocardial cells (for example, thallium-201), it is possible with *myocardial perfusion imaging* to demonstrate ischaemic or infarcted heart muscle. In this case, the distribution of isotope reflects coronary artery blood flow, for an area which is not perfused does not incorporate the radionuclide. The reversibility of ischaemia, as well as the response to exercise or drug therapy may also be evaluated.

Nuclear imaging techniques require sophisticated apparatus and are limited, to a degree, by the radionuclides that can be used and by difficulty in obtaining spatial resolution of structures within the heart. However, in a specialised department equipped for such investigative work, the techniques provide a fast and simple method of investigating circulatory performance, particularly during exercise and when sequential examinations are required.

Computed Tomography

Computed axial tomography (CAT scanning) relies upon a computer to build up an image from the X-ray density measured across multiple 'slices' through the subject. Its application to cardiac investigation has been limited because the X-ray exposure time required is long in comparison to heart movements. However, faster scanners and methods to synchronise data collection with events in the cardiac cycle may yet realise the potential of this technique to produce a three-dimensional picture with accurate spatial resolution of cardiac morphology. At present, its main application is the demonstration of stationary pathology within the cardiovascular system. This includes such things as aortic arch anomalies, aneurysms or dissection of the aorta, and cardiac tumours. Because the X-ray densities of blood and muscle are quite similar, 'enhancement' of the image by injection of contrast material is usually necessary to achieve clear demarcation between intravascular and extravascular structures.

Positron Emission Tomography

In essence, the concepts of nuclear cardiology and computed tomography are joined together and extended to a biochemical level in the application of positron emission tomography to cardiovascular investigation. Here, isotopes that emit positrons are incorporated into the normal metabolic pathways of the heart and observed with cross-sectional imaging. Early research experience suggests that this technique may prove useful for the study of myocardial blood flow and metabolism. However, its complexity makes widespread availability of the technique unlikely.

Magnetic Resonance Imaging

Although still in its infancy as regards application to the cardiovascular system, the use of nuclear magnetic resonance to image the heart or to study muscle physiology appears promising. This technique depends upon using the behaviour of molecular nuclei which have been subject to a magnetic field in order to estimate the density of tissues or concentrations of biochemical substances. As an imaging techniques, it is non-invasive, yields good structural resolution and does not require injection of radionuclides or contrast material into the patient. The instrumentation for clinical work is, at present, cumbersome and expensive, but future refinements probably will bring about greater availability and more widespread application.

Cardiac Catheterisation and Angiography

It is fair to say that this is the investigation which has made the greatest contribution to the elucidation of normal circulatory physiology and the alterations brought about by disease. While non-invasive techniques increasingly complement and replace cardiac catheterisation, it remains the standard with which newer methods of cardiac investigation are compared. With the advent of balloon dilatation of vessels, and devices for the occlusion of abnormal vessels or septal defects, the catheterisation laboratory has become a facility for the treatment as well as the diagnosis of heart conditions.

In general, for the common varieties of congenital heart disease, right heart catheterisation has most to offer in the diagnosis of left-to-right shunts. In right-to-left shunts, the angiocardiogram may be more useful, since the opaque medium is then carried across into the systemic circulation. Septal defects in infants and children often permit investigation of both the left and right sides of the heart from the systemic venous route. The complementary techniques of left heart catheterisation and dye injection studies, particularly as regards coronary artery disease, have added greatly to the information which can be obtained at cardiac catheterisation.

Right Heart Catheterisation

This investigation involves the passage of a flexible, radio-opaque catheter from a peripheral vein through the right heart chambers out into the lung vessels and sometimes through abnormal communications or septal defects. Its passage is guided by fluoroscopy and checked by pressure measurements and blood sampling. At least three sets of direct information can be obtained:

1. Changes of pressure
2. Changes of oxygenation of the blood
3. The demonstration of abnormal communications

This information can be coupled with simultaneous investigations of, say, the cardiac output to supply a great deal of additional derived or indirect data.

Changes of Pressure. The pressures within various heart chambers and associated great vessels are usually expressed in mmHg above an arbitrary zero level or base-line, from which the recording instrument is calibrated. Although pressures have, on occasion, been measured with an ordinary saline manometer, it is more usual to employ an electromanometer. This transforms the pressure changes transmitted through a fluid-filled catheter into electronic impulses which are then amplified so as to activate the recording instrument. Alternatively, the record can be projected on an oscilloscope screen. The normal pressures in the various heart chambers can be memorised by reference to a simple diagram. There are of course fairly wide variations between patients and under various conditions in the same patient.

The pressure in the great veins and right atrium is low and reflects the low intrathoracic pressure which, in some phases of respiration, is negative. The *a, c* and *v* waves are distinguishable in the right atrial pressure record. The right ventricular systolic pressure is generally between 20 and 30 mmHg, with a zero diastolic pressure. Where the diastolic pressure is raised, it may indicate pulmonary regurgitation or a failing right ventricle. The systolic pressure in the pulmonary artery will be the same as in the right ventricle, providing there is no obstruction (functional or organic) at the pulmonary valve or in the right ventricular outflow tract. There is, however, a positive diastolic pressure in the pulmonary artery. This results from pulmonary valve closure as the right ventricular pressure falls. The normal systolic/diastolic pulmonary artery pressure is in the region of 25/10 mmHg. As with aortic regurgitation, pulmonary regurgitation is usually revealed by a wide pulmonary artery pulse pressure, with a raised systolic and low diastolic pressure.

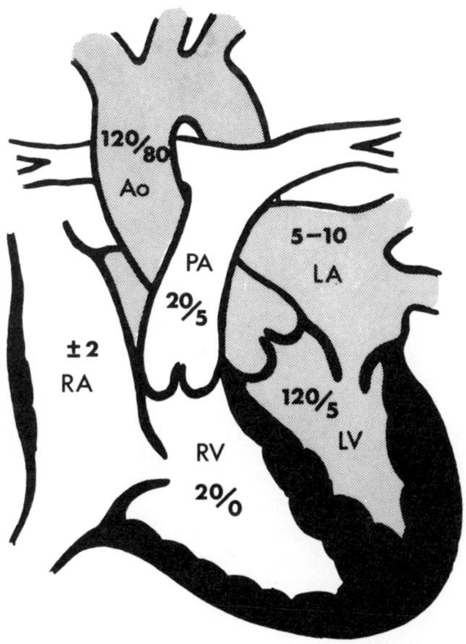

Fig. 4.42. Approximate normal pressures within the heart and great vessels.

In the course of blood-flow through the smaller but more numerous pulmonary arteries and arterioles, there is a progressive fall in pressure such that, in the pulmonary capillaries and the pulmonary veins beyond, the pressure has fallen to 5–10 mmHg. Generally this pressure is also recorded in the left atrium. Measurement of this left atrial pressure can be approximated at right heart catheterisation by wedging the cardiac catheter in a distal pulmonary artery branch, so as to block forward flow in the vessel completely. The pressure then recorded is known as the *pulmonary capillary venous* (PCV) or *wedge* pressure and represents the pressure distal to the blocking catheter, i.e. the left atrial pressure. A simplified modification of this manoeuvre, in which a balloon-tipped catheter is floated into the pulmonary circulation and the balloon is inflated to obtain a wedge pressure, has widespread application in intensive care unit monitoring of patients with heart failure.

The accuracy of the pulmonary capillary wedge pressure in reflecting the true left atrial pressure has been verified on a number of occasions by comparing the pressure obtained with that recorded by direct left atrial needle puncture. The left atrial pressure tracing, however, shows in addition the *a, c* and *v* positive deflections, and the *x* and *y* negative deflections that are observed also in the right atrium.

Measurements of pressures obtained at cardiac catheterisation are particularly useful in the diagnosis of obstructive lesions, especially at the level of the pulmonary valve or the infundibulum of the right ventricle. They are also of use in diagnosing tricuspid stenosis. Through the pulmonary capillary wedge pressure, indication is also given of the left atrial pressure, from which it is possible to estimate the degree of any existing mitral stenosis. Straightforward right heart catheterisation, however, gives no direct information about pressure in the left ventricle or systemic circulation.

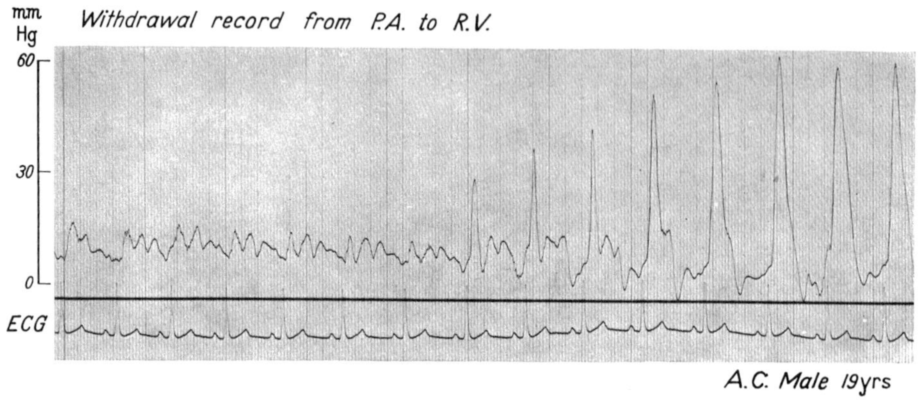

Fig. 4.43. Pressure withdrawal record taken in a case of pulmonary valve stenosis during passage of the catheter from pulmonary artery into right ventricle. Note the drop in diastolic pressure on entering the ventricle.

Pressure measurements are also of help in diagnosing hypertension in the pulmonary arterial system and in assessing its severity. The pulmonary arterial pressure, taken in conjunction with the left atrial pressure and cardiac output, permits calculation of a figure for the pulmonary vascular resistance. Estimation of pulmonary vascular resistance is of considerable importance in assessing the suitability of septal defects and more complex lesions for surgical correction.

When large volumes of blood traverse the pulmonary valve ring, *functional pressure gradients* are common. For example, in an adult with an atrial septal defect there may be a flow amounting to something between 15 and 18 l/min passing through the right heart (a '3-to-1' shunt), and, in these circumstances, the normal pulmonary valve acts as an obstruction to this torrential flow. This flow gradient – often in the region of 20–30 mmHg – disappears on closure of the septal defect. The same phenomenon may be seen in transposition of the great vessels, where increased pulmonary blood flow may cause a pressure difference between the left ventricle and the pulmonary artery in the presence of an anatomically normal outflow tract.

Changes of Oxygen Saturation. In the right atrium, venous blood from the superior vena cava, inferior vena cava and coronary sinus come together and the resultant mixture passes through the right ventricle and pulmonary vessels to the lungs. This blood has a venous oxygen saturation in the region of 65–75%. Where there is a shunt of 'arterial' blood into the right atrium, right ventricle or pulmonary artery, there is a rise of oxygen saturation at the appropriate level.

By convention, a rise in oxygen content of 2 vol. % in the right atrium is considered diagnostic of a left-to-right shunt at atrial level, while a rise of 1 vol. % and $\frac{1}{2}$ vol. % at right ventricular and pulmonary artery levels, respectively, indicates a shunt at ventricular or great vessels level.

By estimating the degree of saturation of the blood in a systemic artery, it is possible to calculate separately the amount of blood flow through the pulmonary vascular bed and the systemic vascular bed. In this way, the volume of the shunt from one circulation to the other can be estimated. Similarly, if the systemic arterial blood is desaturated, it is likely to indicate the presence of a right-to-left shunt of venous blood into the systemic circulation, the magnitude of which also can be calculated.

It should be borne in mind that inferior caval blood may have a higher oxygen saturation than that in the superior vena cava, due to the return of a stream of fairly highly saturated blood from the kidneys. The kidneys act as filters and the volume of blood passing through them is well in excess of their parenchymal oxygen requirements. Consequently, the returning blood in the renal veins may have a relatively high oxygen saturation. This observation is of value when one cannulates the inferior vena cava for cardiopulmonary bypass: if very red (oxygenated) blood returns from the cannula, the tip probably has passed beyond the entrance of the hepatic veins and may obstruct drainage of blood from the liver during cardiopulmonary bypass.

In contrast the myocardium extracts a great deal of oxygen from the blood so that the blood entering the right atrium from the coronary sinus has a lower oxygen saturation (about 40%) than any other blood in the body. If the cardiac catheter in the right atrium samples a stream of blood from the region of the coronary sinus, or, if the catheter tip enters this orifice, the blood sample obtained will have a deceptively low oxygen saturation.

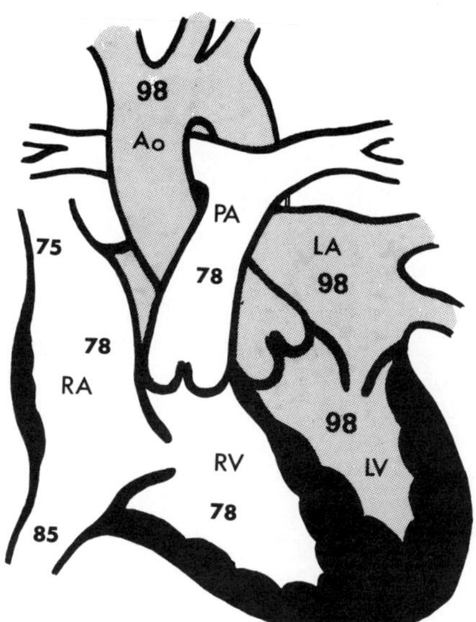

Fig. 4.44. Approximate figures for the degree of oxygen saturation (%) of the blood in the normal heart and great vessels.

Abnormal Passage of the Catheter. In following the passage through the heart and out into the pulmonary arteries it may be seen to take an abnormal course or come to lie in a characteristic position. Such observations can contribute information of diagnostic value. For example, the catheter may cross the atrial septum into the left atrium, confirming the presence of an atrial septal defect or

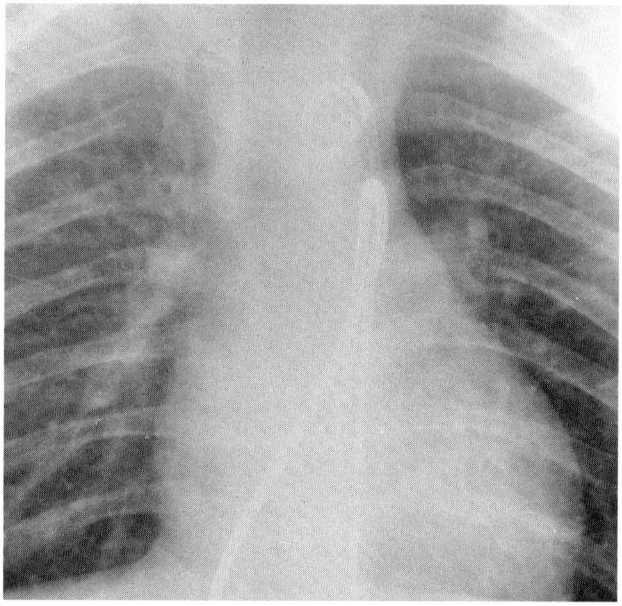

Fig. 4.45. The more opaque catheter has passed through the right heart chambers, pulmonary artery and ductus to enter the descending aorta. A second catheter is seen to have passed retrograde up the descending aorta into the aortic arch.

a persistent foramen ovale. In ventricular septal defect, the catheter may cross into the left ventricle or, more likely, pass out into the aorta. In persistent ductus arteriosus, the ductus is catheterised directly in about 70% of cases where this is attempted. Similarly, the catheter may pass into a pulmonary vein from the vena cavae or the right atrium and establish a diagnosis of anomalous pulmonary venous drainage, or the course of the catheter may suggest transposition of the great vessels.

Left Heart Catheterisation

Catheterisation of the right heart may supply information of pressure and oxygen saturation from all the cardiac chambers except the left ventricle and left atrium. If these have not been entered through a septal defect, it is possible to catheterise them 'retrograde' by passing the catheter proximally from the femoral or brachial arteries. The measurement of the pressure in the left ventricle enables estimation of the diastolic gradient across the mitral valve, the

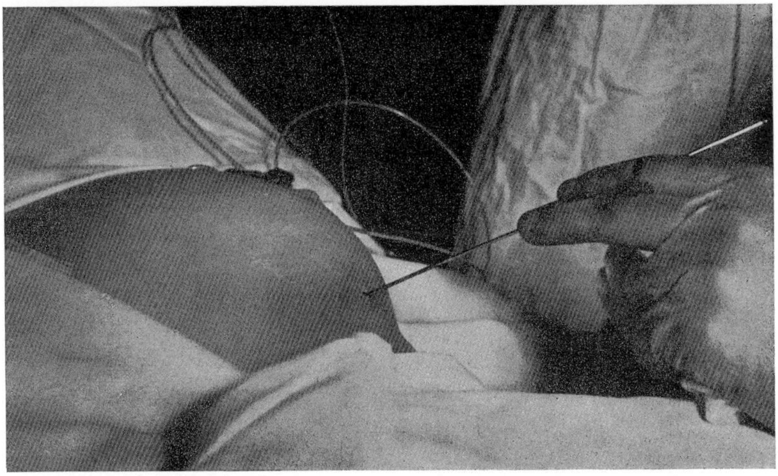

Fig. 4.46. Left ventricular puncture. The needle is inserted into the ventricle at the point at which the impulse is clearly felt. Pressures are recorded by means of an electromanometer.

systolic pressure gradient across the aortic valve and left ventricular function. By inserting a cannula or an indwelling needle into the brachial or femoral artery it is also possible to obtain information about the circulation distal to the left ventricle. Simultaneous pressure measurements here and in the left ventricle, for example, may be useful in documenting obstruction of the left ventricular outflow or coarctation of the aorta.

While largely of historical interest, some of the techniques originally used to gain access to the left atrium and left ventricle may be useful in certain circumstances and illustrate the anatomical relationships of these structures. *Left atrial puncture* was first described by Allison, who entered the left atrium by means of a long needle passed under vision through a bronchoscope. The needle passed through the bronchial wall just lateral to the carina where the tracheal bifurcation straddles the left atrium. The method was extended by passing a long, fine catheter down the needle and through the mitral valve into the left ventricle. By this technique, the validity of pulmonary capillary wedge pressure as a measure of left atrial pressure was confirmed, and mitral valve disease was assessed by synchronous pressure measurements in the left atrium and left ventricle.

An alternative approach to the left atrium was introduced by Bjork of Sweden. He described percutaneous needle puncture of the left atrium from the back, the needle entering about the level of the ninth rib in the right paravertebral area and passing medially beyond the vertebral body. The patient lay on either his left side or, more conveniently, face down, while a thin catheter was passed through the needle into the left atrium and manipulated into the left ventricle during continuous pressure observations. This investigation was associated with a fair incidence of pain, stiffness and morbidity. These landmarks are, however, worth remembering in the examination of patients with stab wounds or other traumatic injuries of the thorax.

Another route to the left atrium was from the suprasternal notch or the supraclavicular fossa. In this case, the needle was passed through the skin and aorta, measuring this pressure *en route*, and also, if possible, through the right pulmonary artery before entering the left atrium.

In aortic valve disease, *left ventricular puncture* was accomplished safely and simply by percutaneous needle puncture of the hypertrophied ventricle at the point where it impinged against the chest wall. In the apex of the heart, there are no large coronary arteries to be damaged. Passing a catheter through the needle into the left ventricle and on across the aortic valve permit withdrawal measurements of pressure across the left ventricular outflow tract. If measurements of the cardiac output are made at the time, the approximate size of the aortic valve orifice can be calculated.

The information obtained at cardiac catheterisation can be of great value in making a diagnosis, but it is subject to certain limitations. These may arise from errors in the technique of blood sampling and analysis, or in the recording of pressure measurements. Furthermore the data received may be incorrectely

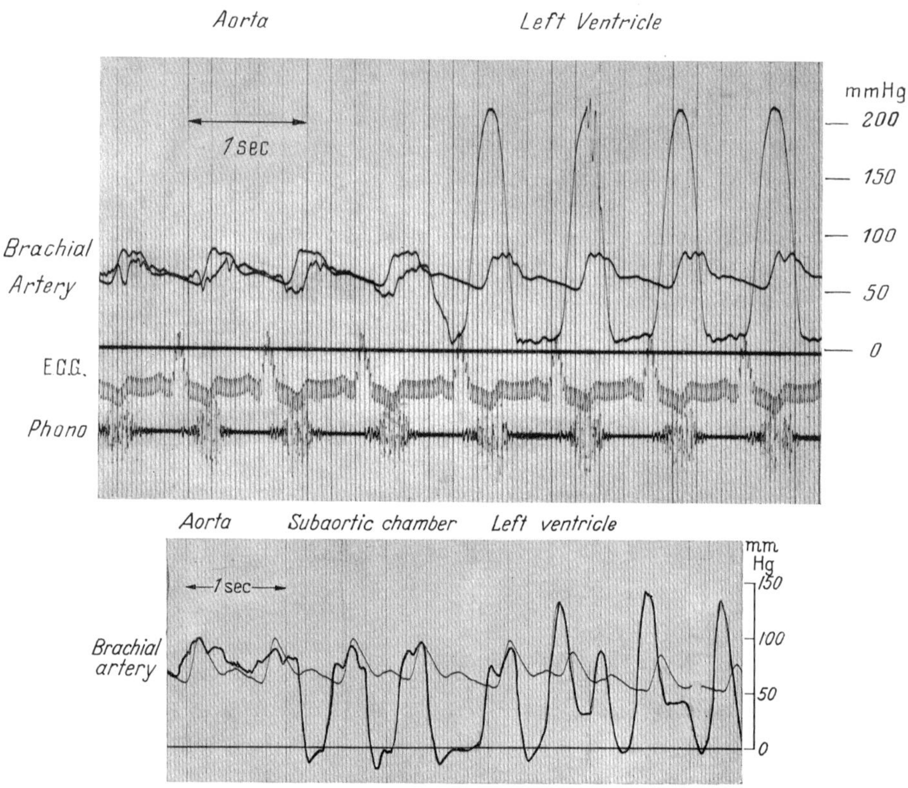

Fig. 4.47. As the catheter passes from aorta to left ventricle, there is a normal drop of diastolic pressure as the valve is passed. A systolic gradient of about 120 mm also becomes apparent. The simultaneous brachial artery trace overlies the aortic and left ventricular records (*upper*). In this case of subvalvar aortic stenosis, the catheter passage across the valve is indicated by the fall in diastolic pressure but the systolic pressure gradient only appears at a lower level. Faint line indicates brachial artery pressure (*lower*).

interpreted. Information is generally collected over a period of a few heart beats during the patient's life. This only reflects the pressures and oxygen saturation of the blood at one brief point in time, under examination conditions, which may be quite abnormal. This applies particularly to an apprehensive or an over-sedated patient at the end of a long and difficult catheterisation.

A sound principle to adopt is that, if the catheterisation results (or the results of other investigations) are totally at variance with the history and observed physical signs, radiography and electrocardiography, they are probably wrong and should be disregarded or at least repeated.

Angiography

This is a technique for visualising the cardiac chambers, the coronary arteries and the great vessels by means of injected contrast medium. As a rule, an injection of an iodine compound is made into the appropriate part of the circulation via a catheter that has been passed into the heart or associated great arteries. In the case of coronary artery studies, the orifice of the vessel is cannulated selectively. For X-ray examination, about 1.5 ml/kg (the dosage varying from 0.75 to 2 ml/kg) total volume of contrast is used. With newer contrast mediums and methods of X-ray recording, such as digital subtraction angiography, a smaller amount may be sufficient.

Using axial projections to profile intracardiac structures or special views that prevent overlap, it is possible to obtain good resolution and a great deal of information about cardiac structure and function. In Fallot's tetralogy, for example, injection of contrast into the right ventricular chamber (a 'right ventricular angiogram') can demonstate the right ventricular outflow tract, the size and number of ventricular septal defects and the relation of the aorta to the ventricular septum.

Aortography (the injection of contrast into the aorta) may visualise a persistent ductus arteriosus, deformity or regurgitation of the aortic valve, collateral vessels to the lung in cases of pulmonary atresia, and aneurysms of the ascending or descending aorta. Selective coronary angiography is, at present, the only means of delineating the site of strictures within the coronary vessels.

Most commonly, X-ray pictures are taken following the injection of contrast and projected onto an image intensifier, which is photographed by a 35 mm camera. This produces a 'cine-angiocardiogram', which, when developed and projected, not only indicates the passage of blood but also gives information about the function of various heart chambers and presence of shunts. Alternatively, in examinations where the structures are not moving, such as aortography, a series of 'cut' X-ray films may be produced by sequential exposure of a number of X-ray plates. Recently, techniques have been developed to electronically code the X-ray image and remove background shadows; this permits visualisation of structures with a smaller injection of contrast material, sometimes via a peripheral vein. The resulting image is recorded on electromagnetic tape and projected on a television screen, the technique being known as *digital subtraction angiography*.

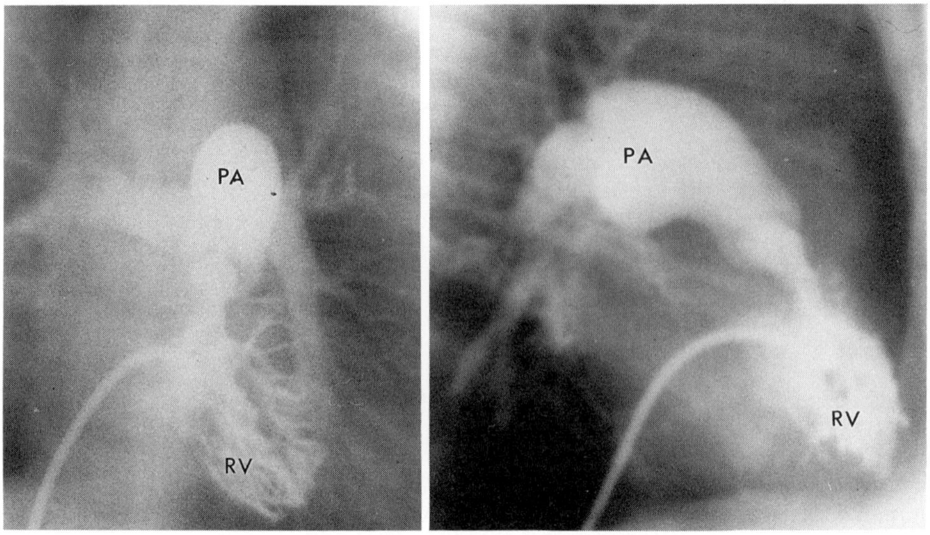

Fig. 4.48. Right ventricular angiograms in the anteroposterior and lateral projections in a case of valvar pulmonary stenosis. The thickened valve domes during systole and there is both post-stenotic dilatation of the pulmonary artery distal to the valve and narrowing of the muscular right ventricle proximal to it.

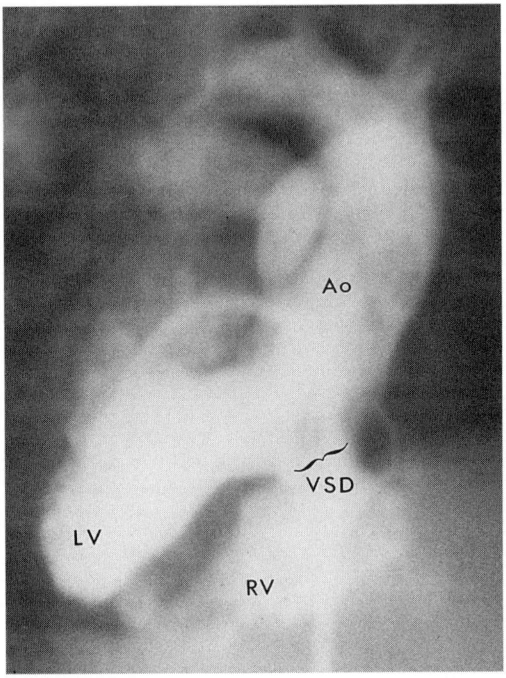

Fig. 4.49. Left ventricular angiogram in Fallot's tetralogy. The catheter has passed up the inferior vena cava, across an atrial septal defect and into the left ventricle through the mitral valve. The aorta over-rides a large ventricular septal defect.

Interventional Cardiac Catheterisation

The invention of several types of devices has permitted permanent alterations to be made to the circulation during cardiac catheterisation. Probably the first of these to achieve widespread usage was the Rashkind septostomy balloon. This is a catheter with a tough, inflatable balloon on the end. It is passed across the patent foramen ovale, usually in a baby with transposition of the great arteries, the balloon is inflated, and the catheter is jerked back into the right atrium. This manoeuvre tears the atrial septum, causing a defect that allows mixing of systemic and pulmonary venous blood.

More recently, a different type of balloon has been used to dilate strictures in the coronary arteries, while larger versions have successfully relieved stenosis of the pulmonary valve and narrowing of systemic and pulmonary arterial branches. Blocking off abnormal vessels is another application, with special balloons or coils that are released from a catheter to occlude collateral vessels in the lung, for example.

Devices for closing the persistent ductus arteriosus or atrial septal defect by catheter placement of an 'umbrella' across the lumen are currently under clinical investigation. Experimental work with lasers suggests that coronary artery stenosis may be amenable to catheter removal using this technique in the future.

All of these manipulations have a small but real morbidity and mortality associated with their use, and only long-term follow-up will establish their place in the management of heart disease. Most are advisedly carried out in centres equipped for cardiac surgery and with a surgical team available to deal with any urgent complications.

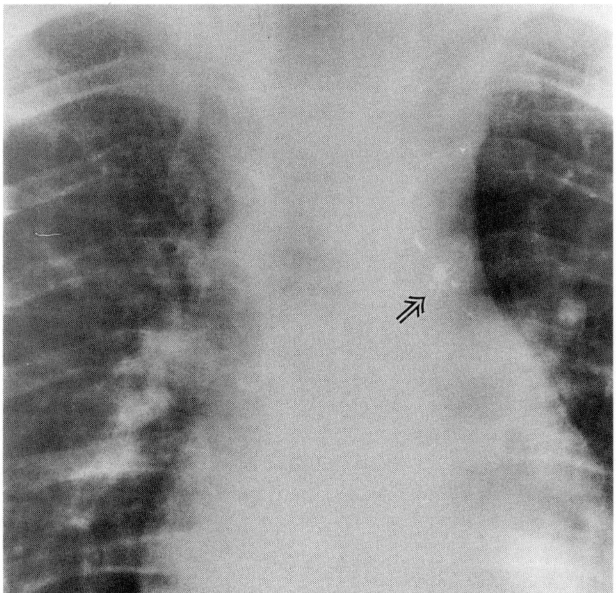

Fig. 4.50. Chest X-ray after catheter closure of a persistent ductus arteriosus showing the umbrella device in the ductus.

Further Reading

Berman DS, Mason DT (eds). Clinical nuclear cardiology. Grune & Stratton, New York, 1981
Elliott LP, Schiebler GL. X-ray diagnosis of congenital cardiac disease, 2nd edn. Charles C Thomas, Springfield, 1979
Garsoh A. Electrocardiography. In: Anderson RH, Macartney FJ, Shinebourne EA, Tynan M (eds) Paediatric cardiology. Churchill Livingstone, London, 1987, pp 235–317
Grossman W (ed). Cardiac catheterisation and angiography, 3rd edn. Lea & Febiger, Philadelphia, 1986
Gruntzig AR. Transluminal dilatation of coronary artery stenosis. Lancet 1978; i: 263
Jefferson K, Reese S. Clinical cardiac radiology, 2nd edn. Butterworths, London, 1980
Kean DM, Smith MA. Magneitc resonance imaging: principles and applications. William Heinemann Medical Books, London, 1986
Rashkind WJ. Transcatheter treatment of congenital heart disease. Circulation 1983; 67: 711–716
Rowlands DJ. The resting electrocardiogram. In Julian DG, Camm AJ, Fox KM, Hall RJC, Poole-Wilson PA (eds) Diseases of the heart. Baillière Tindall, London, 1989, pp 146–213
Silverman NH, Snider AR. Two-dimensional echocardiography in congenital heart diseae. Appleton-Century-Crofts, Norwalk, 1982

Chapter 5

Temporary Support of the Circulation

The primary function of the heart – to pump blood – sustains all other organs in the body. Impairment of this function over a long period of time, or even brief complete loss of cardiac output, may result in damage that leaves the patient with a permanent disability, regardless of ultimate cardiac recovery. In contrast with the broken leg, which can be rested in plaster for 6 weeks awaiting repair and return of function, the heart must continue to work immediately after major injury or cardiac surgery. Thus, measures to enhance, complement or substitute the pumping activity of the heart are encountered frequently in both the medical and surgical practice of cardiology.

Temporary support of the circulation broadly falls into two categories – pharmacological and mechanical.

Pharmacological Support

Pharmacological support embraces a large and growing number of drugs that act directly upon the heart or vascular system. *Inotropic agents* enhance contractility of the heart muscle, albeit at the cost of increased oxygen consumption by the heart itself. They usually are administered by continuous intravenous infusion, titrating the dose to the patients requirements. The commonly used catecholamines (adrenaline, dopamine, dobutamine, isoprenaline) all cause undesirable side-effects of vasoconstriction or tachycardia at very high doses, and for this reason they are often used in combination with each other or a vasodilator drug. The more recently introduced phosphodiesterase inhibitors may be pharmacologically synergistic with the action of the catecholamines and also promote vasodilatation.

The rationale for vasodilatation in the treatment of cardiac failure is to reduce the resistance against which the heart must pump. It should be carefully balanced against critical pressure requirements for perfusion of the cerebral, renal and myocardial circulations. This so-called 'afterload reduction' may be effected by a number of agents that vary in their mechanisms and duration of action as well as in the mode of their administration. Some, such as nitroglycerine or epoprostenol, are particularly effective in the coronary or pulmonary circulations, for example, and may convey added benefit for the management of coronary insufficiency or pulmonary vasoconstriction.

As a general rule, cardiotonic drugs are given for several days or longer, while the heart recovers, and the drugs are then gradually withdrawn as the heart demonstrates improved function by maintaining the circulation at the same or lower filling pressures. When the requirement for pharmacological support increases, it may be due to metabolic derangements (typically acidosis) which render the drugs less effective. But more often this situation indicates progressive damage or failure of the heart muscle.

Mechanical Support

Mechanical support of the circulation ranges from simple compression of the heart (external or internal cardiac massage) to extremely complex pumping devices completely replacing the heart's function. In contrast with inotropic agents, mechanical support does not increase the oxygen consumption of or work done by the heart and, in theory, should optimise its recovery. In practice, however, most techniques of mechanical circulatory support are highly invasive and are accompanied by a significant incidence of complications. Their use is thus reserved for specific indications (such as emergency resuscitation or open heart surgery) or when pharmacological interventions have proved inadequate.

Cardiac massage constitutes the most primitive type of circulatory support. It is used to treat the acute and unanticipated loss of cardiac output, for example during a sudden arrhythmia or during blood loss from abrupt haemorrhage. If perfusion to the brain and coronary circulation can be maintained while measures are taken to remedy whatever precipitated the cardiac decompensation, the outlook may be quite favourable even after 30 or 60 minutes of cardiopulmonary resuscitation. This interval may also permit the organisation of more sophisticated mechanical assistance for problems that cannot be readily reversed. The size of the patient's pupils is observed as an indication of cerebral perfusion (although this sign may be altered by drugs), while the ECG, and particularly the ability to defibrillate the heart, give an indication of blood flow to the cardiac muscle.

The deliberate interruption of cardiac function is a planned event in most open heart operations, in order to achieve satisfactory and safe operating conditions. During this time the circulation is taken over by the 'heart–lung machine'.

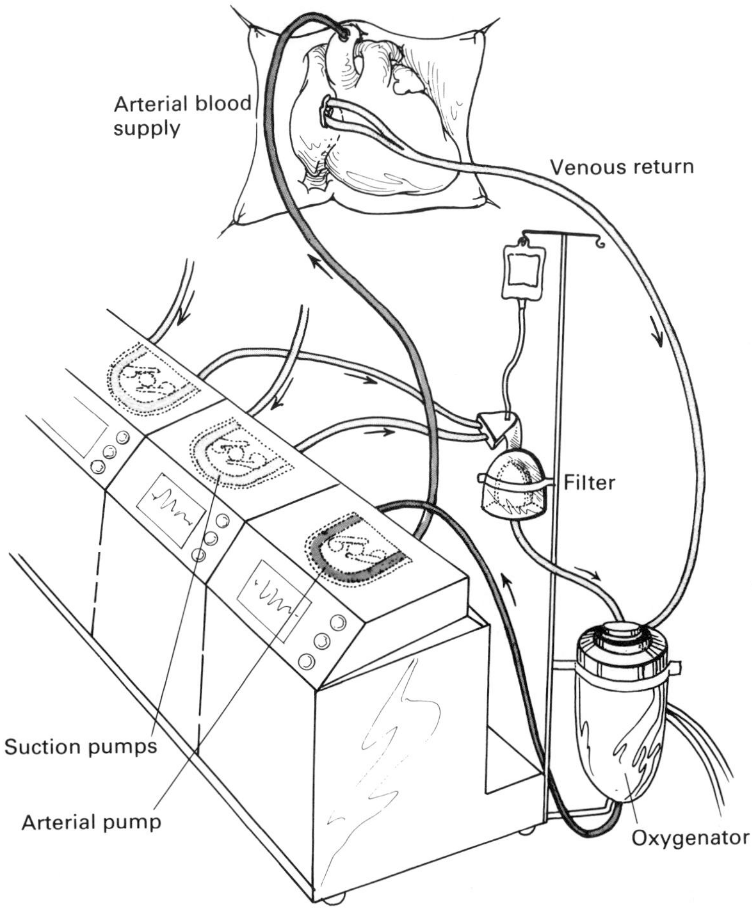

Fig. 5.1. Diagram of a typical heart–lung machine. Blood from the venous side of the circulation is drained into the oxygenator and then pumped back into the aorta.

Principles of Cardiopulmonary Bypass

Although the human heart has two pumping chambers, only one pump is needed to propel the blood in the *heart–lung apparatus*, since the flow of venous blood from the body to the artificial lung or oxygenator is effected by gravity. The oxygenated blood is then pumped into the arterial circulation under positive pressure. A simple type of pump, which milks the blood along the tubing, is used and the blood is delivered into the ascending aorta through a plastic cannula. Alternatively, a pulse may be given to the circuit to simulate cardiac ejection.

The venous blood is collected from the heart by one or two fairly wide tubes in the right atrium or the vena cavae.

Clotting of the blood in the extracorporeal circuit is prevented by the use of heparin administered to the patient in a dose of 70 mg/m^2 or 2.3 mg/kg body weight.

Since blood is being lost continuously from the cut edges of the incisions and the cardiac chambers, it is returned to the circuit by two or more suction pumps. This suction blood is filtered free of particulate matter, and is defoamed or has its bubbles removed in the oxygenator.

By allowing the blood to pass through a heat exchanger connected to a source of hot or cold water, the temperature of the blood and consequently the temperature of the patient's body can be kept normal or manipulated at will.

The *oxygenator* or *artificial lungs* have become progressively simplified and standardised to the point where they are supplied as sterile, disposable units of high efficiency. The commonest is the bubble oxygenator. In this type, oxygen is bubbled through the venous blood to form a froth so that each bubble of oxygen is coated with a thin film of venous blood. Gas transfer occurs very efficiently under these circumstances, and the froth of oxygenated blood then flows over a sponge-like mesh coated with antifoam. This chemical has the property of dispersing bubbles and reconstitutes fully oxygenated blood.

A newer type of oxygenator is the membrane oxygenator, here the blood and gas are separated by a semi-permeable membrane rather like the lung, with no blood–air interface. There is no frothing and consequently less damage to the blood components. This can be an advantage with long perfusions, when the cumulative damage to the blood may be considerable.

Most oxygenators incorporate a filter and a heat exchanger and this simplifies the circuit considerably.

The goal of cardiopulmonary bypass is to provide an adequate flow of fully oxygenated blood to the systemic tissue and vital organs, particularly the brain. At normal temperatures it is estimated that an adequate flow is about 2.2–2.4 l/m^2 body surface area. This requirement is proportionally less at lower body temperatures; at 30°C there is a reduction of approximately 50% in the body's oxygen requirements. Most heart–lung circuits supply an excess of oxygenated blood above the body's basic requirements; this provides a safety factor allowing for periods of reduced flow and unforeseen technical emergencies.

For precise surgery, a dry field and quiet operating conditions are necessary. The rhythmical contractions of the heart are usually eliminated by inducing ventricular fibrillation with a low voltage electrical current, by temporary periods of ischaemic arrest or by the use of a cold cardioplegic solution.

During the period of surgery on the open heart it is vital to *protect the viability and integrity of the myocardium*. This can be achieved by providing flow through the coronary arteries from the aorta or by perfusing the coronary arteries separately with cannulae. The flow of oxygenated blood maintains the contractility of the myocardium so that either the heart's contraction will be continued or active ventricular fibrillation will persist.

If a relaxed asystolic myocardium is preferred, and this offers better operating conditions, the heart's action can be arrested by the injection of a cardioplegic solution into the aortic root or directly into the coronary orifices. The active ingredient of most of these solutions is potassium, which ensures diastolic or flaccid arrest of the heart's action.

Arrest of the heart's action is useful but protection of the myocardium from ischaemic damage can only be reliably achieved by reducing the temperature of the myocardium to perhaps 8–10°C. The combined technique of chemical arrest with local cooling ('cold cardioplegia') can be brought about by injection of the potassium-containing solution at about 4°C; about one litre of solution is injected in the average adult.

In practice it is usual to reduce the temperature of the entire body to 25°C and the myocardial temperature to about 8–10°C. Additional safety margins are provided by local external cooling of the heart by irrigating the pericardial cavity with cold saline at a temperature of 4°C.

Open heart surgery can also be carried out under the theoretically ideal conditions of profound hypothermia with circulatory arrest. This method has been particularly useful in developing infant and neonatal cardiac surgery, but it does introduce some real and potential hazards, including ischaemic cerebral damage and air embolism.

In this technique, the infant is sometimes cooled first by means of ice applied around the body, by core-cooling on bypass or by a combination of surface cooling with a short period of low-temperature perfusion. When the infant's body temperature falls to about 18–20°C or lower, the entire circulation is arrested and the vascular bed is drained into the extracorporeal circuit. This combination of cardiac arrest plus exanguination provides ideal operating conditions.

Rewarming and resuscitation are effected by re-establishing the circulation and blood-stream rewarming through the heart–lung machine.

A compromise technique frequently used today is to combine a conventional extracorporeal circulation with low temperatures and reduced or very low flows. This achieves excellent operating conditions during the time they are needed without introducing the neurological hazards consequent upon a total arrest of the circulation.

An important aspect of the use of the heart–lung machine is to wean the patient safely from the apparatus, the so-called 'coming off bypass'. First it is essential to ensure that all air trapped within the cardiac chambers is eliminated. Attention is directed towards this end well before weaning from the machine by filling the heart slowly with blood while the lungs are gently ventilated. The apex of the left ventricle should certainly be aspirated repeatedly or vented through a wide-bore cannula and air should be aspirated from the left atrial appendage, right superior pulmonary vein and the most anteriorly placed segment of the aortic arch. An alternative technique is to aspirate continuously from the ascending aorta while the heart is allowed to fill and eject any concealed air.

Increasing amounts of blood are slowly redirected from the heart–lung apparatus to the body by progressively closing off the venous line leading to the machine. At the same time the increasing work-load and output of the heart are monitored by watching the level of the systemic blood pressure and the venous or right atrial pressure. As the circulation fills up, the venous pressure rises and, when this is at an arbitrary figure of about 10 mmHg and the blood pressure is adequate, the arterial pump can be stopped. The normal circulation is now re-established. Any remaining blood can be returned slowly and intermittently to the body from the machine. Normally, this is adequate, but where there is doubt about the functional efficiency of the left ventricle, a left atrial pressure is also recorded. A left atrial pressure above about 15–17 mmHg suggests a poor left ventricular function or over-filling of the circulation. The former may be corrected with catacholamine support or, where left ventricular function is severely compromised, by the use of other support techniques.

When the ventricles fail to support the circulation after a heart operation, the initial method of assistance is to keep the patient on the cardiopulmonary bypass machine while any abnormalities in body temperature, serum potassium, acid–base balance and other parameters are corrected. Meanwhile, the empty beating heart is perfused and given a chance to recover from any reversible injury which occurred during the operation. It is often possible after an hour or so of such support to wean the patient slowly from the bypass machine, as the myocardium recovers.

Long-Term Circulatory Support

In some cases, it will still be impossible to wean the patient from the heart–lung machine, despite maximal pharmacological support and a period of recovery. When the heart continues to contract and eject blood, even if inadequately, it is possible to augment its action by intra-aortic balloon counterpulsation. An inflatable balloon is passed into the thoracic aorta and triggered from the

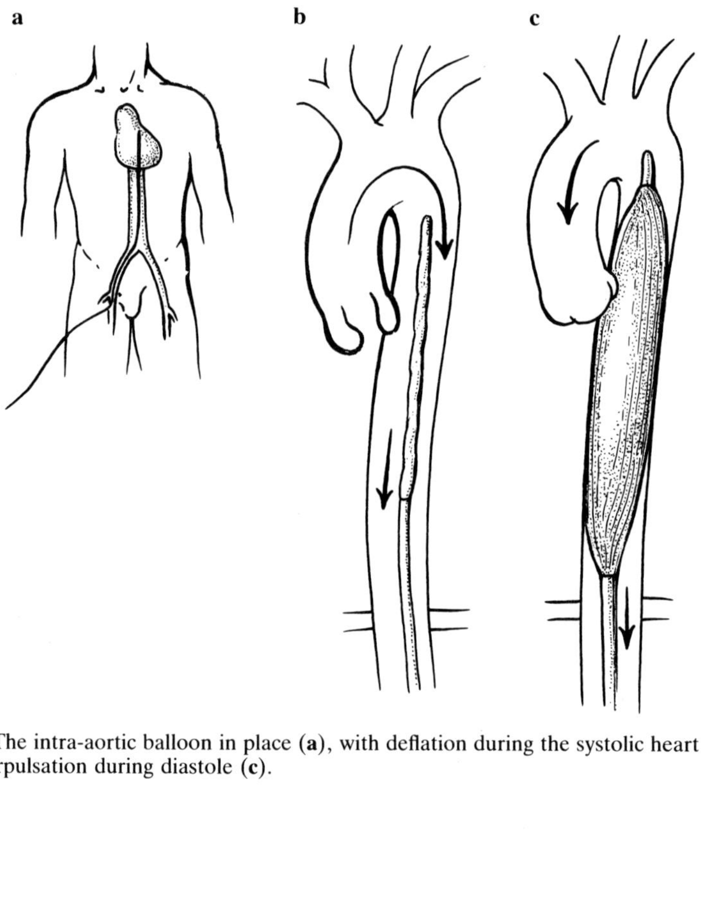

Fig. 5.2. The intra-aortic balloon in place (**a**), with deflation during the systolic heart ejection (**b**) and counterpulsation during diastole (**c**).

patient's ECG or arterial pulse to inflate during diastole. This additional displacement of blood in diastole ('diastolic augmentation') increases both the cardiac output and coronary perfusion. As the balloon collapses it may also create a suction effect that reduces the afterload against which the heart must eject. Overall, counterpulsation may be very effective, provided a basic heart ejection is present to be augmented.

Intra-aortic balloon counterpulsation is also useful for supporting the circulation after myocardial infarction and its complications, the balloon being left in place for several weeks if necessary, to allow the myocardium to recover before undertaking cardiac surgery. Unfortunately, it is of little value in children because the pliable aorta tends to distend, giving no augmentation of pressure or flow.

Where there is no cardiac ejection or forward movement of blood from the heart, or when balloon counterpulsation is ineffective, more sophisticated types of assistance are necessary. The other currently available mechanical circulatory assist devices fall broadly into two groups: ventricular assist devices (VAD) supplement or replace the function of the in situ natural heart, while the total artificial heart (TAH) completely replaces the patient's heart, both functionally and anatomically. Either can be used as a 'bridge' to transplant, i.e. to maintain the circulation for a limited period of days or weeks while a suitable donor heart is organised. But only the VADs conserve the potential for salvage of the patient's own heart.

Ventricular assist devices may support the left ventricle (LVAD), the right ventricle (RVAD) or both sides of the heart (BVAD). In each case, a pump is interposed between the failing ventricle or its respective atrium and the appropriate great vessel. In the context of open heart surgery, this may be achieved simply by connecting a roller pump of the heart–lung machine to a tube draining blood from the left atrium and, on the other side, to the aortic perfusion cannula. This apparatus offers a strictly limited period of circulatory

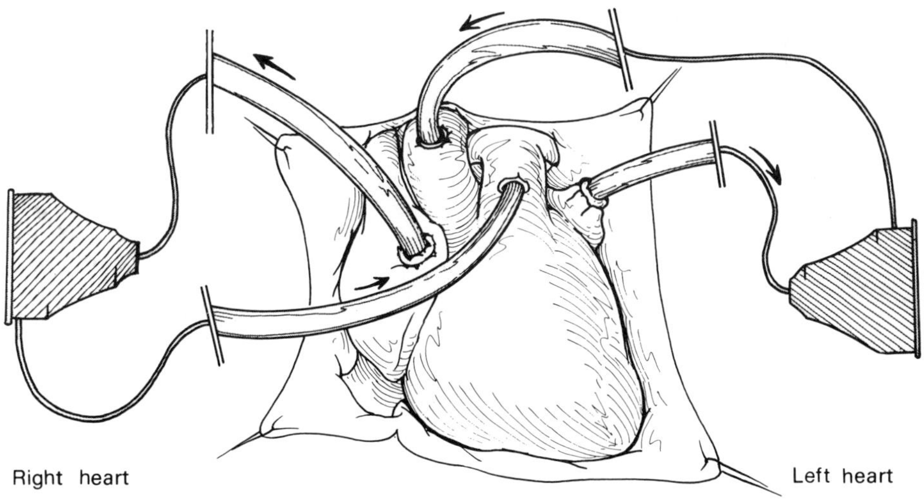

Fig. 5.3. Circuit for biventricular assist. Blood from the left atrium is pumped to the aorta to support the systemic circulation, while a similar centrifugal pump assists the right ventricle by transferring blood from the right atrium to the pulmonary artery.

support, measured in hours, as an emergency expedient. When much longer support is necessary, the cannulae are connected to centrifugal pumps. Although flow is non-pulsatile, these devices show comparatively few complications in the first week of support and have been used as long as 1 month. Often, this type of ventricular assist is combined with intra-aortic balloon counterpulsation.

Pulsatile ventricular assistance can be provided by a slightly more complex apparatus which incorporates inlet and outlet valves and a moveable diaphragm. Driven by a pneumatic system, the pumping sac may be located either outside the chest or within the abdominal cavity. In the former, the assist device is connected to the heart by conduits which pass through the skin, while in the latter (an 'implantable heterotopic prosthetic ventricle'), connecting conduits are passed through the diaphragm to the pump. This type of mechanical assistance can be established without cardiopulmonary bypass in patients who have not undergone heart surgery.

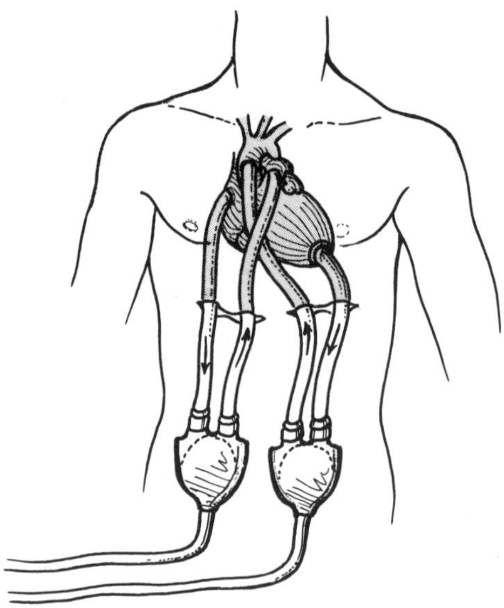

Fig. 5.4. A biventricular assist device positioned outside the chest – extracorporeal or paracorporeal.

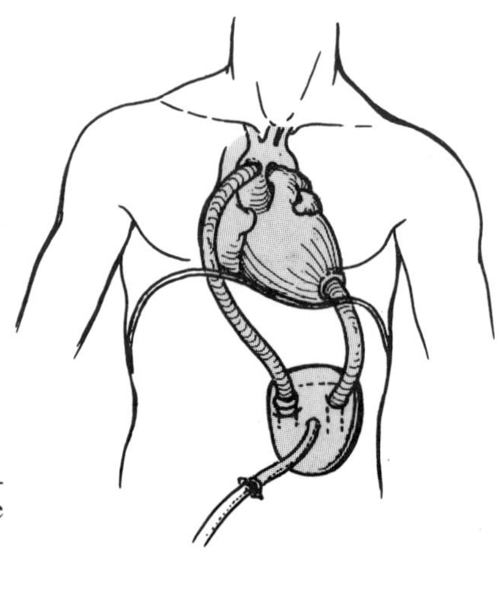

Fig. 5.5. Implantable heterotopic prosthetic left ventricle in the abdominal cavity. The pneumatic drive-line leaves the body subcutaneously.

Blood is propelled around this closed circuit by displacement of the moveable diaphragm in co-ordination with the hearts own action. Modifications replacing the cumbersome pneumatic drive system with an electromechanical driving device could, in theory, make the implantable VAD adaptable to portable battery power and give the patient more freedom of movement. These types of assist devices are better suited to moderately long-term support, either as a bridge to ultimate transplantation of the heart or awaiting ventricular recovery. They have been used successfully for periods as long as 3 months.

The total artificial heart differs from the foregoing in that the natural heart is removed completely, and the mechanical assist device is attached directly to the remnants of the atria and great vessels. Accordingly, there is no longer the prospect of the native heart's recovery and the patient's long-term future depends entirely upon transplantation. The development of an electronically driven motor to compress the blood sacs of the total artificial heart is a recent step towards a completely implantable device that would allow the patient freedom from the driving and monitoring console. Used as a bridge to transplantation, the total artificial heart has been implanted effectively for more than 120 days. At the present time, however, this is a developmental field for scientific investigation.

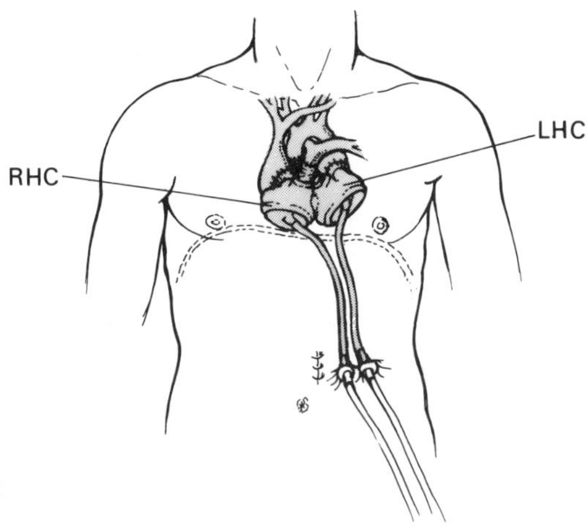

Fig. 5.6. The total artificial heart. RHC, Right heart component; LHR, left heart component.

Ultimately, the driving mechanism may well be compacted and electrically driven or even atomically powered. But, at present, the limitations of the total artificial heart do not lie so much with this aspect of technology as in the bioincompatability of man and machine. Anticoagulation is necessary for mechanical circulatory support, and nearly half of the patients suffer some type of bleeding complication. A more serious, though less frequent, complication is thromboembolism, particularly to the brain. Clot tends to form on the synthetic pump membranes and valves at the blood–machine interface, and is then disseminated into the circulation. New design and materials may prevent such difficulties in future assist devices.

With regard to suitability for subsequent transplantation, infection is also a major disadvantage of mechanical support. This tends to occur where drive lines or conduits pass through the skin; should it progress to involve the mediastinum, removal of the device, like other foreign bodies, may be necessary to erradicate the infection. In addition to having portals of entry, the assisted patient may suffer depression of immunologic function, while the surfaces of some polymers used in the assist devices also predispose to bacterial infection.

Consideration of the complications, the limited availability of donor hearts for transplantation, and the growing number of patients who suffer debilitating heart failure has led to the development of skeletal muscle as a cardiac assist device. By electrical stimulation, it is possible to transform 'fast' skeletal muscle into a 'slow' muscle that does not fatigue (similar to cardiac muscle). The muscle flap is wrapped around the ventricle ('cardiomyopexy'), grafted into the heart ('cardiomyoplasty') or wrapped around the descending thoracic aorta for counterpulsation. A considerable delay (several weeks) is necessary for revascularisation and transformation of the muscle flap and its vascular pedicle. So far, these techniques are largely experimental; potentially, they could play an important role in ventricular assist techniques in the future.

Extracorporeal Respiratory Support

When the problem lies mainly with the respiratory system, specifically the ability of the lung to supply oxygen to the tissues and to eliminate carbon dioxide, the myocardium is likely to also fail eventually as a result of the abnormal blood gases and secondary metabolic disturbances. Early attempts to manage the adult respiratory distress syndrome used a membrane oxygenator with a perfusion pump that removed blood from the venous circulation (right atrium) and returned it to the femoral artery. This was a venoarterial bypass, and the type of support commonly referred to as 'extracorporeal membrane oxygenation' (ECMO). In theory, the circuit takes about half of the cardiac output and should supply oxygen and correct any gaseous deficits, thus maintaining the circulation.

Although ECMO achieved good oxygenation, it proved to be a continuation of heart–lung bypass in that it resulted in cumulative organ damage to the heart, the lungs (which were hypoperfused), the liver and the kidneys. The poor results (only about 15% of patients recovered) may also have been due in part to lung damage from continued positive pressure ventilation, and in part to the fact that the oxygenated portion of the cardiac output did not benefit the important upper half of the body. Accordingly, venoarterial ECMO is no longer used in adults.

However, the application of ECMO techniques to neonates has been considerably more encouraging, possibly because the conditions that cause respiratory failure in the newborn baby (such as meconium aspiration, persistent feotal circulation, diaphragmatic hernia) are potentially more rapidly reversible. Usually, desaturated blood is removed from the right atrium via a cannula that has been passed through the internal jugular vein, and oxygenated blood is returned retrograde through the ligated right internal carotid artery. Occlusion of these vessels is surprisingly well tolerated. However, anticoagulation is still necessary during the time of respiratory support, and bleeding, particularly intracerebral haemorrhage, remains a worrying complication.

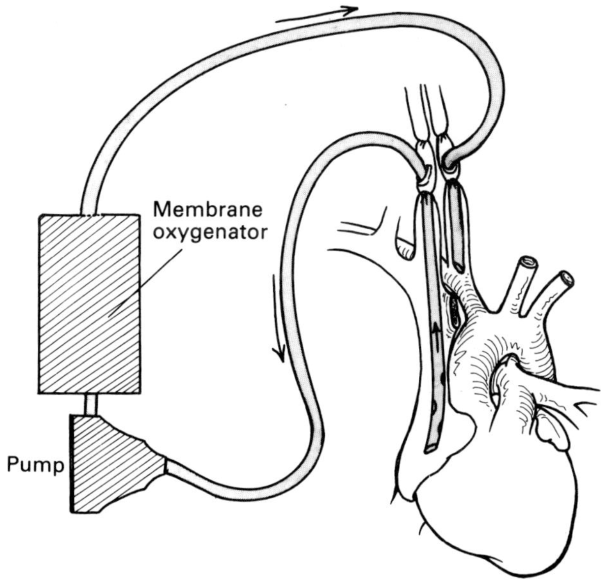

Fig. 5.7. Schematic perfusion circuit for extracorporeal membrane oxygenation in the neonate.

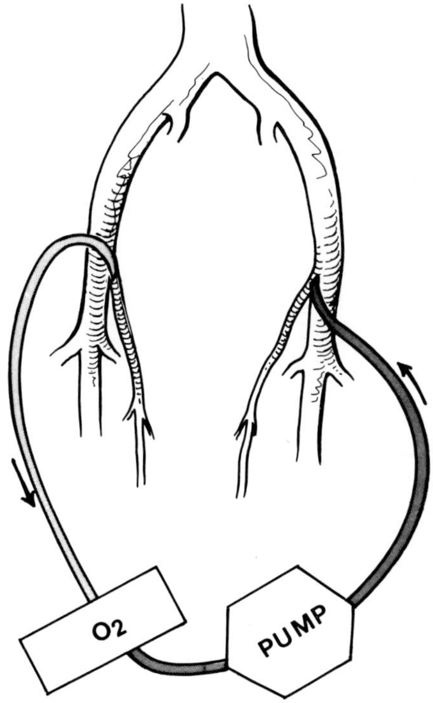

Fig. 5.8. Veno-venous extracorporeal CO_2 removal circuit for adult respiratory support.

In view of the very poor prognosis of 'shock lung' or the adult respiratory distress syndrome (more than 90% of the patients fail to survive) new techniques have been explored to support the respiratory system in adults. Reasoning that the main problem lay with carbon dioxide elimination rather than oxygenation, a veno-venous bypass was introduced – extracorporeal CO_2 removal ($ECCO_2R$). In this low-flow system, something between 20% and 30% of the cardiac output is withdrawn from the femoral vein, passed through the membrane oxygenator and pumped back into the opposite femoral vein fully oxygenated. The technique is minimally invasive (recently developed cannulae have been placed percutaneously through the saphenous vein) and causes little change in central haemodynamics. Blood-flow is maintained through the lungs, which may now be gently inflated at low levels of inspired oxygen and minimal pressure, giving them an opportunity to recover. Generally, a response is seen after 1–2 days of treatment if the patient is going to survive, but much longer respiratory support (usually between 1 week and 30 days) is necessary for pulmonary recovery. About half of the patients can now be salvaged by this technique.

Further Reading

Acker MA, Stephenson LW. Skeletal muscle: a potential power source for cardiac assist devices. NIPS 1987; 2: 223–6

Altieri FD, Watson JI. Implantable ventricular assist systems. Artif Organs 1987; 11: 237–246

Gattinoni L, Presenti A, Mascheroni D, et al. Low frequency positive pressure ventilation with extracorporeal CO_2 removal in severe acute respiratory failure. JAMA 1986; 256: 881–886

Gibbon JH Jr. Application of a mechanical heart and lung apparatus to cardiac surgery. In: Recent advances in cardiovascular physiology and surgery. University of Minnesota, Minneapolis, 1953, pp 107–113

Opie LH, Chatterjee K, Gersh BJ, et al. Drugs for the heart, 2nd (expanded) edn. W.B. Saunders Company, Philadelphia, 1987

Ross DN. Hypothermia. II. Physiological observations during hypothermia. Guy's Hosp Rep 1954; 103: 116

Sethia B, Wheatley DJ, Taylor KM. Short review: the current status of bypass. Support Systems 1983; 1: 271

Chapter 6

Congenital Heart Disease

Introduction

Fundamental to the successful surgical management of congenital heart defects is an accurate preoperative diagnosis. This is achieved through an open mind which contains knowledge of the conditions that may be encountered, a thorough clinical examination and the intelligent interpretation of appropriate special investigations. For convenience, congenital lesions are frequently subdivided according to the presence or absence of cyanosis, recognising also that there is an important intermediate group of conditions in which cyanosis may become intermittently apparent on exercise or exertion.

In broad terms, the principles of management follow rather different lines for cyanotic and acyanotic defects, and within the latter group, for those with left-to-right shunts as opposed to those with obstructive lesions. Such a classification is thus relevant and clinically useful. However, increasingly detailed anatomical studies have now made available a large amount of morphological information which further facilitates the surgical repair of complex heart defects. Diagnosis has also become more accurate through the development of terminology to describe cardiac anatomy in a precise, logical and complete manner.

Nomenclature and Sequential Segmental Analysis

A description of cardiac morphology may be likened to the drawing of a map. Firstly, a set of definitions is agreed upon such that the 'explorer' (or morphologist) can identify the particular feature of the territory under consideration. Armed with the knowledge of what constitutes a lake or a mountain or a river, for example, it is then possible to describe the terrain, and, having noted all the constituent parts, to produce a symbolic picture of the area. As greater knowledge becomes available, more detail is added to the map, which eventually becomes a self-explanatory guide for those who are familiar with the definitions and symbols employed. To plan a journey then, one reads the map and finds that the road passes through the mountain, follows the river to a lake, etc. Similarly, *sequential chamber analysis* follows the pathway of blood flow through the heart, using details of anatomy as descriptive signposts.

Several concepts underlie the system of sequential chamber analysis. The first of these is that every heart has three attributes by which it is characterised, each of these being independent of the other two. These are (1) chamber morphology, (2) the way in which segments of the heart are joined to each other, i.e. connections, and (3) the three-dimensional spatial orientation of the various components, i.e. relationships. Morphology is based on anatomical definition of structures and allows their identification. Connections, in congenitally malformed hearts, tend to have an important influence on haemodynamics and physiology, while positions and relations determine access to the heart and some aspects of surgical correction.

The second concept is that all characteristics – morphology, connections, relations and associated malformations – must be established for each heart, regardless of how simple or complex it may be. While such a system may initially appear cumbersome and perhaps, in many cases, unnecessary, there is much to commend it. In addition to encouraging precise communication, sequential chamber analysis helps the surgeon to develop a logical approach to complex malformations and also alerts him to various details of morphology (such as the distribution of the conducting system) which may be encountered at operation. A valuable exercise for the surgeon is to satisfy himself preoperatively that each segment of cardiac anatomy has been demonstrated and that he appreciates the implications for surgical repair.

Finally, it will be apparent from the terminology employed that this system of nomenclature is completely divorced from embryology and developmental anatomy. In part, this is because the relationship between many congenital heart malformations and the development of the heart is complex and incompletely understood, and, in part, because diagnosis and treatment are most effectively based upon observable fact rather than speculation as to the aetiology of the malformation. In only a very small number of congenital heart defects (such as anomalies of pulmonary venous connection) does knowledge of the relevant embryology facilitate clinical diagnosis or surgical management.

Morphology

Certain structural characteristics make possible the identification of the cardiac chambers and great vessels regardless of where they are found or to what they are attached. Thus, the morphological right atrium has a blunt, broad-based appendage, a sulcus terminalis, and, when an atrial septum is present, an oval fossa with its limbus. The morphological left atrium, in contrast, possesses a long, narrow appendage without a terminal sulcus and has the flap-valve side of the oval fossa.

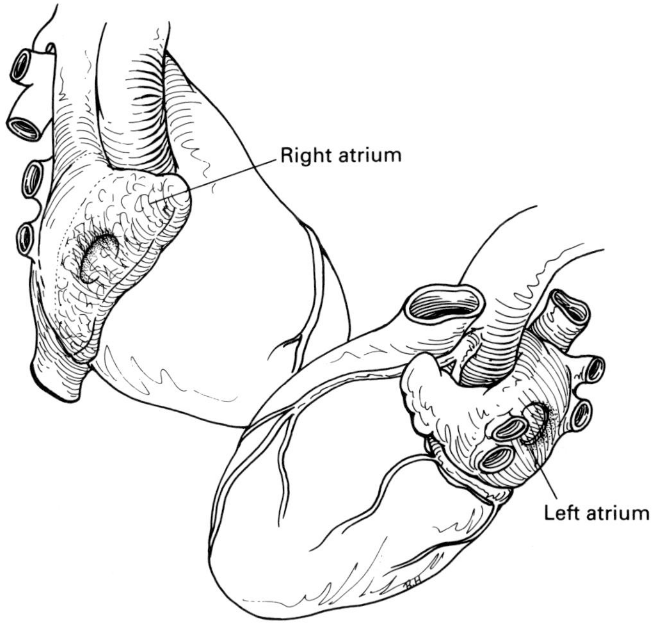

Fig. 6.1. The morphological features of the right and left atria.

Ventricular chamber type is determined by the trabecular portion of the septum and apex: in a morphological right ventricle, coarse trabeculations are apparent on angiography or gross examination, while those of the morphological left ventricle are fine and delicate. Occasionally, when only one ventricular chamber is present, the trabeculations are unlike either a 'left' or 'right' ventricle, and the chamber is then said to have indeterminate morphology.

As regards the great vessels, the aorta usually gives off at least one coronary artery and branches to the systemic circulation, whereas the pulmonary artery supplies branches to the lungs. Formerly, a ventricular chamber was defined in terms of having an inlet valve and an outlet valve, a chamber lacking the former being an 'outlet chamber' and one lacking both, a 'trabeculated pouch'. However, it is now considered more useful to describe the relative sizes of the ventricular chambers along with the presence or absence of valvar (inlet and outlet) and muscular (inlet, trabecular and outlet) components.

Connections

Connections simply define the way in which segments of the heart are joined to each other. There are thus connections between the atria and the ventricles (the 'atrioventricular' connection) and between the ventricles and great vessels (the 'ventriculoarterial' connection).

Each connection has two features which need to be known: (1) the *type* of connection indicates which atrium is connected to which ventricle, while (2) the *mode* of connection refers to the type of valve found at the junction. Again it will be apparent that a connection exists and is described independent of where the cardiac chambers lie within the chest or in relation to one another.

Types of Connection. Given that nearly every heart has two atrial chambers, the types of atrioventricular connection may be subdivided according to whether each atrium connects (actually or potentially) with a separate ventricular chamber ('biventricular atrioventricular' connection), both connect to the same ventricular cavity ('univentricular atrioventricular' connection) or one connection is absent ('absent left' connection or 'absent right' connection).

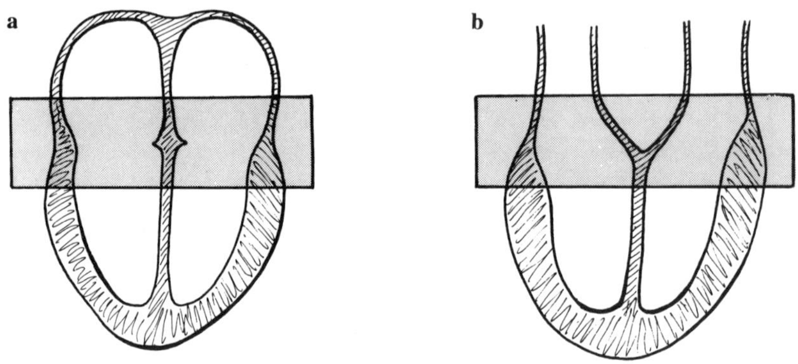

Fig. 6.2. The atrioventricular connections (**a**) and ventriculoarterial connections (**b**).

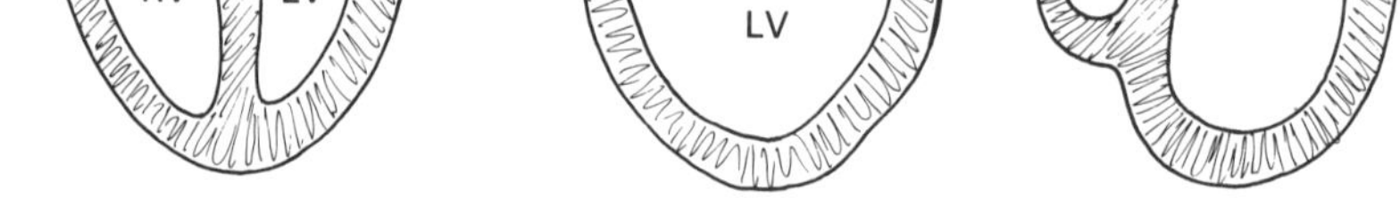

Fig. 6.3. Examples of atrioventricular connections; 'biventricular' (**a**), 'absent right' connection (**b**), and 'univentricular' connection (**c**). After R.H. Anderson, Royal Brompton Hospital.

The biventricular atrioventricular connections are further subdivided according to the morphology of the two joined chambers. When the atrium and ventricle are of like morphology (that is, a morphological right atrium connected to a morphological right ventricle and a morphological left atrium connected to a morphological left ventricle), the connection is said to be *concordant*. If each connects with the morphological opposite chamber, it is *discordant*. When isomeric atria are present (two morphological right or morphological left atria) the half-concordant, half-discordant connection is called 'ambiguous'. When the

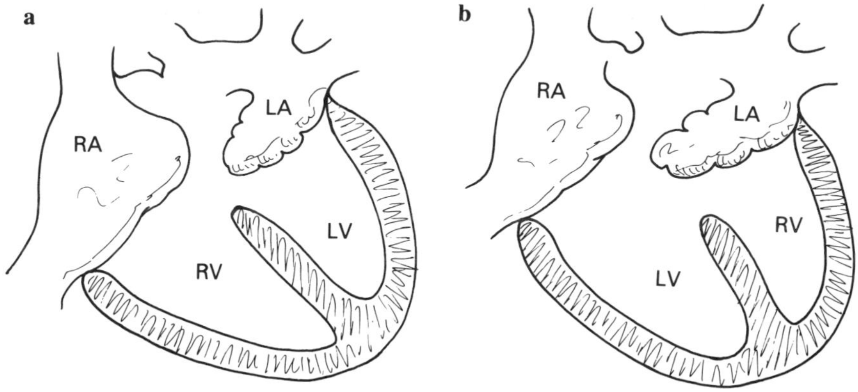

Fig. 6.4. Concordant (**a**) and discordant (**b**) atrioventricular connections.

morphological left ventricle gives off the aorta and the morphological right ventricle gives off the pulmonic trunk, the connection is 'concordant'. The pulmonic trunk arising from the left ventricular chamber and aorta from a right ventricular chamber produces a discordant connection (commonly known as 'transposition'), while both great vessels coming from either ventricle gives rise to a double outlet connection.

The final possibility, that of single outlet, again has four more subgroups. These are a *common* arterial trunk (giving off coronary, systemic and pulmonary

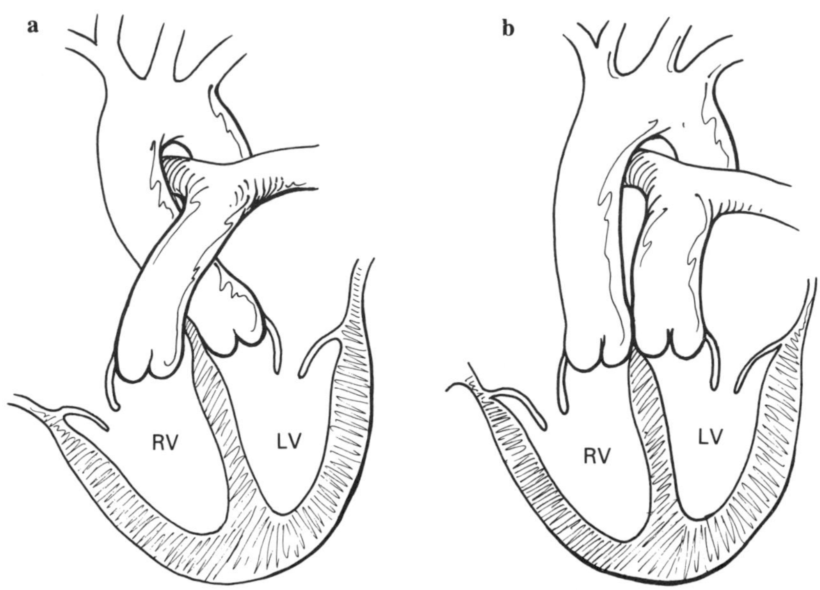

Fig. 6.5. Concordant (normal, **a**) and discordant (transposed, **b**) ventriculoarterial connections.

branches, traditionally called truncus arteriosus), a *solitary* arterial trunk (differentiated from the common arterial trunk by the absence of pulmonary branches within the pericardium), a *single* pulmonary trunk (with aortic atresia) and a *single* aortic trunk (with pulmonary atresia).

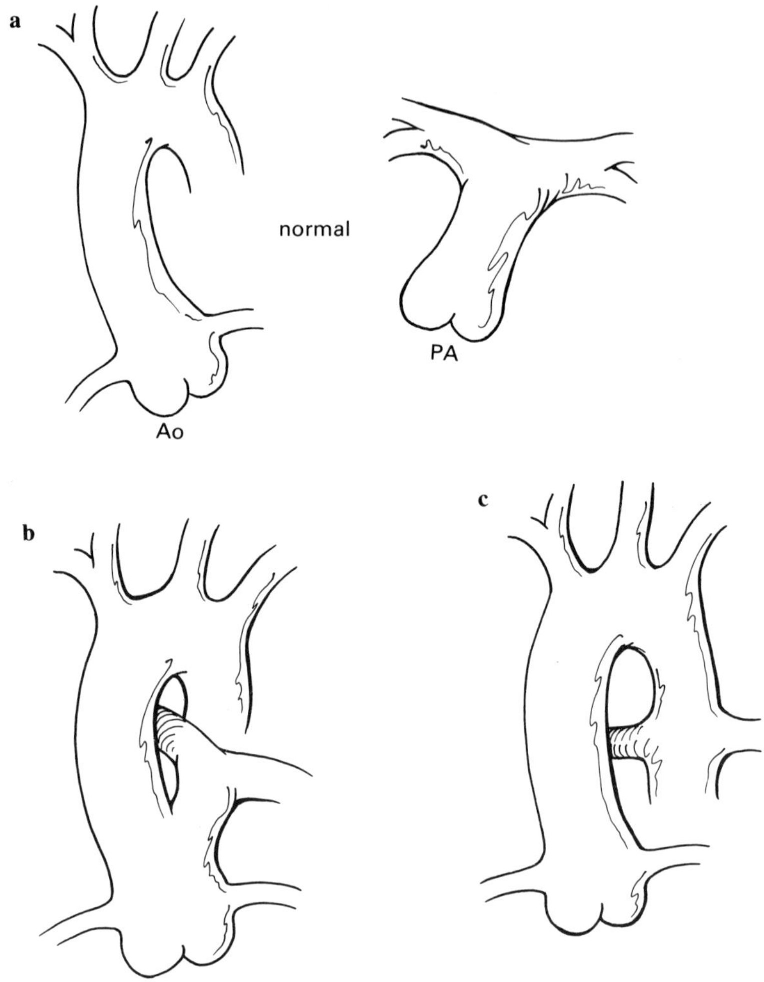

Fig. 6.6. Normal great arteries (**a**). The common arterial trunk gives off branches to the coronary, systemic and pulmonary circulations within the pericardium (**b**), in contrast with a solitary arterial trunk (**c**) where the latter are extrapericardial.

Modes of Connection. The modes of connection at the atrioventricular position are more variable than between the ventricles and the great arteries. In both cases, there may be two perforate valves or one perforate and one imperforate valve. And, in either position, a perforate valve may lie partially over both ventricular chambers and thus 'over-ride' the ventricular septum. In this situation, the mode of the connection determines its type, for the over-riding valve is by convention assigned to whichever ventricle receives its larger portion. Thus, the atrioventricular connection may produce a *double inlet* ventricle by virtue of an over-riding left or right atrioventricular valve and, similarly, a *double outlet* ventricle, may arise due to over-riding of the aortic or pulmonary valves. The atrioventricular connection may be guarded, in addition, by a single, common valve shared between the two atria and ventricles, or by a valve whose tension apparatus is found in both ventricular chambers and thus is called a 'straddling' valve.

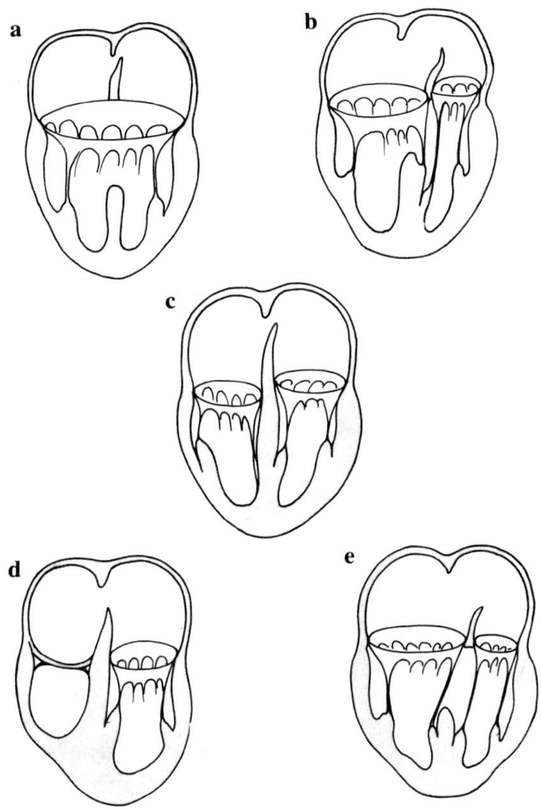

Fig. 6.7. Modes of atrioventricular connection. The centre figure illustrates a normal heart with a perforate valve leading to each ventricle (**c**). The abnormal situations, shown clockwise from the upper left corner, are a common valve (**a**), a straddling right A-V valve (**b**), an over-riding A-V valve (**e**), and an imperforate right AV valve (tricuspid atresia, **d**). After R.H. Anderson, Royal Brompton Hospital.

Positions and relations

These characteristics define the location of the heart within the chest and the spatial orientation of its parts in relation to one another. As previously noted, 'dextrocardia' indicates that the apex of the heart points to the right, 'levocardia'

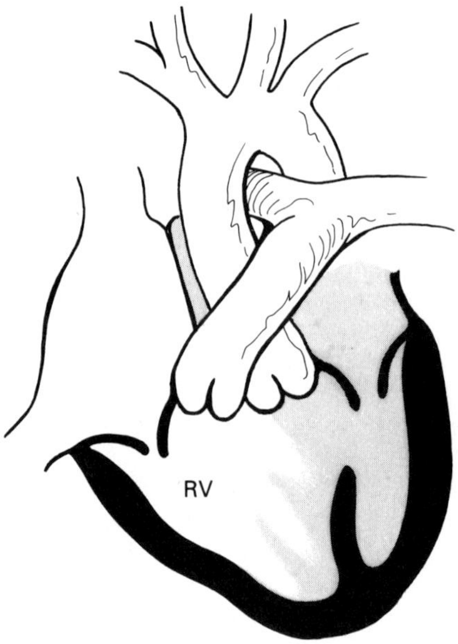

Fig. 6.8. Double outlet right ventricle. Both the aorta and pulmonary artery arise from the right ventricle.

to the left, and 'mesocardia' indicates that the apex is central or not identifiable. More precise indications of cardiac position can be given again, using the terminology of sequential chamber analysis. Both the heart and the other organs in the body have a left side and a right side. Normally, the left lung has two lobes with the main bronchus lying below the pulmonary artery, and the spleen and stomach are found in the left side of the abdomen. The right lung has three lobes and a bronchus that lies above the pulmonary artery, with the liver to the right side in the abdomen. When the morphological right atrium lies on the right side of the heart and the morphological left atrium on the left side, it is called *situs solitus*.

Since there is usually concordance or agreement between the arrangement of the atria and other viscera, one can infer the presence of situs solitus in the heart by observing the position of the stomach bubble and arrangement of the bronchi on the chest X-ray. Rarely the viscera and atria occupy mirror image positions (that is, a morphological left atrium on the right side and a morphological right atrium of the left), i.e. *situs inversus*. It follows that the apex of the heart normally points to the left with situs solitus and to the right with situs inversus.

In addition to normal and inverted atria it is possible to have a heart in which both appendages resemble that of a right atrium or a left chamber. This is called *isomerism*, a condition that is frequently associated with complex cardiac malformations. In right isomerism there are usually two 'right' lungs and the spleen is absent, while left isomerism tends to have a left bronchial arrangement in both lungs and multiple spleens. The atrial arrangement and thus situs can also be inferred from echocardiographic positions of the great vessels in the abdomen.

Spatial relationships generally are designated in two or, occasionally, three dimensions. Thus, the normal aorta lies to the right and slightly posterior to the

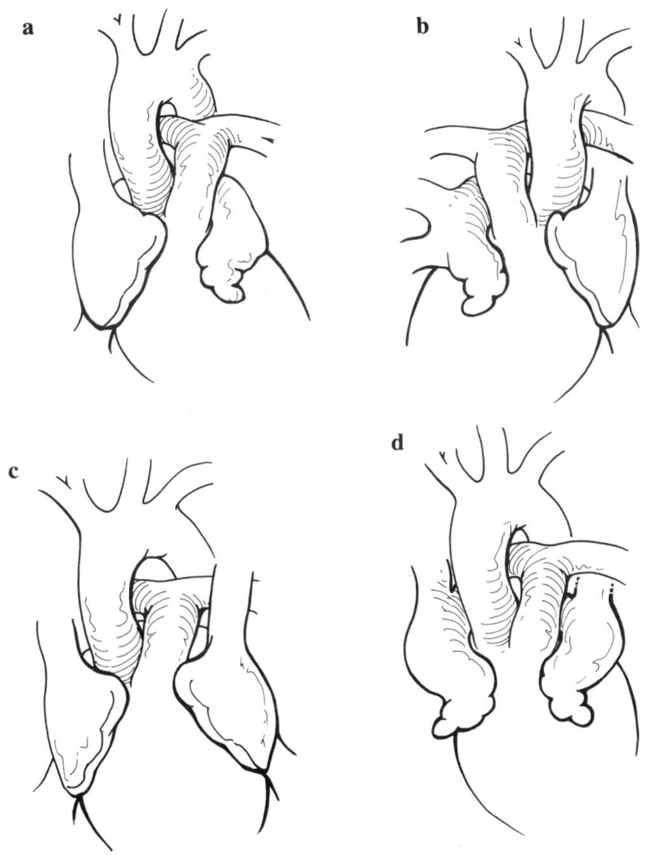

Fig. 6.9. Types of atrial arrangements. **a** Solitus, usual arrangement. **b** Inversus, mirror image. **c** Right atrial isomerism. **d** Left atrial isomerism.

pulmonary artery, while the left ventricle lies to the left and posterior to the right ventricle. Terms such as, for example, 'upstairs-downstairs' or 'over-and-under' ventricles indicate that the chambers have a superior–inferior relationship.

Within this framework of morphology, connections and relations, the details of cardiac structure and any defects which are present may be filled in. These are generally organised according to the chamber or connection in which they occur and following the flow of blood through the heart from venous to arterial side. At atrial level such anomalies would include the sites of pulmonary and systemic venous drainage as well as defects in the interatrial septum, followed by a description of the atrioventricular connection. The topology of the ventricle (right-handed or left-handed) is established when this is not obvious from the atrioventricular connection, and abnormalities within the ventricles, such as septal defects or dominance of one chamber, are noted. Finally, the ventriculo-arterial connection is described, along with the morphology of the aortic arch and the branch pulmonary arteries. Mention of any positional abnormalities and spatial relationships of importance should then complete the cardiac diagnosis.

Cyanotic Congenital Heart Disease

It will be recalled that 5 g of reduced haemoglobin/100 cc blood is necessary to produce clinically apparent cyanosis and thus corresponds to an arterial saturation of about 85%. There are three general groups of heart defects which produce central cyanosis.

1. A right-to-left shunt, usually with reduced pulmonary flow, is the commonest situation. Tetralogy of Fallot is a familiar example of this type of defect.
2. Parallel systemic and pulmonary circulations, as seen in uncorrected transposition of the great vessels ('transposition physiology'), causes profound cyanosis often with increased pulmonary blood flow.
3. Defects in which both the systemic and pulmonary venous return must pass through the same cardiac chamber ('common mixing') include, for example, total anomalous pulmonary venous connection, single ventricle and tricuspid atresia, in which variable proportions of oxygenated desaturated blood usually give rise to some degree of cyanosis.

Central cyanosis caused by heart malformations must always be differentiated from that caused by lung problems, especially in young infants. The so-called hyperoxia or nitrogen washout test is a useful (but not infallible) investigation for this purpose. The patient breathes 100% oxygen for 5–10 minutes, following which a sample of blood is taken from the right radial artery. If the Po_2 has risen above 160 mmHg, cyanotic heart disease is unlikely to be the cause of the patient's hypoxia. This is because shunting or mixing of desaturated blood within the heart will still lower the saturation of fully oxygenated blood from the lungs in cyanotic heart defects, whereas the hypoxia of pulmonary origin is usually reversed by increased oxygen entering the blood as it passes through the lungs.

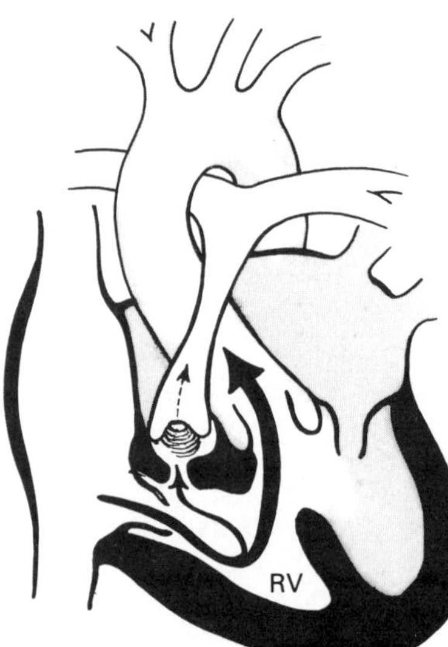

Fig. 6.10. Cyanosis in tetralogy of Fallot is due to desaturated (blue) blood passing from the right ventricle to the left side of the heart.

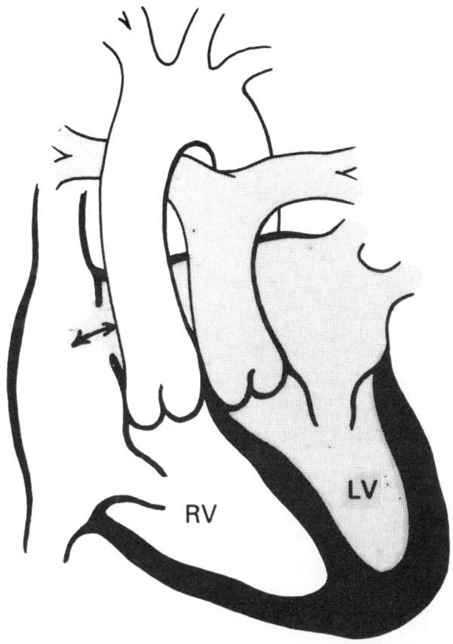

Fig. 6.11. Transposition produces cyanosis because blood from the body passed back to the aorta (blue, desaturated blood), while oxygenated blood remains in the pulmonary circuit.

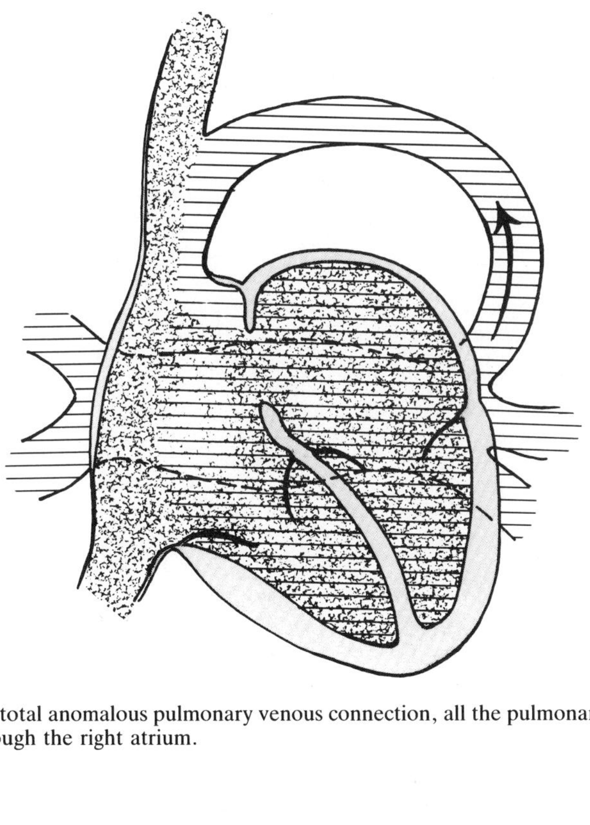

Fig. 6.12. In total anomalous pulmonary venous connection, all the pulmonary and systemic blood must pass through the right atrium.

Tetralogy of Fallot, Pulmonary Stenosis or Pulmonary Atresia with Ventricular Septal Defect

(Atrioventricular concordance; ventriculoarterial concordance or biventricular aortic origin; ventricular septal defect; right ventricular outflow obstruction)

These conditions have in common a communication between two ventricular chambers and some degree of obstruction to blood reaching the lungs from the right ventricle. They encompass a spectrum of malformations. The most common example is Fallot's tetralogy, which comprises about 10% of all congenital heart defects. In tetralogy of Fallot, there is a large ventricular septal defect with narrowing of the right ventricular outflow tract and displacement of the aorta, such that it over-rides the septal defect. Right ventricular hypertrophy, the fourth feature of the tetralogy, is simply the result of increased pressure in the right ventricle as a result of the pulmonary stenosis and ventricular septal defect. The term 'pentalogy of Fallot' has been applied when there is a co-existing atrial septal defect, but it serves no useful purpose.

With extreme obstruction of right ventricular outflow, continuity between the right ventricle and pulmonary artery is lost, resulting in tetralogy of Fallot with pulmonary atresia. There is no clear demarcation between this condition and pulmonary atresia with ventricular septal defect, although the arrangement of the pulmonary blood supply may be more variable and complex in extreme examples of the latter condition, and the right ventricular outflow may lack an infundibular component.

At the other end of the spectrum are examples of Fallot's tetralogy where the infundibular obstruction is mild and the pulmonary arteries are well developed. Because such patients have very little clinical evidence of arterial desaturation,

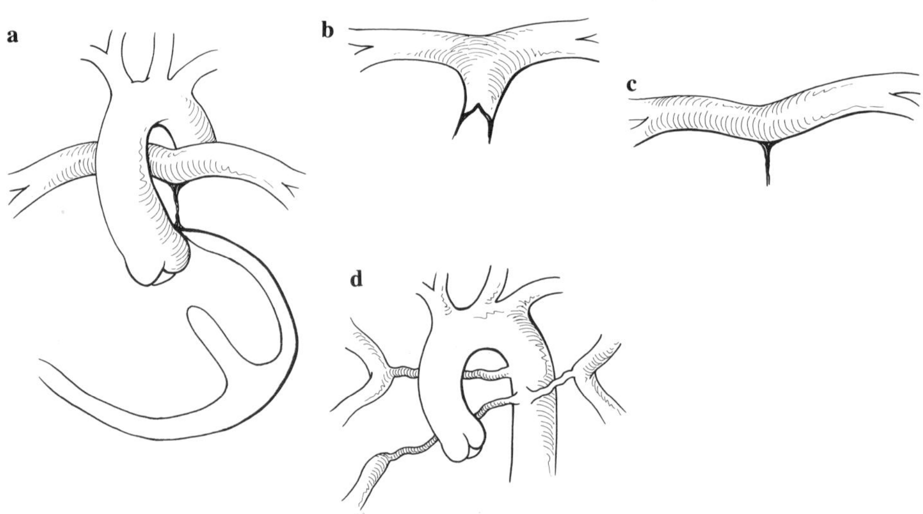

Fig. 6.13. Types of pulmonary arteries found in pulmonary atresia with ventricular septal defect: Pulmonary atresia/VSD. There is no continuity between the right ventricle and pulmonary arteries (**a**). Valvar atresia (**b**). Absence of main pulmonary artery (**c**). Major aorto pulmonary collateral arteries (**d**).

they have been called 'acyanotic Fallot's'. However, the presence of a large ventricular septal defect with aortic overriding justifies their inclusion within the definition of Fallot's tetralogy. These patients should be differentiated from patients with other types of ventricular septal defect with pulmonary stenosis, who also tend to have good development of the pulmonary vessels and a variable degree of cyanosis. In the latter group, there is no anterior displacement of the infundibular septum. Although right ventricular outflow obstruction may be severe as the result of a narrowed valve or muscle within the ventricular chamber, the ventricular septal defect is not necessarily large or related to the aorta.

Anatomy. Remembering that the hallmark of classical tetralogy of Fallot is a large septal defect with an over-riding aorta and infundibular pulmonary stenosis, it is possible to characterise the anatomical variations within this group of malformations according to these three features.

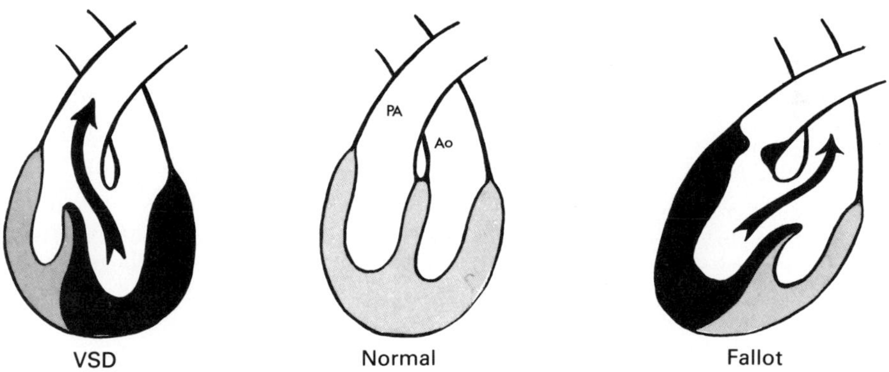

Fig. 6.14. Anatomical features of Fallot's tetralogy contrasted with simple ventricular septal defect.

The ventricular septal defect usually extends from the membranous septum towards the infundibulum of the right ventricle and, in children, has a diameter of 15–20 mm. One border is formed by the annulus of the tricuspid valve and another by the aortic valve. Occasionally, a small rim of muscles separates the defect from the tricuspid valve such that it is surrounded entirely by muscle and thus is less close to the conduction tissue. Less commonly, a deficiency of the infundibular portion of the septum brings the septal defect immediately below both great vessels ('subpulmonary' ventricular septal defect or 'doubly committed subarterial' defect). Additional septal defects in the trabecular part of the septum are not uncommon.

The degree of aortic overriding is quite variable. The vessel may arise entirely from the left ventricle (ventricular septal defect and pulmonary stenosis) or completely from the right ventricle (double outlet right ventricle). By anatomical convention, the valve is assigned to the ventricle which underlies half or more of its circumference, but in tetralogy of Fallot it is sometimes held that 90% of the aorta should arise from the right ventricle to qualify as a double outlet connection.

The levels of obstruction to right ventricular outflow also are variable. Most commonly in Fallot's tetralogy there is narrowing of the muscular infundibulum as the result of anterior septal displacement, with additional enlargement of septal or parietal extensions of the septomarginal trabeculation. A less common site of muscular obstruction is lower down within the right ventricular cavity. Here abnormal muscle bundles may divide the ventricle into a low pressure and a high pressure chamber, the so-called double-chambered right ventricle. About three-quarters of patients with tetralogy also have obstruction at the level of the pulmonary valve. This may be due to a small valve ring or fusion of the valve cusps. In the most severe cases there is obstruction distally within the pulmonary arteries themselves, either in the form of generalised underdevelopment or localised stenoses. In some patients the artery will be only a few millimetres in diameter, while in others it may be solid, absent in part or represented by a fibrous strand. Complete blockage may occur at any of these levels – infundibulum, valve or artery – producing 'pulmonary atresia'. In cases of pulmonary atresia the blood flow to the lungs must enter distal to the obstructed segment, usually from collateral vessels or occasionally via a patent arterial duct.

Other major cardiac defects occur upon occasion in association with the anatomical features of Fallot's tetralogy. These include complete atrioventricular septal defect, aortopulmonary window and vascular rings.

Haemodynamics. As the result of the large ventricular septal defect, both ventricles are in free communication and it is usual to find equal pressures in the right and left ventricles in patients with Fallot's tetralogy. Rarely, right ventricular pressure is higher than left as the result of fibrous tissue from the tricuspid valve partially occluding the ventricular septal defect. Such cases of 'flap-valve' ventricular septal defect may be confused clinically and haemodynamically with pulmonary stenosis and intact ventricular septum.

In the presence of a large ventricular communication, the ventricles discharge their contents into the aorta and pulmonary artery during systole in inverse proportion to the obstruction encountered at each outflow tract. When the resistance to flow offered by the pulmonary stenosis exceeds that of the peripheral systemic vessel, blood from both ventricles flows preferentially into the aorta that offers the pathway of least resistance. Because this stream of blood is a mixture of both the right and left ventricular contents, it produces the clinical features of cyanosis. Only a small portion of the cardiac output takes the course into the pulmonary artery. The lungs are consequently poorly vascularised and the total quantity of blood taking up oxygen is small.

As the venous return from the body is delivered to the right ventricle and most of it passes across the ventricular septal defect into the aorta, the right ventricle dominates the circulation. The left ventricle on the other hand receives only the small amount of blood returning from the poorly vascularised lungs and generally plays a subsidiary role. In very severe tetralogy of Fallot, the left ventricle may be poorly developed.

The degree of cyanosis in patients with Fallot's tetralogy is variable. As the right-to-left shunting of blood depends upon the relative resistances to flow in the systemic and pulmonary circulations, changes in these resistances will result in varying arterial oxygen saturation. On the right side, the infundibulum and muscular outflow have a variable degree of tonus. With increasing muscle

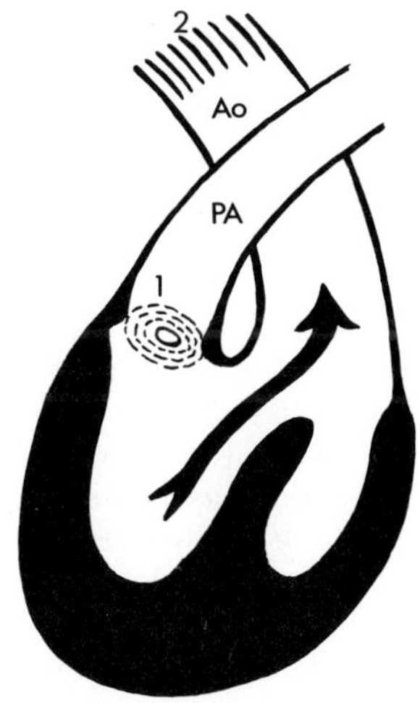

Fig. 6.15. Variations in tonus as the infundibular stenosis deflects a greater or lesser proportion of blood into the aorta. 1, Infundibular muscle; 2, aorta.

hypertrophy or constriction, more of the right ventricular blood shunts into the aorta producing increasing cyanosis. As the muscle relaxes more blood is able to flow into the lungs with a consequent reduction in cyanosis.

Less attention has been paid to the systemic peripheral resistance in Fallot's tetralogy. It is probable that squatting increases the peripheral resistance and in this way diverts more blood to the lungs for oxygenation. Conversely, exercise is known to cause systemic vasodilatation, and this is one of the reasons for increasing cyanosis on physical exertion in these patients.

Clinical Features. The outstanding sign is cyanosis which, as the result of increasing infundibular muscle obstruction, generally becomes apparent during the first year of life. An asymptomatic heart murmur may have been noticed previously. On the rare occasion when there is severe cyanosis at birth, this usually indicates poorly developed pulmonary arteries or pulmonary atresia with insufficient flow through a ductus arteriosus or collateral vessel. Rarely, patients with Fallot's tetralogy or pulmonary atresia with ventricular septal defect will present at around 3 months of age with heart failure and signs of a large left-to-right shunt. This may be due to minimal infundibular obstruction (acyanotic tetralogy) or massive blood flow through major aortopulmonary collateral arteries (MAPCAs).

Although cyanosis is often marked and is the feature responsible for bringing the child to the notice of the doctor, it is not the only source of disability. Tiredness and breathlessness result from hypoxia due to inadequate delivery of blood to the lungs for oxygenation, and it may severely limit exercise capacity. In the infant this is seen as inability to feed, while the toddler easily becomes exhausted with attempts to increase physical activity. Older children may even become bedridden or confined to a wheelchair with untreated tetralogy of Fallot. When cyanosis is severe and dyspnoea and fatigue are disproportionately slight, some other condition, such as transposition of the great vessels, should be suspected.

Cyanotic 'spells' or 'attacks' indicate an intermittent critical reduction in pulmonary blood flow. In their fullest form, the child appears more deeply cyanosed than usual, cries with pain and then becomes pale; this is followed by loss of consciousness. These episodes represent nearly complete obstruction to blood flow through the right ventricular infundibulum and a phase of gross right-to-left shunting. The murmur of pulmonary stenosis may disappear completely during such an attack. The resulting hypoxia causes myocardial and cerebral ischaemia with consequent chest pain, low cardiac output and fainting. Such episodes are of serious prognosis and may result in permanent brain damage.

Squatting is characteristic of older children with Fallot's tetralogy, and the diagnosis should be accepted with reservation unless this is present. The squatting attitude usually is assumed after exertion, but, in more severe cases, the child may squat even at rest in bed. The position adopted is that of fully flexed knees with the buttocks close to or actually touching the ground.

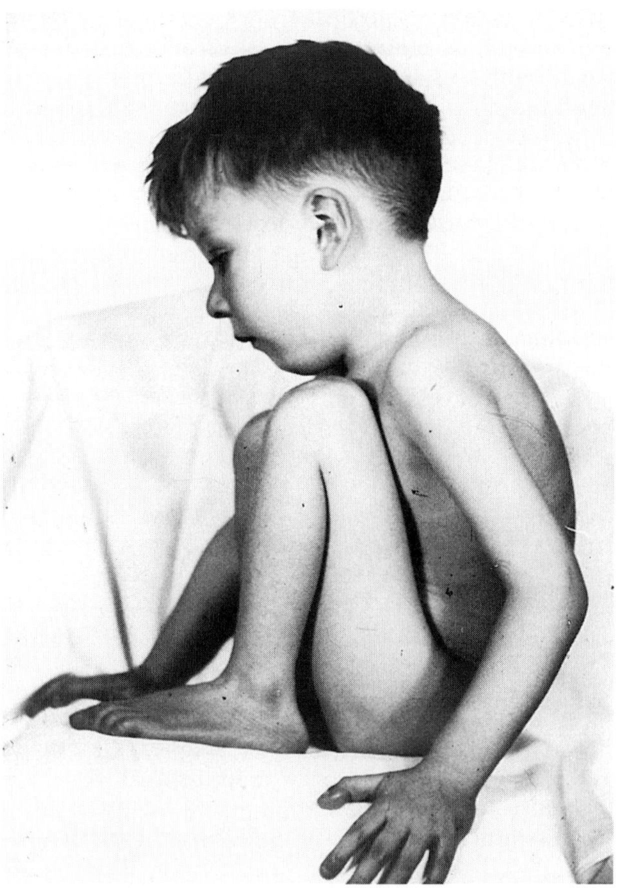

Fig. 6.16. Squatting in tetralogy of Fallot.

All cyanotic children with right-to-left shunts, including those with Fallot's tetralogy, are liable to the complications of cerebral thrombosis and paradoxical septic embolism. They may present, therefore, with focal neurological signs, features suggestive of intracranial infection or the manifestations of a cerebral abscess.

On physical examination the child is often underdeveloped physically, with thin legs and poor musculature, although infants tend to be well nourished. Clubbing is always present after about 6 months of age and its severity usually is related to the degree of cyanosis. The peripheral circulation is good, with warm extremities and prominent veins, particularly on the back of the hands. This contrasts with the poor peripheral circulation in patients with pulmonary stenosis and intact ventricular septum or a restrictive ventricular septal defect, a helpful point in making this important differential diagnosis.

The arterial pulses are full, reflecting a normal cardiac output. Even more importance is attached to the jugular venous pressure: with severe pulmonary stenosis this may be prominent. However, the presence of an accentuated *a* wave, particularly in association with an enlarged liver, suggests an obstructed right ventricle without a ventricular septal defect, or possibly tricuspid atresia.

The cardiac impulse is right ventricular in type but generally is not particularly striking. A thrill is often palpable over the outflow tract in about the third left interspace. The absence of a thrill, thought to arise from the site of the pulmonary stenosis, does not rule out a diagnosis of Fallot's tetralogy but rather suggests the possibility of associated pulmonary atresia.

On auscultation, one hears a fairly harsh systolic murmur, which is of ejection type over most of the precordium but maximal over the site of the pulmonary stenosis. The murmur is usally short, as would be expected, because the right ventricle can eject its blood also through the large ventricular septal defect. Separate closure of the pulmonic valve cannot usually be distinguished; this is due to limited movement and deformity of the cusps together with the low diastolic closing pressure in the pulmonary artery. A continuous murmur, often best appreciated posteriorly, indicates the presence of collateral vessels. An immediate diastolic murmur is found occasionally in older patients who have developed aortic regurgitation or in the subset of patients with tetralogy and absent pulmonary valve syndrome.

Special Investigations. The packed cell volume and haemoglobin should be recorded in every patient since polycythaemia is the rule in cyanotic heart disease and, like clubbing or cyanosis, reflects the severity of the condition. An exception of this rule is the young infant, who may not yet have acquired polycythaemia. Its absence in other patients should suggest the possibility of anaemia.

The chest radiograph reveals poorly vascularised, 'oligaemic' lung fields. There may be assymetry, such that the vascular pattern is more evident in one lung than the other, a feature which should be confirmed by angiography. Some of the most severe cases have apparently good vasculature in the region of the hilum, but, on closer inspection, the shadows are seen to be broken up and reticulated. This appearance represents a dense network of fine collateral vessels surrounding the major bronchi. The cardiac silhouette in Fallot's tetralogy is usually described as bootshaped ('coeur en sabot'), which is caused by the high blunt apex of the hypertrophied right ventricle and the concave bay in the usual

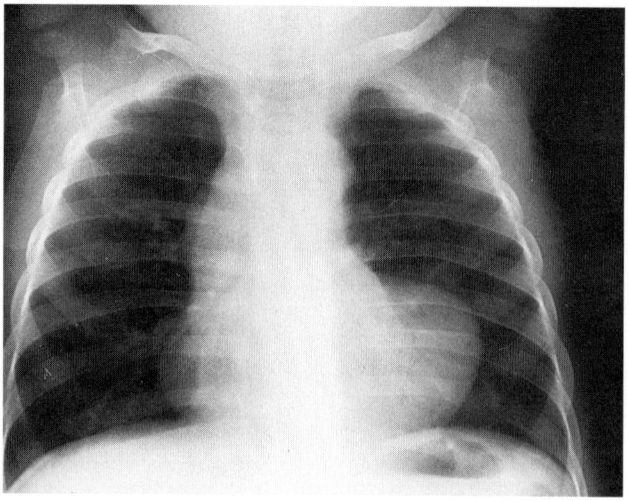

Fig. 6.17. Chest X-ray in Fallot's tetralogy.

position of the pulmonary artery. With pulmonary stenosis and ventricular septal defect, the cardiac shadow may be unremarkable but there is not infrequently post-stenotic dilatation of the main pulmonary artery. Massive enlargement of the main and branch pulmonary arteries is virtually diagnostic of tetralogy with absent pulmonary valve. The aortic knuckle is usually prominent and, in about one-quarter of all patients with Fallot's tetralogy, lies to the right of the trachea (right aortic arch).

The ECG demonstrates right axis deviation and moderate right ventricular hypertrophy. Right ventricular strain patterns and prominent P waves are unusual, because right ventricular pressure generally is not higher than systolic. Left axis deviation should alert one to a diagnosis of tricuspid atresia.

In classical tetralogy, cardiac catheterisation confirms the presence of equal right and left ventricular peak systolic pressures, and indicates the degree of pulmonary stenosis and the level of systemic arterial oxygen saturation. With ventricular septal defect and pulmonary stenosis, right ventricular pressure may be less than systemic, while severe pulmonary stenosis with a restrictive ventricular septal defect occasionally causes pressure in the right ventricle to exceed that in the left. An atrial septal defect, a patent foramen ovale or a patent ductus arteriosus may be crossed by the catheter.

Angiography with injection into the right and left ventricles and the ascending aorta is the most useful investigation. It should demonstrate the level and severity of right ventricular outflow obstruction, the anatomy of the pulmonary artery, the position of the ventricular septal defect, the presence of additional septal defects, and the origin of the aorta and coronary arteries.

When there is pulmonary atresia, the source of pulmonary blood flow to each lung segment must be established, usually by additional injections of contrast into the aorta, ductus or collateral vessels. A retrograde pressure injection through a catheter wedged in a pulmonary vein may be necessary to visualise 'true' (i.e. derived from the embryonic sixth aortic arch) pulmonary arteries that have not been otherwise demonstrated.

a

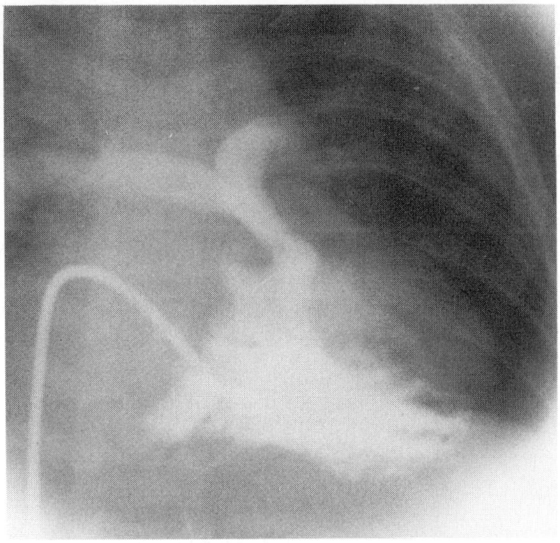

b

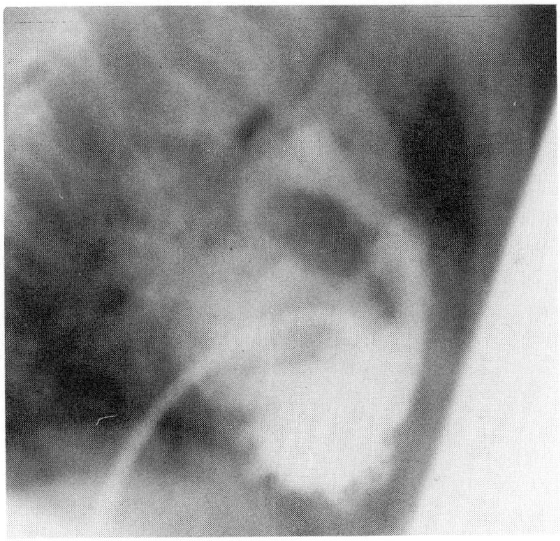

Fig. 6.18. Antero–posterior (a) and lateral (b) views of right ventricular angiogram in Fallot's tetralogy.

The side of the aortic arch, anomalies of brachiocephalic vessels, and patency of any previously constructed systemic pulmonary anastomoses should also be observed. While some of this information may be obtained from echocardiography, particularly with colour Doppler studies, it is still generally accepted that angiography is essential to demonstrate the complete pulmonary arterial tree.

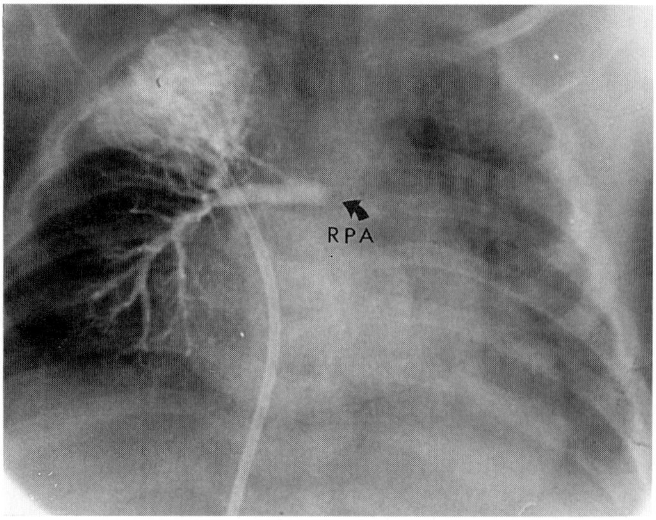

Fig. 6.19. Pulmonary artery visualised retrograde by injection of dye into a pulmonary vein.

Differential Diagnosis. Before accepting a diagnosis of Fallot's tetralogy, other causes of cyanotic congenital heart disease should be excluded. Babies with pulmonary stenosis or atresia, intact ventricular septum and reverse atrial shunt present with severe cyanosis and sudden deterioration during the first days of life, as a result of ductus closure. The right ventricle in these patients is under considerably greater tension than the left; this is usually reflected in elevation of the venous pressure, liver enlargement, a heaving right ventricular impulse and marked right ventricular dominance with 'strain' on the ECG. Patients with transposition of the great arteries tend to present earlier with profound cyanosis at birth, but here the lung fields are well vascularised.

In tricuspid atresia, the ECG is useful, as right atrial enlargement with left ventricular dominance and left axis deviation should be observable. Echocardiography and/or cardiac catheterisation are usually necessary to establish the diagnosis with certainty.

Indications for Operation. At any age, severe or increasing hypoxia that cannot be controlled by drug therapy (beta-blocking agents or, if a patent arterial duct is present, prostaglandins) is an indication for surgical intervention. Patients who suffer cyanotic spells are at risk of death or cerebral damage during these attacks, and operation then becomes an urgent necessity. In cases with pulmonary atresia, surgery is very occasionally required to control congestive heart failure resulting from massive flow through collateral vessels. More commonly, procedures are undertaken to promote growth of the pulmonary arteries or to 'unifocalise' pulmonary blood flow in asymptomatic or complex cases. Apart from these special circumstances, a diagnosis of Fallot's tetralogy, ventricular septal defect and pulmonary stenosis, or pulmonary atresia with ventricular septal defect may now be considered an indication for elective operation, in view of the very good results of surgery and the very poor long-term outlook for untreated patients.

Principles of Treatment. The ultimate goal of surgery in this group of conditions is to achieve complete anatomical and physiological correction by relief of the right ventricular outflow obstruction and closure of the ventricular septal defect. The means by which this ideal is achieved for any individual patient will depend upon a number of factors. Closure of the ventricular septal defect means that the entire cardiac output must flow through the lungs and be pumped into the systemic circulation by the left ventricle. This will be possible only if the obstruction to pulmonary flow can be adequately relieved without excessive damage to the coronary arteries or ventricular muscle, and if the pulmonary arteries and left ventricle are sufficiently developed to cope with the increased volume of blood that will pass through them. In some cases it will be possible to perform complete correction in the first instance, while other patients will require one or more preliminary surgical procedures to improve the chance of successful repair subsequently.

The choice between complete primary correction or a palliative operation must take into account the age and condition of the patient, the experience and facilities of the surgical team and a number of anatomical details. These so-called risk factors, i.e. factors that can be shown to be associated with an unsuccessful surgical outcome, have been derived by reviewing very extensive surgical experience. They vary somewhat from one institution to another and also change with the passage of time and the acquisition of new knowledge.

In general, the mortality for complete correction tends to be higher when the pulmonary arteries and left ventricle are underdeveloped, when there is an abnormal distribution of the right or left pulmonary artery branches, or when the packed cell volume exceeds about 45%. Correction at a young age and small size, particulary when a transannular patch or valved extracardiac conduit are needed, has also been associated with increased operative mortality. For these patients, a palliative procedure is carried out to relieve symptoms and to bring about a more favourable situation for later correction.

Palliation of Fallot's tetralogy or pulmonary atresia with ventricular septal defect generally involves augmentation of pulmonary blood flow by one of several methods. In complex cases, it may be necessary also to join up arteries that supply isolated parts of the lung ('unifocalisation') or to close off collateral vessels whose perfusion is not necessary. In an individual patient, the exact procedure or combination of procedures is chosen both to bring about optimum development of the pulmonary circulation and to be easily reversed or taken down through a median sternotomy at the time of complete repair.

Complete correction is done as the primary procedure in patients with suitable anatomy or as a secondary procedure following a palliative operation. Intra-operatively, the circulation is maintained by means of a heart–lung machine for at least half an hour and often considerably longer. Infants and patients with excessive development of collateral vessels are cooled to 20°C or lower, so that the pump flow may be reduced or stopped altogether to facilitate exposure. Any major collateral vessels and previously constructed systemic–pulmonary anastomoses are controlled soon after the start of cardiopulmonary bypass to prevent cardiac distension and flooding of the lungs. Right ventricular outflow obstruction is relieved by the removal of muscle bundles and by opening up the stenotic valve. In some cases, a patch of pericardium or other material has to be used to widen the right ventricular infundibulum ('subannular patch') or across the outflow tract onto the pulmonary artery ('transannular patch'). The latter

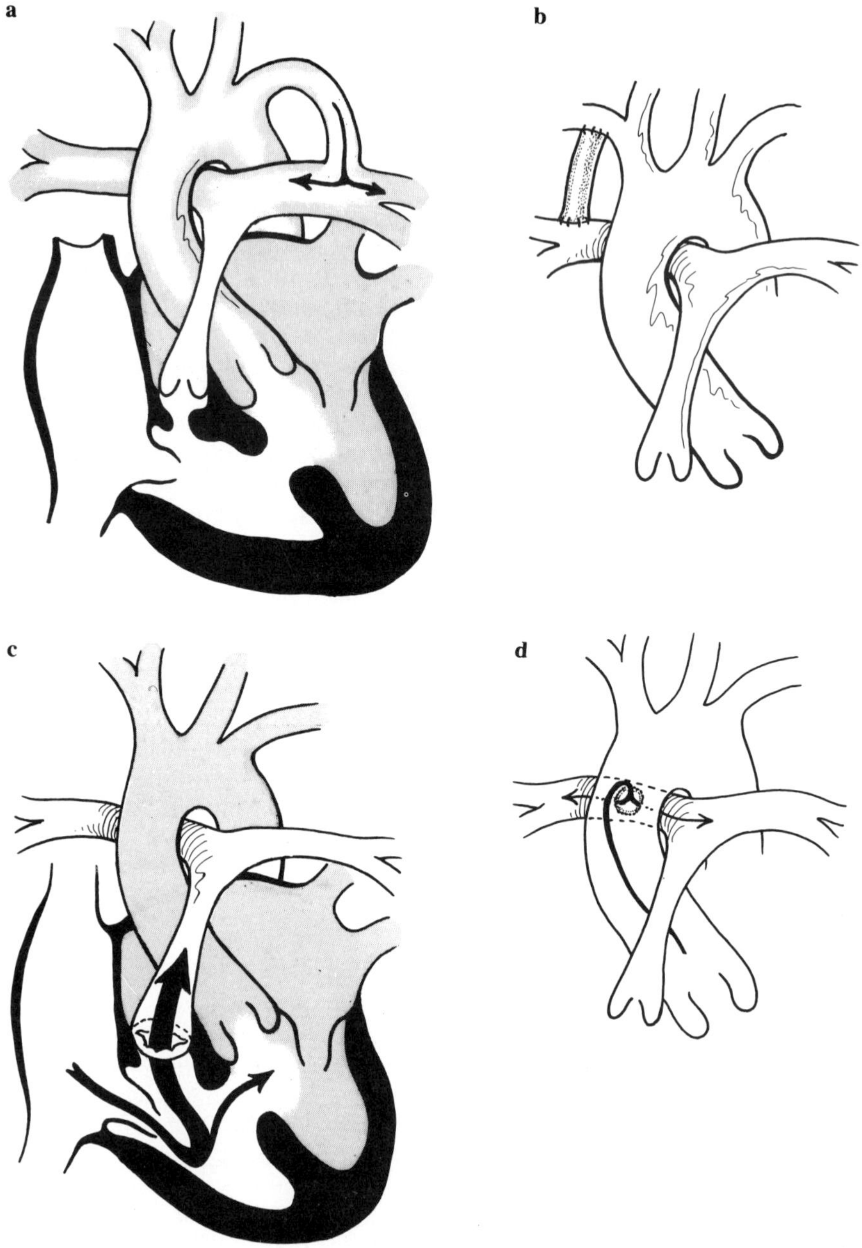

Fig. 6.20. Commonly-used types of systemic–pulmonary anastomoses, each of which diverts some blood from the systemic circulation to the lung arteries: Blalock operation (**a**). Modified Blalock operation (**b**). Waterston operation (**d**). The classical Brock operation, which promotes flow through the right ventricle to the lungs (**c**).

renders the pulmonary valve incompetent which, although well tolerated in the short term, may require pulmonary valve replacement later in life. When there is pulmonary atresia, a valve-bearing tube ('valved extracardiac conduit') is used to connect the right ventricle to the pulmonary arteries. The ventricular septal defect is closed with a Dacron patch, and any atrial septal defect is closed with a patch or direct suture.

Results. The early survival among patients undergoing complete repair of Fallot's tetralogy should now exceed 95%, and operative mortality approaches zero in many centres throughout the world. Straightforward cases of pulmonary atresia with ventricular septal defect also have around 5% early mortality, although the risk with repair may be as great as 25%–40% when there are complex pulmonary arterial problems. Similarly the risk of correction for Fallot's tetralogy increases in the presence of major associated anomalies (e.g. aortopulmonary window, complete atrioventricular septal defect,) and some of the more difficult subsets, such as the absent pulmonary valve syndrome, have a very high mortality in infancy. Provided that the ventricular septal defect is closed and right ventricular outflow obstruction relieved, survivors of complete correction generally have excellent late results.

Pulmonary Atresia with Intact Ventricular Septum

Pulmonary atresia occurring without a ventricular septal defect produces a condition very different from either the Fallot-like group of anomalies, on the one hand, or pulmonary valve stenosis, on the other. The connections between atria, ventricles and great vessels are concordant but there is complete obstruction to blood flow at the pulmonary valve level. Although present, the right ventricle tends to be small, and more severe examples are sometimes described as 'hypoplastic right heart syndrome'. By definition, the tricuspid valve is present and patent. While it is a rare malformation (pulmonary atresia with intact ventricular septum accounts for about 1% of patients born with congenital heart defects), this lesion is among the more common to cause cyanosis in the new-born.

Anatomy. The pulmonary valve consists of imperforate fibrous tissue with variable development of ridges in the position of the commissures. Although the valve annulus is small and may be separated from the right ventricular cavity by muscle, the main and branch pulmonary arteries generally have normal development and distribution. Severe hypertrophy with a variable degree of hypolasia of the right ventricle is the rule, often with complete loss of trabecular or infundibular portions. Occasionally, however, the ventricle is massively dilated. The tricuspid valve shows a spectrum of anomalies, from thickening and fusion of the cusps to an Ebstein-like malformation. The ventricular septum is closed, and the presence of an interatrial defect is mandatory for maintenance of the circulation. A patent arterial duct nearly always constitutes the sole source of pulmonary blood flow. Most cases have some myocardial fibrosis, which may involve the left ventricle as well as the right, and in some cases abnormal communications ('sinusoids') are present between the right ventricle cavity and the coronary arteries.

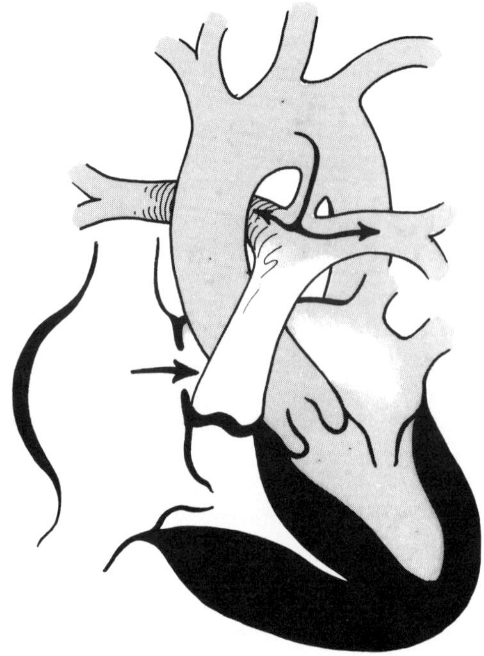

Fig. 6.21. Morphologic features of pulmonary atresia with intact ventricular septum.

Patients who have a pinpoint orifice at the pulmonary valve may exhibit many of these anatomical features, but their clinical prognosis tends to be rather better and, accordingly, they are classified as severe, critical pulmonary stenosis.

Haemodynamics. The completely obstructed and severely hypertrophied right ventricle works at a pressure exceeding that in the left ventricle. There usually is some degree of regurgitation through the tricuspid valve and, when present, sinusoids also decompress the right ventricle slightly by conducting desaturated blood retrograde into the coronary arteries. This may further impair muscle function. Due to the diminished capacity of the right ventricular cavity and its thick inelastic wall, an increased pressure results in the right atrium. This causes blood to shunt from right to left across the atrial septum, returning the systemic venous blood to the left side of the heart and producing cyanosis. Blood reaches the lungs through the patent ductus arteriosus.

Clinical Features. The usual presentation is cyanosis on the 1st or 2nd day of life. With closure of the ductus, the hypoxia becomes profound and is complicated by a metabolic acidosis. Examination usually discloses a single second heart sound but, unlike pulmonary atresia with ventricular septal defect, the cardiac impulse is dominated by the left ventricle. When a sick infant is first examined, there is frequently an absence of cardiac murmurs. Only later, when the cardiac output improves, do murmurs of tricuspid regurgitation and/or a patent ductus arteriosus become apparent. In older patients, an accentuated *a* wave may be seen in the jugular venous pulse and signs of tricuspid regurgitation, such as liver pulsation, are not uncommon.

Special Investigations. The chest X-ray shows normal or reduced vascularity of the lungs, with a concavity in the position of the pulmonary artery. When the heart shadow is large, this is usually the result of right atrial dilatation.

The ECG is dominated by left ventricular forces, even at birth, and soon after, enlargement of P waves suggest right atrial hypertrophy. Patients who have been severely hypoxic or those with multiple sinusoids may demonstrate changes of myocardial ischaemia.

The diagnosis of pulmonary atresia with intact ventricular septum can be fairly accurately established by real-time echocardiography, although a slightly patent pulmonary valve or a small ventricular septal defect cannot always be excluded. A good impression of the size of the right ventricular cavity and tricuspid valve, as well as some measure of ventricular function, may also be gained from this investigation. Cardiac catheterisation and angiography will confirm atresia of the pulmonary valve and visualise the degree of right ventricular development as well as the presence of sinusoids, the degree of tricuspid regurgitation and patency of the ductus arteriosus. It has been suggested that catheterisation is an unnecessary hazard for these sick babies, but others hold that surgical treatment can best be planned with a detailed knowledge of ventricular and pulmonary arterial morphology provided by angiography. At present, there is no conclusive evidence that skilful invasive studies by an experienced cardiologist are detrimental. At the same time, refinements of echocardiography, particularly Doppler and colour-flow mapping, continue to improve accuracy and resolution. It is thus largely up to the surgeon to decide whether he has sufficient information to embark upon treatment.

Differential Diagnosis. In addition to excluding the Fallot-like conditions, it is important to differentiate between tricuspid atresia and Ebstein's malformation of the tricuspid valve. Tricuspid atresia may occur with pulmonary atresia, and in these cases the right ventricle will be entered at catheterisation through a ventricular septal defect rather than the tricuspid valve. Ebstein's malformation may be difficult to exclude: indeed, it occasionally accompanies pulmonary atresia with intact ventricular septum. Right ventricular angiography is helpful, and it should be possible to pass the catheter across the pulmonary valve in cases of isolated Ebstein's malformation.

Indications for Operation. A case of pulmonary atresia with intact ventricular septum should be regarded as one of surgical urgency. Even though pulmonary blood flow through the ductus may be sustained by administration of intravenous prostaglandin, the situation is precarious until a reliable source of pulmonary perfusion is established. Without treatment about half of the patients die within a fortnight of birth and survival for more than a year is rare.

Principles of Treatment. Surgical management is governed by the immediate necessity of ensuring adequate pulmonary blood-flow as well as the eventual desirability of decompressing and developing a right ventricle, and separating the pulmonary and systemic circulations. Pulmonary valvotomy alone generally gives insufficient augmentation of blood flow because the muscle-bound ventricle and small tricuspid valve still consitute an obstruction to forward flow. Usually, valvotomy is combined with a systemic pulmonary anastomosis (see Tetralogy of Fallot) or continued administration of prostaglandin. Alternatively a systemic–pulmonary anastomosis is performed without valvotomy, the right ventricle being opened up at a subsequent operation. If the right ventricle and tricuspid valve develop adequately, complete correction is made by reversing the shunt operation and closing the atrial septal defect. When the ventricle remains underdeveloped, a direct connection is made between the right atrium and pulmonary arteries (the Fontan operation – see Tricuspid Atresia) with closure of the atrial septal defect.

Results. Eighty to ninety per cent of patients will survive the initial palliative shunt or valvotomy when prostaglandin is available to resuscitate the baby preoperatively, and surgery can be carried out in a unit experienced in the care of neonates. The results of subsequent correction depend on development of the pulmonary arteries and right ventricle, and on ventricular function. Mortality for either biventricular correction or the Fontan operation is 15%–20%. The long-term survivors generally have a good exercise capacity.

Transposition of the Great Arteries (Atrioventricular concordance with ventriculoarterial discordance)

In this condition, the aorta and pulmonary artery arise from the morphologically inappropriate pumping chamber; that is, the aorta from the right ventricle and the pulmonary artery from left ventricle. A number of other cardiac defects may be found in association with transposed great vessels. Of patients presenting with cyanosis in the first months of life, about one-quarter will be found to have transposition of the great arteries.

Anatomy. The precise developmental mechanism leading to transposition is uncertain but probably involves both an abnormality in conotruncal septation and maldevelopment of the infundibular muscle beneath the great vessels. The aorta usually lies anterior and to the right of the pulmonary artery, but the two great vessels may assume any spatial relationship. It is important to remember that coronary arteries arise only from the aortic sinuses that 'face' the pulmonary valve, regardless of their position.

In transposition of the great vessels, it is the aortic valve which is supported completely by a muscular conus, while the pulmonary valve is usually in continuity with the mitral annulus and at a lower level. The right ventricle tends to be thicker than normal, while the left ventricle becomes thin and compressed into a 'banana-shaped' chamber. Generally, the atria and atrioventricular valves are unremarkable, although the tricuspid valve may be smaller than average and abnormal insertion of the mitral valve in the subpulmonary area may produce left ventricular outflow obstruction.

Cases in which there is no other haemodynamically important abnormality are called 'simple' transposition. When another major cardiac defect is present, the transposition is said to be 'complex'. The most common associations are ventricular septal defect, patent ductus arteriosus and left ventricular outflow obstruction, either singly or in combination. Both simple and complex cases of transposition are examples of 'complete' transposition. This should be differentiated from 'corrected' transposition, in which associated atrioventricular discordance brings about a physiological correction of the circulation.

Haemodynamics. The systemic and pulmonary circulations operate in parallel, with desaturated blood from the venae cavae passing from the right atrium to the right ventricle and thence into the aorta. Oxygenated blood from the left atrium flows to the left ventricle and back to the lungs. Such a state, with two independent circulations, is incompatible with life, unless there is some communication that allows mixing of oxygenated and deoxygenated blood. This may be at atrial level (atrial septal defect), ventricular level (ventricular septal defect) or great vessel level (patent ductus arteriosus).

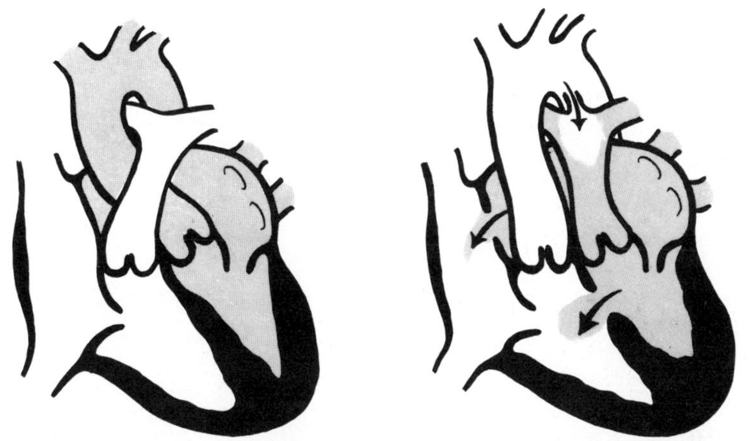

Fig. 6.22. Transposition of the great vessels showing available sites of mixing.

The pulmonary blood flow is at least normal and often excessive, particularly in the presence of a ventricular septal defect or patent arterial duct. In this situation, pulmonary arterial pressure may be elevated and obstructive pulmonary vascular changes develop rapidly.

The basic haemodynamics are modified by associated lesions. Left ventricular outflow obstruction, whether valvar or subpulmonary in location, tends to reduce pulmonary blood flow. When a ventricular septal defect is also present, this may protect the lungs and give an additional benefit of encouraging oxygenated blood to shunt from the left to the right ventricle. However, outflow obstruction in the presence of an intact septum causes elevation of left ventricular pressure and profound hypoxia.

Clinical Features. Cyanosis is frequently present at birth and nearly always apparent during the first day of life. Rapid deterioration follows thereafter, as the patient develops tachypnoea and metabolic acidosis. When an atrial or ventricular septal defect is present, or the ductus remains patent, the infant may present a few weeks later with signs of congestive heart failure and a lesser degree of cyanosis.

Apart from cyanosis, physical signs in the infant are rather non-specific. A short ejection systolic murmur along the left sternal edge is present in about half the patients. Most have a parasternal right ventricular impulse and normal splitting of the second heart sound. This latter feature helps to differentiate the cyanotic patient with transposed great arteries from cases of Fallot's tetralogy.

The occasional patient who survives to childhood without treatment will usually be found to have a ventricular septal defect with pulmonary stenosis or a degree of pulmonary vascular disease limiting pulmonary blood flow. Compared with a case of Fallot's tetralogy, the intensity of cyanosis is disproportionately great in relation to the degree of disability. Even though the child is markedly blue and clubbed, he may be active about the ward. Hypercyanotic attacks or 'spells' occur infrequently, and squatting is not a common clinical feature of transposed great vessels.

Special Investigations. At birth the ECG may be within normal limits, only later showing the development of right ventricular dominance. The small vascular pedicle, which results from superimposition of the aorta and pulmonary artery

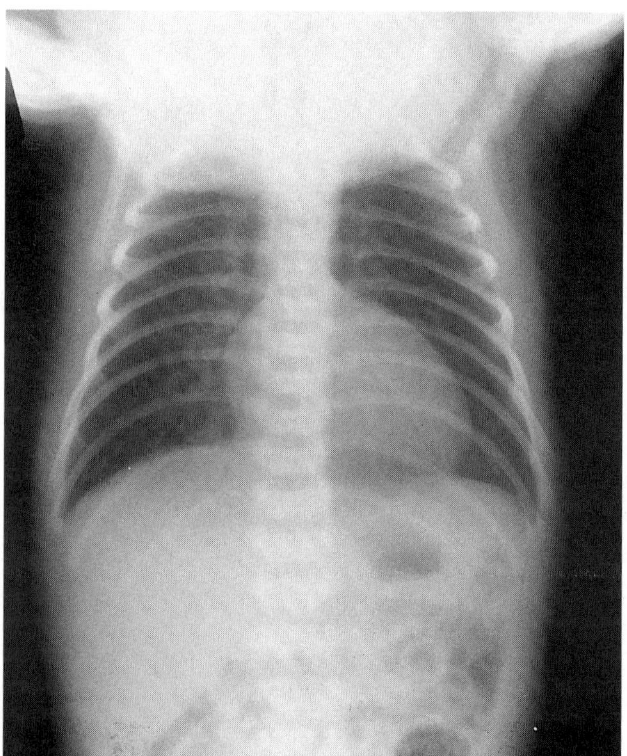

Fig. 6.23. Chest X-ray of an infant with 'simple' transposition of the great vessels.

on chest X-ray, causes the heart shadow to resemble an 'egg on its side'. Lung vascularity is either normal or increased.

The diagnosis of transposed great arteries can be established with certainty by real-time echocardiography. This will demonstrate the abnormal origin of the great vessels as well as the presence of atrial or ventricular septal defects, coarctation of the aorta, a patent ductus arteriosus, left ventricular outflow obstruction and abnormalities of the mitral or tricuspid valves.

Cardiac catheterisation is carried out to perform an atrial septostomy and, the condition of the patient permitting, to quantitate intracardiac shunts and pressures. Because the systemic and pulmonary circulations are essentially parallel and separate, any shunt that occurs between them must be bidirectional. Thus, a portion of oxygenated blood from the pulmonary circuit is exchanged (at atrial, ventricular or great vessel level) for an equal volume of blood from the systemic circuit; this blood constitutes the effective pulmonary blood flow. Blood that stays in the pulmonary circuit contributes nothing to systemic arterial saturation and accordingly is ineffective in oxygenating the patient. The systemic arterial saturation measured at catheter, then, is a reflection of how adequately blood is 'mixing' in the two circulations.

Angiography may be carried out at the initial catheterisation or deferred to a subsequent investigation, depending upon the patient's condition and the proposed plan of management. An injection of contrast into the right ventricle demonstrates the position of the aorta and any septal defects, while an aortogram should visualise the coronary arteries and, if present, a persistent ductus arteriosus or coarctation of the aorta. A left ventricular injection shows the outflow tract of that ventricle, particularly the presence of subvalvar pulmonary obstruction, and any abnormalities of the pulmonary arteries.

Differential Diagnosis. Usually, other types of cyanotic heart disease will be excluded by echocardiography and/or cardiac catheterisation. In cases of complex transposition, however, the relationships among atrioventricular valves, great vessels and septal defects may be difficult to establish with certainty. Some cases will resemble double outlet right ventricle and others will approach the spectrum of 'single ventricle' or 'univentricular atrioventricular' connection.

Indications for Operation. Hypoxia is the chief indication for surgical intervention, although elective anatomical correction is also performed routinely during the neonatal period. In the presence of major associated defects, operation may be needed also to control heart failure, relieve obstruction of the aorta (coarctation), protect the lungs from excessive blood flow or bring about development of a cardiac chamber. The clinical counterparts of these physiological indications are severe cyanosis, failure to thrive (infants) or growth retardation (children) and limitation of exercise capacity.

Principles of Treatment. In the critically ill new-born infant, the primary aim is to increase the mixing of arterial and venous blood in order to relieve hypoxia and correct any metabolic acidosis. In the short term, pharmacological dilatation of the ductus arteriosus by infusion of prostaglandin will achieve this until an atrial septal defect can be created by balloon septostomy (Rashkind's procedure;

see Chap. 4). In this procedure the cardiologist passes a balloon-tipped catheter through the femoral or umbilical vein and across the patent foramen ovale. When the balloon is inflated and jerked back into the right atrium, a large tear is made in the atrial septum, ensuring an atrial septal defect. Even when a ventricular septal defect or patent ductus arteriosus is present, more complete mixing will take place at atrial level. From this point, management is individualised according to the specific anatomy of the patient, the philosophy of the physicians and surgeons caring for the baby, and the facilities and expertise available to the surgical team.

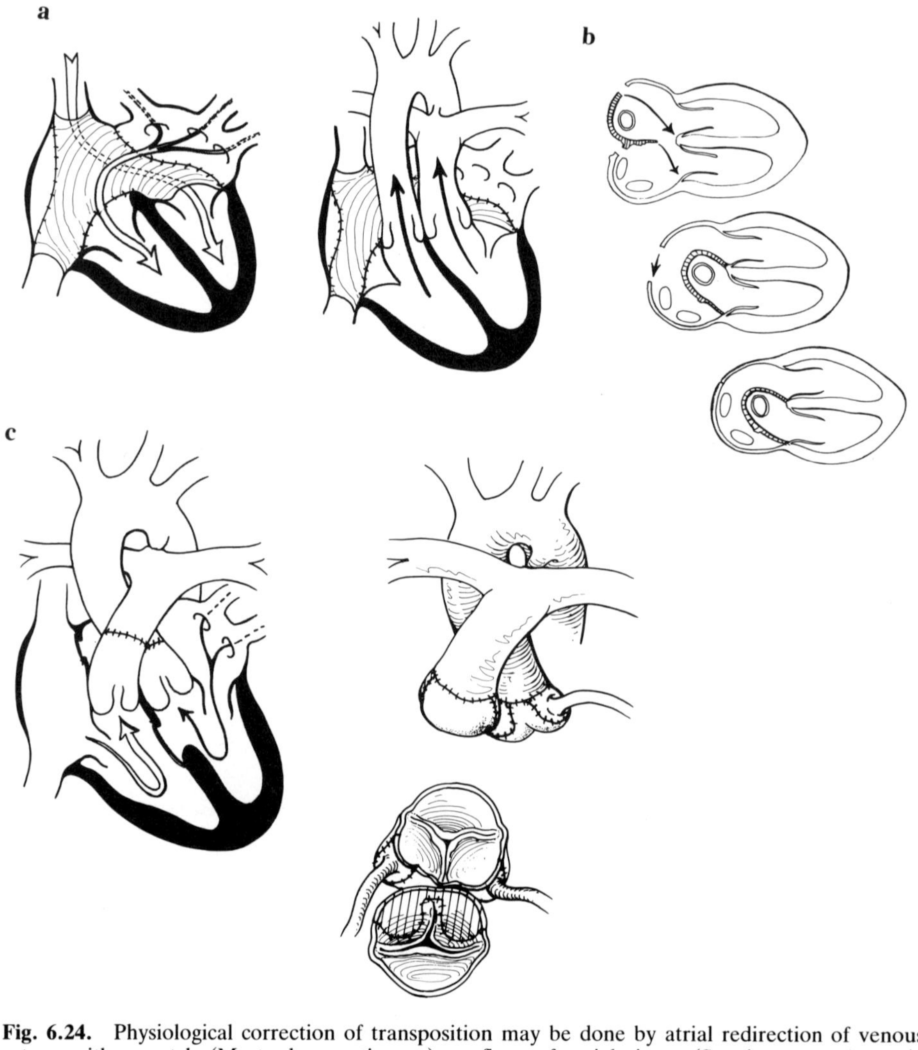

Fig. 6.24. Physiological correction of transposition may be done by atrial redirection of venous return with a patch (Mustard operation, **a**) or flaps of atrial tissue (Senning operation, **b**). Anatomical correction involves switching the great vessels to the appropriate ventricle (**c**).

In patients with simple transposition, an early choice must be made between *anatomical* correction by transfer of the great vessels with reimplantation of the coronary arteries, or *physiological* correction by redirection of the venous blood at atrial level. The former requires a left ventricle capable of supporting the systemic circulation as well as a normal pulmonary valve and an unobstructed left ventricular outflow tract. The arterial switch operation for anatomical correction of simple transposition must thus be done in the first few weeks of life, before the normal fall of pulmonary resistance causes left ventricular pressure to decline with accompanying loss of muscle mass. The occasional patient in whom a large patent duct arteriosus or dynamic obstruction to left ventricular outflow maintains a raised pressure in the left ventricle, may remain a candidate for the arterial switch operation somewhat longer. Atrial redirection of venous return, on the other hand, accepts the right ventricle as the systemic pumping chamber and can be carried out an any age. Usually it is done between 3 and 12 months of age. Either a patch of pericardium (Mustard operation) or infolding of the patient's own atrial and septal tissues (Senning operation) is used to direct the caval blood across the mitral valve and the pulmonary venous blood across the tricuspid valve.

In patients with transposition and ventricular septal defect, management depends primarily upon the presence or absence of restriction to pulmonary blood flow. When the lungs are subjected to the full force of systemic pressure as well as increased flow and hypoxia, there is a tendency to develop both congestive heart failure and pulmonary vascular disease early in life. For such patients, the choice lies between palliative banding of the pulmonary artery to reduce pulmonary pressure and flow, even at the cost of increased cyanosis, and primary anatomical correction, usually involving the arterial switch operation with closure of the atrial and ventricular septal defects. Banding is a closed procedure and can be followed by complete correction and pulmonary artery debanding (which must be done with cardiopulmonary bypass) sometime between 1 and 4 years of age.

Patients who have restriction of pulmonary blood flow are protected from the development of pulmonary vascular changes. Indeed, if the left ventricular outflow obstruction is severe or complete (pulmonary atresia), a systemic pulmonary anastomosis (see Tetralogy of Fallot) may be necessary to provide adequate oxygenation. In most of these cases, it will be possible to direct blood from the left ventricle through the ventricular septal defect and into the aorta by creating an intraventricular tunnel. The pulmonary artery, which still arises from the left ventricle, is closed off proximally and connected to the right ventricle with a valved conduit. This procedure, the Rastelli operation, also achieves a type of anatomical correction, as the left ventricle supplies the systemic circulation, and the right ventricle the pulmonary circulation. Because the mediastinum needs a sufficient space for the conduit, elective repair is usually carried out at 4 to 6 years of age.

Nearly all patients with untreated transposition of the great arteries, with or without a ventricular septal defect, eventually develop pulmonary vascular disease. In these cases, a palliative arterial or venous redirection may improve the patient's oxygenation and capacity for exercise. It is necessary, however, to leave the ventricular septal defect open or, in the case of simple transposition, to create a communication between the ventricles, as a 'safety valve' for the hypertensive lungs.

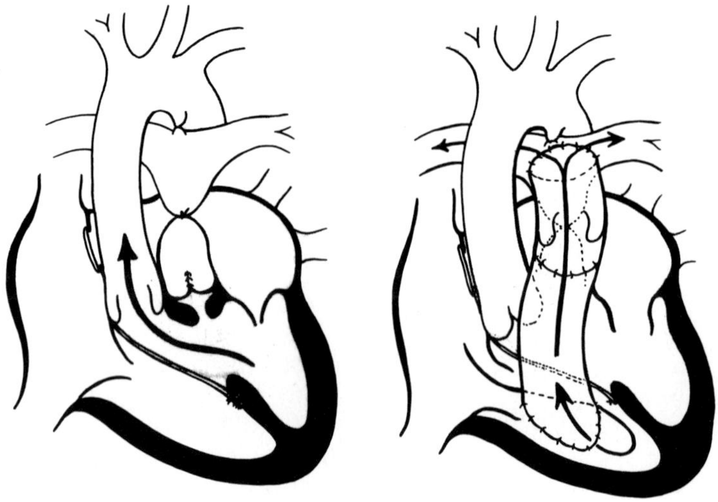

Fig. 6.25. Rastelli operation for transposition of the great vessels with ventricular septal defect and pulmonary stenosis.

Results. There remains considerable variability in the results of the various procedures for both simple and complex transposition of the great vessels: this is probably due, in part, to recent changes in surgical management. Early survival after the Mustard or Senning operation is more than 95% in most units, while similar results also have been achieved with the neonatal switch operation. Following atrial redirection, there is also a small but significant late mortality of about 1% per year due to baffle obstruction, caval obstruction, tricuspid valve regurgitation or right ventricular failure, some cases needing reoperation. While the anatomical correction may achieve better long-term ventricular function, late results are still awaited. In complex cases, the Rastelli operation now carries a risk of about 10%, as does the switch operation with septal defect closure. In most cases, conduit replacement is eventually necessary after a Rastelli procedure, while some patients managed by arterial switch procedure may require further operation to relieve supravalvar or subvalvar pulmonary obstruction. The late survival and exercise tolerance in both groups of patients appears to be good.

Tricuspid Atresia (Absent right atrioventricular connection; right atrioventricular valve atresia; univentricular atrioventricular connection)

The absence of a communication between the right atrium and the ventricular chamber produces one type of 'univentricular atrioventricular' connection. In such hearts, the only outlet from the right atrium is an atrial septal defect. The left atrium is normally connected to a morphological left ventricle. Tricuspid atresia is a rare malformation comprising between 1% and 3% of congential heart defects.

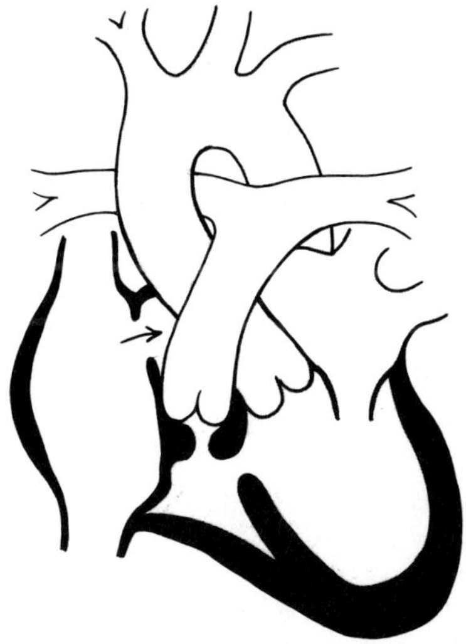

Fig. 6.26. Tricuspid atresia.

Anatomy. The tricuspid valve is usually completely absent, a muscular floor having taken its place in the right atrium. Less commonly, a membrane of fibrous tissue completely occludes the valve orifice and, in some of these cases, it may be possible to identify remnants of valve structure. The left atrium, left ventricle and mitral valve generally are normal, although enlarged as the result of increased blood flow through them. There is nearly always a ventricular septal defect leading to a small right ventricle. An atrial septal defect is obligatory for return of systemic venous blood to the circulation.

Based on the origin of the great arteries, tricuspid atresia may be divided into two types. About two-thirds of the cases have concordant ventriculoarterial connections, i.e. the aorta arises from the left ventricle and pulmonary artery from the right. In these patients there tends to be some limitation of pulmonary blood flow sooner or later, as the result of infundibular or valvar pulmonary stenosis or a restrictive ventricular septal defect. Accordingly, the pulmonary arteries may be smaller than normal. In the remaining one-third of cases, a somewhat better developed right ventricle gives off the aorta and the pulmonary artery arises from the left ventricle (ventriculoarterial discordance). These cases tend to have increased pulmonary blood flow as well as large pulmonary vessels. Associated coarctation of the aorta and subaortic obstruction are not uncommon.

Haemodynamics. Since all of the systemic and pulmonary venous return must pass through the left atrium, tricuspid atresia is, in the first instance, a common-mixing type of cyanotic heart lesion. Most cases also have a reduced pulmonary blood flow contributing further to arterial desaturation. Pressure in the right atrium exceeds that in the left, which maintains the patency of the foramen ovale and allows right-to-left shunting at atrial level. When the ventricular septal defect is large, right and left ventricular pressures will be equal, and flow into the systemic and pulmonary circulations will be governed by their relative resistances. These may include anatomical obstructions such as pulmonary stenosis or aortic coarctation.

There is, thus, a broad spectrum of haemodynamic abnormalities found in patients with tricuspid atresia. In those without pulmonary stenosis at birth, the normally elevated vascular resistance in the lungs maintains a more or less balanced circulation for several weeks. When the resistance declines, there follows a marked increase in pulmonary flow, an increase in systemic oxygen saturation and volume overloading of the left ventricle. The subsequent spontaneous development of infundibular pulmonary stenosis or restriction in the size of the ventricular septal defect again limits pulmonary blood flow, with a corresponding reduction in oxygen saturation. In patients who have pulmonary stenosis from birth, the same events cause additional restriction of pulmonary perfusion and profound hypoxia.

Clinical features. From the above, it will be apparent that the clinical presentation depends largely upon the patient's pulmonary blood flow and this may change considerably during the circulatory evolution. Concordant connection of the great vessels generally is accompanied by cyanosis from birth; it is not unusual for this to become more severe, sometimes with spells, between 12 and 18 months of age. In patients with unrestricted pulmonary blood flow, cyanosis is minimal and the clinical picture is dominated by signs of a hyperdynamic circulation with pulmonary congestion. A systolic murmur is nearly always present, and patients with excessive pulmonary flow may also have a mitral diastolic flow murmur. A loud second sound suggests elevation of pulmonary arterial resistance, while a pansystolic murmur at the apex indicates mitral regurgitation. These findings are of particular importance if a Fontan type of procedure is contemplated. When coarctation of the aorta, patent ductus arteriosus or subaortic stenosis are associated with tricuspid atresia, the clinical presentation tends to be modified.

Special Investigations. The chest X-ray is non-specific and may show either an enlarged heart with pulmonary plethora or a small cardiac shadow with oligaemic lung fields.

The ECG in patients with tricuspid atresia usually has tall, peaked P waves consistent with right atrial hypertrophy. Concordant connection of the great vessels tends to produce left axis deviation and left ventricular dominance, while a normal or right axis may be found in patients with transposed great arteries.

Two-dimensional echocardiography demonstrates an absence of the right atrioventricular connection, with the atrial septum bowing right to left. The size of the ventricular chambers and the origin and size of the great vessels may be shown also, while Doppler studies will detect the presence of any mitral regurgitation or flow through the ductus. At cardiac catheterisation, the right ventricle is entered only through the ventricular septal defect. Ideally, pressures and saturations in each cardiac chamber and great vessel are measured in order to make accurate calculations of shunts and resistances, but many times it is not possible to enter the pulmonary artery either from the right ventricle or through a systemic pulmonary anastomosis. Angiography demonstrates the size and morphology of the ventricular chambers and pulmonary arteries, the left ventricular ejection fraction and the relationships of the great vessels.

Differential Diagnosis. Patients with tricuspid atresia and pulmonary atresia may be difficult to distinguish from those with pulmonary atresia, intact ventricular septum and a small tricuspid valve. A catheter can usually be passed across the tricuspid valve in these cases, and right ventricular angiography will confirm the presence of an intact ventricular septum with regurgitation through the valve.

Cases of double inlet left ventricle with pulmonary stenosis also mimic tricuspid atresia, but here the presence of a second atrioventricular valve can be demonstrated echocardiographically. Severe cases of Ebstein's malformation can also be identified on echocardiography. However, complete fusion of the valve leaflets very occasionally produces an imperforate Ebstein valve with complete obstruction of the right atrioventricular junction, a condition which is properly classified within the group of absent right connection.

Indications for Operation. When pulmonary stenosis is present, cyanosis tends to progress steadily and augmentation of pulmonary blood flow becomes necessary, usually during the first 2 years of life. Conversely, those patients with increased pulmonary blood flow suffer congestive heart failure and develop pulmonary vascular disease. Surgery is needed early in life to reduce pulmonary flow, usually by banding the pulmonary artery. Occasionally the atrial defect is restrictive, which causes a picture of low cardiac output. Enlargement may be possible by balloon septostomy (see Transposition of the Great Arteries) in infants, but surgical enlargement is likely to be necessary at an older age. Given suitable haemodynamics and good anatomy, a corrective Fontan-type of operation should be carried out electively after about 2 years of age.

Principles of Treatment. The ultimate objective for patients with tricuspid atresia is separation of the systemic and pulmonary circulations, so that the systemic blood is fully oxygenated and the left ventricle is relieved of its volume overload. Because there is effectively only one ventricular pump, this must be used to support the systemic circulation. Blood is conveyed to the lungs directly from the vena cava or right atrium, or through the small, subpulmonary outlet chamber (the original Fontan operation). In the absence of a ventricular pumping chamber on the right side of the heart, the flow of blood into the lungs and hence to the left side of the heart will depend upon the resistance in the pulmonary vessels, competence of the mitral valve and left ventricular function. These requirements should also be kept in mind when carrying out a palliative procedure in order to maximise the chances of a successful Fontan operation in the future.

Results. The risk of pulmonary artery banding for tricuspid atresia ranges from 5% to 30% and probably reflects the preoperative condition of some cases as well as the frequent occurrence of coarctation and subaortic stenosis. Shunt operations presently carry a risk of 0–10%, again reflecting a mortality of surgery in the very sick neonate. With optimal anatomy and haemodynamics, the Fontan operation is generally accomplished with less than 10% mortality. Although late follow-up is still being assessed, few late deaths occur among survivors of a Fontan procedure after an initial 6 month period, and they may maintain their level of exercise tolerance indefinitely. However, there does appear to also be a late phase for both death and reoperation in some patients, beginning about 6 years after the Fontan procedure.

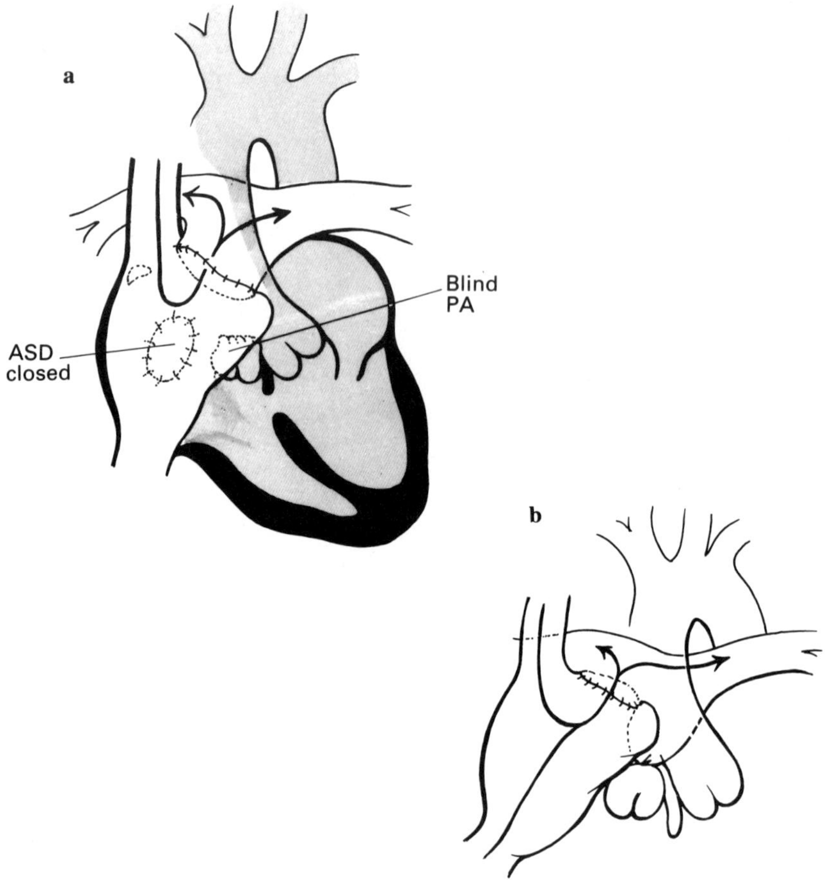

Fig. 6.27. Two types of Fontan operation. The right atrial appendage can be connected to the divided pulmonary artery (anterior 'atriopulmonary' connection, **a**) or a direct 'posterior atriopulmonary' anastomosis may be made between the back of the atria and the undivided right pulmonary artery, **b**).

Total Anomalous Pulmonary Venous Connection

This is a condition in which none of the pulmonary veins are connected directly to the left atrium. Instead, they drain to the right atrium or to a common chamber or trunk which then drains to the right atrium. There is an obligatory atrial septal defect to allow oxygenated blood to return to the left atrium. Total anomalous pulmonary venous drainage may occur in association with a ventricular septal defect or other more complex malformations.

Anatomy and Embryology. During development the pulmonary veins in the lung fail to make contact with the embryonic left atrium, retaining instead their connection to precursors of the systemic veins. Depending upon which connection persists, the anomaly is classified. as *supracardiac*, *infracardiac*, or *intracardiac*. Most commonly the persistent channel is a left superior vena cava which, in turn, drains into the left innominate vein and right superior vena cava. Alternatively, the veins may drain to the coronary sinus, a descending vein that passes to the liver and thence drains to the inferior vena cava, the right superior vena cava, the azygos vein or the right atrium itself. Some of the veins may drain to one site and some to another, a 'mixed' connection.

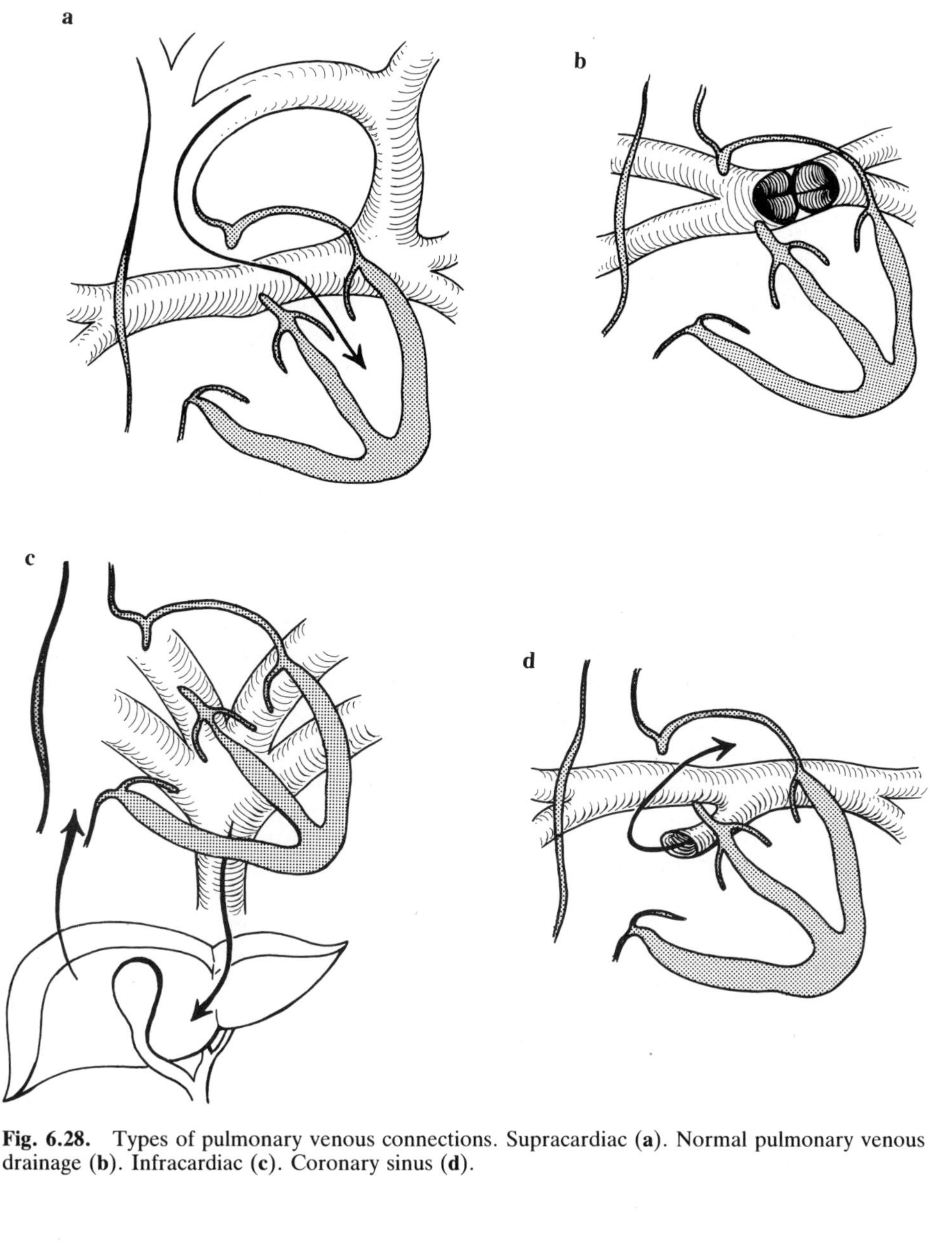

Fig. 6.28. Types of pulmonary venous connections. Supracardiac (**a**). Normal pulmonary venous drainage (**b**). Infracardiac (**c**). Coronary sinus (**d**).

Usually, there is a common posterior chamber (the so-called pulmonary venous confluence) which receives most of the pulmonary veins behind the pericardium. The left atrium is small, and the right sided chambers are enlarged. An atrial septal defect is virtually always present and the ductus arteriosus is nearly always patent.

Haemodynamics. All oxygenated blood from the lungs returns to the right atrium. Its transfer to the left side of the heart is effected through an atrial septal defect or patent foramen ovale. With complete mixing in the right atrium, some desaturated blood must necessarily be carried across from the right atrium, which accounts for the slight degree of cyanosis in these cases.

Depending upon the route of drainage, the connecting channel may be obstructed. This causes back pressure in the lungs and elevation of pulmonary arterial pressure.

Clinical Features. Infants born with this anomaly are likely to die within the first few months of life. This is usually due to pulmonary venous obstruction and low cardiac output. Tachypnoea is the cardinal feature, later accompanied by failure to thrive. Cyanosis and clubbing are not marked until later in childhood, should a large atrial defect and unobstructed venous drainage permit survival long enough for pulmonary vascular disease to become established. Physical signs in infancy are unimpressive, and the diagnosis is easily overlooked or confused with lung disease. In childhood, findings resemble those of an uncomplicated atrial septal defect with a hyperdynamic right ventricle, pulmonary ejection systolic murmur and widely split second sound.

Special Investigations. The chest X-ray may be diagnostic, particularly in cases of total anomalous pulmonary venous drainage to a left superior vena cava. Here, the heart shadow is variously described as the 'cottage-loaf', 'figure-of-eight' or 'snowman'. This shape is due to the distended left ascending vein and superior vena cava, which form a loop around the base of the heart. Pulmonary venous congestion produces a ground-glass haziness to the lung fields, while plethora causes prominent lung markings. (To some people, this combination is suggestive of a snowman standing in the midst of a snow storm.) The heart itself is usually small or only minimally enlarged.

The ECG has the features of right ventricular dominance, as in atrial septal defect.

Echocardiography shows signs of right ventricular volume overload. Failure to visualise the entrance of pulmonary veins into the left atrium is suggestive of total anomalous pulmonary venous connection, but the diagnosis should be accepted with reservation unless the pulmonary venous confluence, each pulmonary vein and the connecting channel are all clearly demonstrated. In drainage to the coronary sinus, the orifice of this structure will be considerably enlarged.

Cardiac catheterisation and pulmonary angiography are diagnostic. The catheter will not enter the pulmonary veins from the left atrium but may be passed into them around the left superior vena cava or through the coronary sinus. At the point of the pulmonary venous connection, a high (>95%) oxygen saturation will be encountered, while lower (around 80%–85%) saturations are found in the aorta and pulmonary artery. The venous phase of a high-quality pulmonary angiogram shows the anatomy of the venous drainage as well as any site of obstruction.

Differential Diagnosis. The most difficult differentiation in the neonate is between total anomalous pulmonary venous connection and pulmonary causes of tachypnoea (pulmonary infection, meconium aspiration). While the hyperoxia test may be helpful, echocardiography and/or cardiac catheterisation usually are necessary to establish the diagnosis. Other causes of pulmonary venous 'obstruction' (mitral stenosis, cor triatriatum) also must be excluded. Cyanosis, plethoric lung fields and cardiac enlargement in older children suggest Eisenmenger's syndrome or, possibly, transposition of the great arteries. This will usually be clarified by echocardiography or cardiac catheterisation.

Indications for Operation. The diagnosis of total anomalous pulmonary venous connection is sufficient reason to undertake operation. Infants with obstructed drainage (which is the rule in infracardiac cases) rapidly succumb to low cardiac output, and older children with a large shunt of blood from the lungs to the right atrium eventually develop pulmonary vascular disease. Approximately 90% of unoperated patients die during the first year of life.

Principles of Treatment. There is no effective medical or surgical palliation for this condition and, therefore, complete correction is done regardless of the patient's age or size. A wide anastamosis is made between the pulmonary venous confluence and the left atrium, and the connecting vein and atrial septal defect are closed. It is usually necessary to use deep hypothermia and total arrest of the circulation to carry out the procedure, particularly in small infants.

Results. Despite advances in infant cardiac surgery, there remains a hospital mortality of 15%–20% for correction of total anomalous pulmonary connection, due in part to the poor preoperative condition of many patients. The operative mortality is lower for cardiac (coronary sinus, right atrium) types and higher for infracardiac and mixed lesions. Late recurrence of venous obstruction is rare but nearly always fatal. Occasional reoperation is necessary for residual septal defects or patent communicating channels, but most survivors have normal subsequent cardiac growth and development.

Ebstein's Malformation

This is a rare condition in which the tricuspid valve is malformed and displaced downwards into the right ventricle. The right ventricle is abnormally developed, particularly the inflow part, which may be of thin muscle or transparent fibrous tissue with small islands of heart muscle surrounding the coronary vessels. Frequently a patent foramen ovale or secundum atrial septal defect is present with resulting cyanosis.

Anatomy. The tricuspid valve shows a spectrum of malformations, often with thickening and distortion of its leaflets. The septal leaflet and, usually, the posterior leaflet are displaced into the ventricle, dividing it into a proximal, atrialised portion and a distal, ventricular portion. Occasionally, fusion of the leaflet results in an imperforate valve. The right atrium is enormously enlarged. There may be associated right ventricular outflow obstruction or ventricular septal defect.

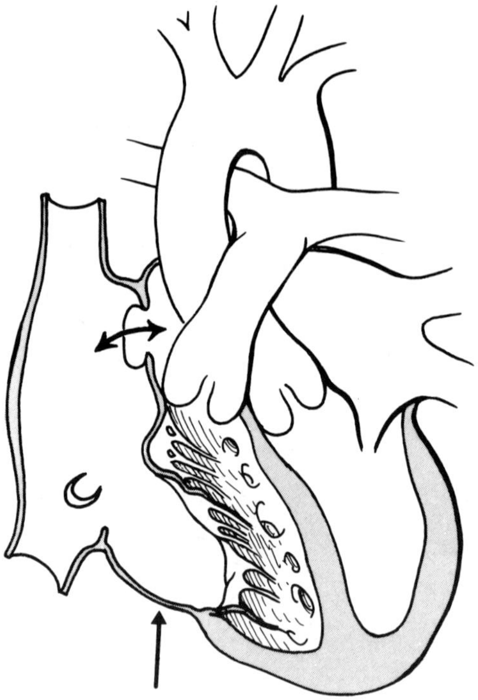

Fig. 6.29. Ebstein's malformation of the tricuspid valve. *Double-headed arrow* indicates atrial septal defect; *single-headed arrow*, the atrialised right ventricle.

Haemodynamics. The malformed valve is incompetent and may also have an element of stenosis. Combined with right ventricular muscle dysfunction, this causes elevation of right atrial pressure. The aneurysmal right atrium may pulsate paradoxically. In the presence of an atrial septal defect, there is generally a right-to-left shunt, which may be considerable and cause severe cyanosis.

Clinical Features. Infants usually present with cyanosis, arrythmias or heart failure. Older patients complain of dyspnoea and fatigue, and are liable to attacks of paroxysmal tachycardia. There may be cyanosis, clubbing and polycythaemia, although a few patients remain asymptomatic; rarely, there is a left-to-right shunt with symptoms of congestive heart failure. The cardiac output is low as a result of impaired right ventricular function. The arterial pulse is small and peripheral cyanosis may be present. The venous pressure may be normal or elevated, and, occasionally, large jugular waves of tricuspid regurgitation are seen. A striking freature is the quiet feel of the precordium, presumably due to cushioning by the large right atrium. On auscultation, there may be a pansystolic murmur of tricuspid regurgitation and a curious diastolic scratching noise caused by flow of blood across the deformed leaflets; this impression of a diastolic scratch strongly favours the diagnosis. The first heart sound is widely split.

Special Investigations. The ECG shows a bizarre right bundle branch pattern with small R waves in the right chest leads, P pulmonale and sometimes a prolonged P-R interval.

The chest X-ray is very characteristic with a large, clearly defined cardiac silhouette, dilated right atrium, small pulmonary artery and aorta, and oligaemic lung fields.

The definitive investigation is real-time echocardiography which will show the morphology of the valve, the size and contractility of the functional right ventricle and presence of septal defects. Doppler studies can also estimate the degree of tricuspid stenosis or regurgitation and, indirectly, right ventricular pressure. Cardiac catheterisation adds little to the diagnosis and carries a small but definite risk of inducing a fatal arrythmia; it may be useful if quantification of shunts and right ventricular pressure are desirable.

Differential Diagnosis. The cyanosed Ebstein's malformation is distinguished from pulmonary stenosis with a reversed interatrial shunt by the absence of giant *a* waves in the venous pulse, a heaving right ventricle, a pulmonary systolic thrill and a long murmur in the latter condition. The chest X-ray and ECG should distinguish between Ebstein's malformation and tricuspid atresia. Acyanotic patients may be confused with pericardial effusion, particularly on the chest radiograph. However, the bizarre ECG and normal venous pressure, along with realtime echocardiography, should differentiate cases of Ebstein's disease.

Indications for Operation. Congestive heart failure carries a grave prognosis, as most patients die within 2 years of its onset, and thus constitutes an indication for operation. Severe or increasing cyanosis with tricuspid regurgitation and increasing heart size also indicate the need for surgery. Some patients will require operation with electrosurgery for life-threatening arrythmias, particularly in association with the Wolff–Parkinson–White syndrome.

Principles of Treatment. In the rare patient with a left-to-right shunt, closure of the atrial septal defect will by itself relieve the volume of overload of the right heart. More commonly, surgery is aimed at restoring competence to the tricuspid valve by reconstruction or replacement, and the atrial defect is repaired at the same time. If operation is required to divide accessory conduction pathways, the valve and septal defect are also repaired. The value of ventricular plication to reduce the atrialised portion is uncertain.

In neonates, the natural fall of pulmonary vascular resistance will lead to an improvement in cyanosis and tricuspid regurgitation as right ventricular pressure declines. Oxygenation can usually be improved by ventilation and maintenance of ductal patency with prostaglandin. Surgery, which carries a prohibitive mortality at this age, should be avoided.

Results. The mortality for repair or replacement of the tricuspid valve and closure of the atrial septal defect in relatively well patients (New York Heart

Association Class II or III) is about 5% but increases dramatically to 20% for those with Class IV symptoms. This probably reflects right ventricular dysfunction, which may also be a contributory factor in the 10%–15% late mortality for this condition.

Uhl's Anomaly

This extremely rare condition is mentioned to differentiate it from Ebstein's malformation. Whereas both may present with cyanosis and an enlarged right heart, the tricuspid valve has a normal attachment in Uhl's anomaly. The right ventricular myocardium, however, is completely absent, producing a paper-thin or 'parchment' right ventricle. The left ventricular myocardium is normal.

Eisenmenger's Syndrome

Unlike the foregoing, this term relates to a number of separate conditions which have in common cyanosis due to increased pulmonary resistance (pulmonary hypertension and pulmonary vascular disease). Any left-to-right shunt may be reversed as the result of a high pulmonary resistance. Eisenmenger's original

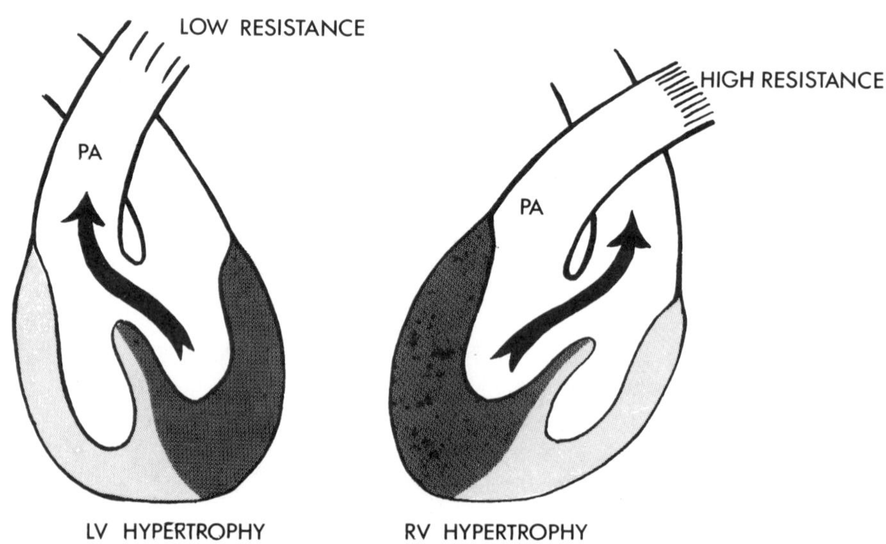

Fig. 6.30. Effect of pulmonary vascular resistance on the left-to-right shunt in ventricular septal defect.

description was based upon a ventricular septal defect, but it is convenient to include the reversal of any of the left-to-right shunting conditions, because the underlying mechanism (i.e. increased pulmonary resistance) is the same in all. The syndrome can, therefore, arise in the context of:

Ventricular septal defect
Persistent ductus arteriosus
Aortopulmonary window
Atrial septal defect
Atrioventricular septal defect
Any other lesion that normally permits left-to-right shunting

Anatomy. The cardiac anomaly is identical with those causing left-to-right shunts in the presence of a normal or moderately raised pulmonary vascular resistance. The important anatomical changes are in the lung vessels.

Macroscopically, these are grossly distended proximally as the result of high pressure and there may be atheromatous changes in their walls. The calibre of the vessels narrows rapidly distally, and casts or injection specimens of these lungs show a 'pruning' of the normal, finer, peripheral subdivisions, the picture being somewhat like the branches of a tree in winter.

Microscopically, the smaller vessels and arterioles show a narrowing of their lumen with thick walls, medial hypertrophy and intimal proliferation. These are the changes found in severe pulmonary hypertension. Initially, they may be reversible; but, later, both the morphological and haemodynamic changes become fixed.

Haemodynamics. In a ventricular septal defect, the direction and volume of the shunt across the defect is dependent upon the resistance of the systemic and pulmonary vascular beds. Where the pulmonary resistance is greater than the systemic resistance, desaturated right ventricular blood will shunt across the defect into the aorta.

In cases of atrial septal defect, it is unusual to encounter a high pulmonary resistance early in life, but after 35 years of age thrombosis tends to occur in the enormously distended lung vessels. This also increases the pulmonary vascular resistance, and the shunt through the atrial septal defect may eventually reverse.

The high pulmonary resistance in younger age groups, notably in cases of ventricular septal defect, may represent a retention of the fetal pulmonary vascular pattern. It seems likely that the high vascular resistance is fixed from birth in some patients, as they never develop signs or symptoms of a left-to-right shunt and are found to have severe vascular damage by one year of age. Fortunately, this situation is rare.

In some cases of ductus arteriosus, probably the critical size being a diameter of more than one centimetre, there is also a high pulmonary vascular resistance which may eventually result in reversal of flow.

Clinical Features. Patients with Eisenmenger's syndrome will have all the features of pulmonary hypertension. Dyspnoea on effort is usually marked and there may be a history of haemoptysis, syncope and angina. Central cyanosis is present together with clubbing of the fingers. Initially, cyanosis may occur on effort only. Differential cyanosis and clubbing of the toes only may suggest a diagnosis of shunt reversal through a ductus arteriosus. Dyspnoea is said to be less severe in these patients since the unsaturated blood enters the aorta beyond the cerebral vessels.

An *a* wave may be prominent on examination of the jugular venous pulse. Other features of pulmonary hypertension are a heaving right ventricular impulse and, often, a palpable pulmonary valve closure. Thrills may not be striking. Similarly, murmurs will be variable or insignificant, depending upon the degree of shunting. For example, the continuous murmur of a persistent ductus arteriosus will be lost and may be simply represented by a short systolic murmur. An ejection sound is common, and the closure of the pulmonary valve imparts a loud, ringing quality to the second sound. This sound is not infrequently followed immediately by the long diastolic murmur of pulmonary regurgitation.

Special Investigations. The chest radiograph is useful, particularly in relation to the lung fields. The characteristic picture is one of great enlargement of the main pulmonary arteries (like drooping moustaches) and there is a variable degree of plethora in the intermediate zone of the lung fields. Distally, the pulmonary vasculature diminishes abruptly such that the peripheral third of the lung fields are 'clear'.

The cardiac contour may be non-specific but should show the features of right ventricular hypertrophy and prominence of the main pulmonary artery.

The ECG confirms the right ventricular hypertrophy, often with the addition of a strain pattern over the right ventricular leads and prominent right atrial P waves.

Cardiac catheterisation is of importance in differentiating this group of conditions from other causes of cyanotic heart disease or pulmonary hypertension. It is necessary to decide whether the pulmonary resistance is fixed or could be manipulated by drugs or oxygen. However, it is of less value in distinguishing the various members of the group. Pulmonary regurgitation is often present so that shunts above the aortic and pulmonary valves may seem to be at ventricular level. The passage of the catheter across a communication may be helpful in demonstrating the underlying anatomy of the condition, but, more often, this has already been seen on echocardiography. If the vascular resistance is high and cannot be lowered by administration of 100% oxygen, there is a very real danger of cardiac arrest after angiography. Accordingly, contrast injection must be omitted in some cases, relying upon real-time echocardiography for details of morphology.

Differential Diagnosis. All the other causes of cyanotic heart disease must be excluded. In this regard, it is important to recall that rare, associated conditions will sometimes produce cyanosis in an otherwise uncomplicated septal defect. These include such things as: a Venturi effect causing right ventricular blood to pass to the aorta through a ventricular septal defect; drainage of a left superior vena cava to the left atrium; pulmonary arterovenous fistula and pulmonary collapse. The other signs of pulmonary hypertension, however, will not be present in these conditions.

It is also important to exclude obstructive left heart lesions, which may produce severe pulmonary hypertension but rarely have an intracardiac shunt. These include mitral stenosis and cor triatriatum, which should be apparent on echocardiography.

Indications for Surgery. Conservative procedures – closure of the ductus or septal defect – should be undertaken only if the pulmonary hypertension is reversible. This usually can be demonstrated at cardiac catheterisation, but if there is any doubt a lung biopsy should be performed. In the absence of transposed great vessels, irreversible pulmonary vascular disease is unlikely in the first year of life and the presence of pulmonary hypertension makes closure of the defect a surgical urgency.

In some cases, the pulmonary resistance is high but lung biopsy shows potentially reversible changes. Such patients can undergo operation with only a slightly increased risk and probably benefit from arrest of the pulmonary vascular disease as well as protection from paradoxical embolus. Long-term follow up of this group, however, is sparse.

When there is severe, established pulmonary vascular disease, with no left-to-right shunt during administration of pulmonary vasodilators, the defect acts to decompress the pulmonary circulation and convey blood, albeit desaturated, to the systemic circulation. Closure is then highly dangerous, and such patients are candidates for heart–lung or possibly lung transplantation.

Principles of Treatment. Treatment should aim, in the first instance, at preventing the development of Eisenmenger's syndrome, by the early diagnosis and repair of cardiac defects with large left-to-right shunts or pulmonary hypertension.

In patients with potentially reversible pulmonary vascular changes, an effort should be made to reduce the pulmonary resistance at the time of operation in order that the defect can be closed with safety. Preoperatively, bed rest and sedation may be helpful, while anticoagulation may prevent or limit thrombosis within the pulmonary vascular bed. In the early postoperative period, factors which raise pulmonary vascular resistance – hypoxia, catecholamines, acidosis, protamine sulphate, blood transfusion – should be avoided. Epoprostenol, a potent vasodilator, may be beneficial in preventing or reversing pulmonary arterial spasm. Planning the surgical procedure in such a way as to minimise cardiopulmonary bypass time and aortic cross-clamping time, as well as to avoid a right ventriculotomy, may also help to conserve right ventricular and pulmonary function.

Heart–lung or lung transplantation is generally reserved for cases where no conservative operation is possible and life expectancy is less than 1 year. There is some evidence that the symptoms of pulmonary hypertension may be reduced by long-term infusion of epoprostenol.

Acyanotic Congenital Heart Lesions: Obstructive Group

The general effects of cardiac obstruction have already been mentioned. When the right or left ventricle is obstructed, it is important for the clinician to be able to assess which chamber carries the obstructive burden and its severity.

Among the obstructive lesions we include aortic, pulmonary and mitral valve stenosis, as well as subvalvar or supravalvar obstructions. In addition, obstructive lesions may co-exist with a left-to-right shunt. The combination of a ventricular septal defect with some degree of pulmonary stenosis is not uncommon, such that even the classification of the obstructive and shunting conditions merge. Greater degrees of pulmonary stenosis in association with a ventricular septal defect bring one, in turn, to the cyanotic group of lesions.

Although it is important to recognise and remember this merging of patterns so as to maintain a flexible attitude in diagnosis, it is of more practical value to the surgeon to have a number of clear-cut clinical pictures in mind.

Pulmonary Stenosis

In this condition, there is incomplete obstruction to the flow of blood from the right ventricle in association with a normal (or essentially intact) ventricular septum. The term 'pulmonary stenosis with normal aortic root' has been used to differentiate this malformation from the pulmonary stenosis with ventricular septal defect or Fallot's tetralogy, but it is more important to emphasise the absence of a ventricular septal defect. Valvar pulmonary stenosis accounts for about 10% of congenital heart defects.

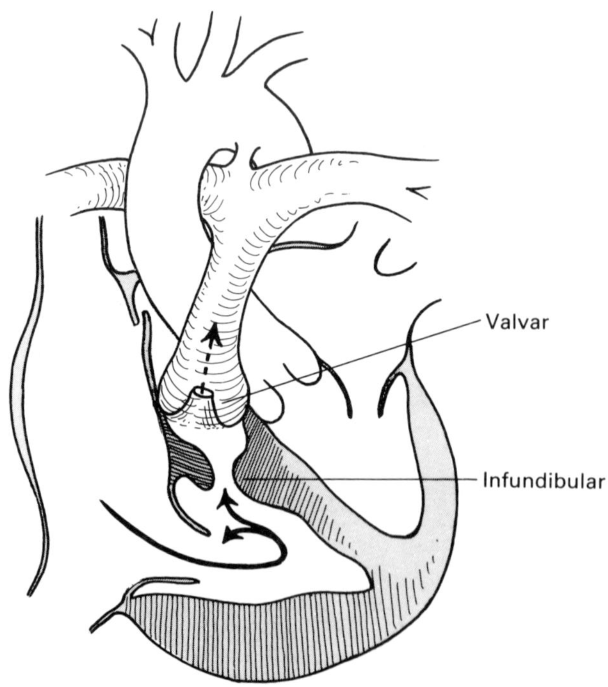

Fig. 6.31. Pulmonary stenosis may occur at valvar or infundibular level, or within the right ventricular cavity.

Anatomy. In the majority of cases, the obstruction is at valve level. Usually three commissures are fused to form a shallow dome with a small central orifice about 2.5–5.0 mm in diameter. In other cases, usually associated with Noonan's syndrome, the valve is dysplastic with greatly thickened leaflets and a small annulus. Intermediate degrees of development are seen in some cases, with two cusps or an elongated eccentric cone, sometimes adherent to the side of the pulmonary trunk. Beyond the valve obstruction, there is local post-stenotic dilatation of the pulmonary artery. A patent foramen ovale or atrial septal defect is often associated.

Less commonly, the obstruction is entirely below the valve and consists of a fibromuscular infundibular stenosis. In a few cases, abnormal muscle bundles proximally divide the right ventricle into two approximately equal-sized portions, the 'double-chambered right ventricle'. Obstruction may occur also more distally in the pulmonary arteries themselves; this is seen in the rubella syndrome.

Haemodynamics. The right ventricle is burdened by its obstructed outlet, and ventricular pressure increases to a level which will overcome the obstruction and maintain the cardiac output. This results in a pressure gradient across the valve. It is not uncommon for the right ventricular pressure to exceed 100 mmHg, while the pulmonary artery pressure is likely to be normal or below normal, in the region of 10–15 mmHg. As a response to this increased work, the right ventricle develops concentric muscular hypertrophy. This may become severe and interfere with relaxation in diastole, therefore impeding ventricular filling and causing elevation of right atrial pressure. This may, in turn, lead to a right-to-left shunt across the patent foramen ovale. When right ventricular hypertrophy is marked, secondary infundibular muscular hypertrophy may also develop and lead to functional infundibular stenosis. It is thus a common experience to find that, following adequate relief of severe valve obstruction, a significant muscular obstruction remains in the right ventricular outflow.

Clinical Features. In ordinary circumstances symptoms are not prominent and infants or young children present with a systolic murmur only. However, when symptoms arise in infancy, the obstruction is usually severe. In advanced cases, there may be syncope or ischaemic pain on exertion – a form of right ventricular angina.

On examination, patients with pulmonary valve stenosis tend to be well nourished and appear healthy. Some are said to have round, moon-like faces with ruddy cheeks, but the lips are pink and there is no cyanosis or clubbing unless there is a reversal of the atrial shunt. The arterial pulse is not remarkable, but the venous pulse may show a giant *a* wave, due to the vigour of the right atrial contractions. Pressure over the liver accentuates this venous pulsation. In addition, there may be a precordial bulge and a sustained heave over the obstructed right ventricle. At the same time, a long systolic thrill is felt over the pulmonary valve area. This combination of a giant *a* wave, thrill and a right ventricular heave is almost diagnostic of valvar pulmonary stenosis.

In the absence of tricuspid regurgitation or a ventricular septal defect, the right ventricle has to propel its entire contents through the stenotic orifice. Consequently, the systolic murmur is of long duration and continues well beyond the aortic component of the second heart sound. This is due to the fact that right ventricular ejection continues after the unobstructed left ventricle has completed its ejection. The late closure of the stenosed pulmonary valve is not generally audible. This combination of an aortic sound lost in the murmur, with a very soft or inaudible pulmonary element, gives the impression of 'absent' second sound at the base, a useful point of differentiation from Fallot's tetralogy in which there is usually a short, harsh murmur and a loud aortic second sound.

Special Investigations. The lung fields will be normal or oligaemic, and there is post-stenotic dilatation of the pulmonary artery in cases of valve stenosis. The heart size is normal, but there may be signs of right atrial enlargement or hypertrophy of the right ventricle. When ventricular failure appears, the heart may become enlarged, as seen in severely disabled infants.

The ECG will show the tall, spiked P waves of right atrial hypertrophy in addition to evidence of right ventricular hypertrophy, often with a strain pattern. The degree and progression of the strain pattern has been found useful as a guide in assessing the severity of the obstruction.

Right ventricular hypertrophy can be detected by echocardiography, which will also locate the site of the obstruction. The gradient across the valve can be estimated reliably from Doppler studies.

Cardiac catheterisation is not essential but documents the right ventricular pressure and the gradient across the stenosis. It is possible also to ascertain the level of the obstruction by measuring the pull-back gradient. Where the right ventricular pressure is higher than that in the femoral artery, it suggests a closed ventricular septum and makes the diagnosis almost certain. Angiography will confirm the site of obstruction, but only in peripheral pulmonary arterial stenosis does it add to the echocardiographic diagnosis.

Differential Diagnosis. Pulmonary stenosis may have to be distinguished from an atrial septal defect, although the two lesions can occur together. Both may have an ejection systolic murmur and thrill to the left of the sternum. However, in atrial septal defect, the pulmonary component of the second sound is clearly audible and widely separated from the aortic component. Also, there is no variation with respiration. The lungs fields are well vascularised in atrial septal defect.

Aortic stenosis may be suggested by the ejection systolic murmur at the base of the heart, but the clinical and electrocardiographic features should point unmistakably to the left ventricle.

In conditions such as acyanotic Fallot's tetralogy or ventricular septal defect with pulmonary stenosis, diagnostic difficulties may arise. In some cases of pulmonary stenosis, it is almost impossible to exclude the presence of a small ventricular septal defect, even at cardiac catheterisation. When right ventricular pressure is higher than systemic, a closed ventricular septum is likely; the presence of a functionally or anatomically small defect does not materially influence management of the patient and is therefore only of academic concern.

A useful clinical point to bear in mind is the finding of a right-sided arch with pulmonary stenosis. This almost always means that there will be a ventricular septal defect present, as a right-sided aortic arch is not usually found in uncomplicated pulmonary stenosis.

Indications for Operation. Like other cardiac obstructions, the decision for treatment depends upon the severity of the stenosis. The presence of symptoms, an increased heart size, or a right ventricular strain pattern on the ECG all signify severe obstruction.

The presence of cyanosis brought about by the reversal of the shunt through an atrial communication means there is considerable buildup of right ventricular pressure and calls for urgent surgical relief.

In Europe, a right ventricular strain pattern on the ECG, particularly if it is increasing, has been considered sufficient indication for surgery. The precise haemodynamic indications for operation are uncertain, but most centres recommend intervention if the right ventricular pressure exceeds 75 mmHg. It is probably a mistake, however, to be too influenced by an arbitrary figure.

Principles of Treatment. The treatment of pulmonary stenosis by Brock and Sellors marked the beginning of direct surgery upon the heart. Closed valvotomy was performed then by passing valvulotomes and dilating instruments through the narrowed valve orifice.

More recently, the options for relief of valvar stenosis have extended to include balloon dilatation, which appears to split the fused commissures. In dysplastic valves or infundibular muscle obstruction, an open operation is still necessary to excise the obstructing tissue. Closure of an associated atrial septal defect also requires open heart surgery, and, for these cases, the valvar stenosis is relieved at the same time. The goal in all cases is to restore a normal right ventricular pressure. For isolated valvar obstruction, particularly in the young infant, operation may be done under inflow occlusion. Cardiopulmonary bypass is usually employed in older patients or when a septal defect requires closure.

Results. Mortality for treatment of pulmonary stenosis, whether by operation or balloon valvuloplasty, approaches zero, although there remains a small risk in the critically ill infant. Late results are generally good, and the need for reoperation extremely rare. Infundibular hypertrophy tends to regress after relief of the valvar obstruction.

Congenital Aortic Stenosis

Obstruction to left ventricular outflow may occur below the aortic valve ('subvalvar'), at the level of the valve ('valvar'), or distal to the valve ('supravalvar'). There may also be a combination of obstruction at all three levels ('multi-level' outflow obstruction) or a generalised underdevelopment of the left ventricular outflow tract. The commonest of these is valvar aortic stenosis, which accounts for about 5% of congenital heart defects.

Anatomy. In aortic valve stenosis, there is a fusion of the valve commissures which may be imperfectly developed. The valve often has two cusps instead of three or incomplete liberation of the commissures. Frequently the cusps are thickened and have pedunculated nodules of fibrous tissue on their ventricular aspect. By adulthood, there may be considerable calcification present, usually starting in the nodular areas and often extending both below the valve and into the aortic wall. In some instances, the calcium is even replaced by a bony matrix.

Localised or 'discrete' subvalvar stenosis may be an acquired lesion due to the build-up of fibrous tissue on a malformed outflow tract. The fibromuscular diaphragm usually encircles the outflow tract and may have finger-like extensions onto the mitral or aortic valve leaflets.

Supravalvar obstruction is rare. The obstruction begins at the top of the sinutubular junction, with a waist-like constriction just above the valve leaflets, at the point where the commissures fuse with the aortic wall. The coronary arteries, arising below the obstruction, may be enormously dilated. The aortic wall is thickened and, in the more diffuse form, may be narrowed as far distally as the left subclavian artery. In some cases the lesion is familial (Williams syndrome), while in others it occurs in association with hypercalcaemia and mental retardation.

Tunnel type obstruction refers to a diffuse underdevelopment of the outflow tract and usually involves multi-level obstruction. The subaortic area is long and narrow, the aortic annulus is small, the valve is thickened and usually has two cusps. The ascending aorta is not enlarged, in contrast with the post-stenotic dilatation of isolated valvar aortic stenosis.

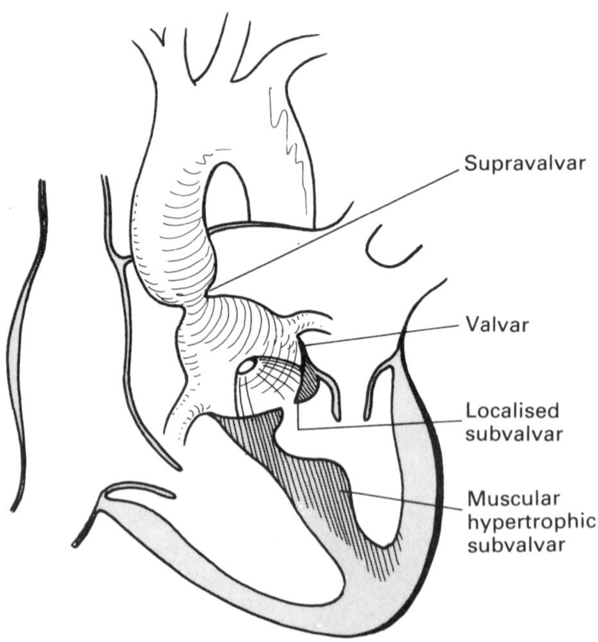

Fig. 6.32. The possible levels of aortic obstruction: hypertrophic muscular, localised subvalvar, valvar and supravalvar.

Secondary muscular hypertrophy may occur with any type of aortic stenosis and is often severe, encroaching upon the ventricular cavity. In aortic valve stenosis, there is characteristically post-stenotic dilatation of the aorta. A degree of valve regurgitation may occur also in valvar and subvalvar lesions.

Haemodynamics. Obstruction of the left ventricle is a more crippling burden on the heart than right ventricular obstruction. The left ventricle undergoes a progressive and massive hypertrophy in order to maintain the cardiac output and systemic arterial pressure. Measurements of the systemic blood pressure in aortic stenosis are not always particularly informative, as the pressure is likely to be maintained at about 100–110 mmHg, although the pulse pressure is narrow. Left ventricular pressure, at rest may be 200 mmHg, however, and rise even further with exercise.

The left ventricle, like the right, has enormous reserves which are quietly exhausted without necessarily producing symptoms. When symptoms do arise, it is no longer an early phase of the disease but rather the dissipation of compensating mechanisms. Deterioration then tends to be rapid, as the result of concentric ventricular hypertrophy which reduces the ventricular cavity and limits filling. At the same time the hypertrophied muscle contributes to further, functional subvalvar obstruction. Concurrently, the massive left ventricle has an increased coronary blood requirement in the face of impaired cardiac output, prolonged systole and impeded diastolic filling. All these factors contribute, ultimately, to impaired coronary blood flow and left ventricular failure.

Clinical Features. Broadly speaking, there are two distinct types of presentation. The infant with critical aortic stenosis may suddenly collapse with metabolic acidosis, severe heart failure and absence of all pulses. This often corresponds to the time of ductus closure but may occur also a few hours after birth. A murmur frequently cannot be heard due to the low cardiac output and later becomes audible after resuscitation.

The more usual presentation is an asymptomatic heart murmur on routine examination. The classical symptoms of breathlessness, syncope and angina are uncommon in childhood but may be found upon exertion or in young adults. Breathlessness comes about as the result of congestion of the lungs and is thought to represent a 'failing' left ventricle. In this respect it is, therefore, an important symptom. Orthopnea and paroxysmal nocturnal dyspnoea are even more unfavourable features.

The stenosed valve may result in a reduced and fixed cardiac output. This may account for syncope on exertion, although mechanisms of reflex vasodilatation may also be contributory.

Angina is a feature of relative coronary insufficiency resulting from the gross hypertrophy of the myocardium. In cases of supravalvar obstruction, tethering of a valve cusp across a commissure may also directly obstruct coronary blood flow. In older patients, predominance of anginal symptoms raises the question of concomitent coronary artery disease. Anginal pains may be difficult to recognise in a young patient, when they sometimes manifest themselves as abdominal pains or a 'stitch', or as pain in the neck and jaw.

The pulse is characteristically slow-rising or anacrotic. The venous pressure is not raised unless there is associated right heart failure, and this is a grave feature. The left ventricular impulse has a sustained thrusting quality, but the heart should not be clinically enlarged unless aortic stenosis is complicated by ventricular dilatation or significant aortic regurgitation.

A systolic thrill is generally palpable over the aortic valve area and is conducted into the neck; it may be felt only on full expiration with the patient sitting up. The systolic murmur is harsh in quality and heard just after the first sound, coincident with opening of the valve. In valvar stenosis, the murmur is preceded by an ejection click, which is a useful point in differentiating other types of left ventricular outflow obstruction. The murmur is followed, as a rule, by a single or 'inaudible' second sound. When the valve is rigid or when it is distorted by a jet through a subaortic diaphragm, there may be a diastolic murmur due to its inability to close.

Special Investigations. The ECG will show a pattern of left ventricular hypertrophy, often with 'strain' over the left ventricular leads.

The chest radiograph shows a small heart unless there is associated aortic regurgitation or left ventricular failure. In addition, there may be evidence of calcification of the valve cusps and post-stenotic dilatation of the ascending aorta, the latter being a feature of valve stenosis and is rarely marked in subvalvar obstruction.

The identification of valve calcification is of the greatest importance in diagnosing aortic valve stenosis. In any case of congenital aortic stenosis over 25 years of age, calcification can generally be demonstrated and, when present, confirms an obstruction at valve level. Conversely, when calcification is absent in this age group, the diagnosis is more likely to be a subaortic obstruction.

Real-time and Doppler echocardiography should demonstrate both the level and severity of left ventricular outflow obstruction, as well as the extent of left ventricular hypertrophy or dilatation. Cardiac catheterisation may be indicated to obtain an accurate gradient in borderline cases, and to perform left ventricular and coronary artery angiography.

Differential Diagnosis. The systolic murmur of mitral prolapse with regurgitation is sometimes confused with that of aortic stenosis, but, in the former, the pulse has a sharper upstroke and the left ventricular thrust is hyperdynamic in quality. The mitral regurgitation murmur is usually best heard out toward the axilla and, unlike the delayed ejection type aortic stenosis murmur, starts with the first heart sound and continues throughout systole.

Pulmonary stenosis is distinguished by the location of the thrill and right ventricular dominance, both clinically and electrocardiographically.

Indications for Operation. As the onset of symptoms in aortic stenosis indicates an advanced lesion, every effort should be made to assess the severity of the obstruction and to relieve it before irreversible myocardial damage has occurred.

Syncope, angina and breathlessness are all features demanding surgical intervention. The presence of left or, more particularly, right ventricular failure increases the risk of operation but is not necessarily a contraindication. In symptomatic infants, operation is a surgical emergency.

When the patient is asymptomatic, the ECG is important. Left ventricular hypertrophy with 'strain' (T wave inversion over the left ventricular leads and ST depression) indicates severe obstruction. In other cases, a measured gradient of more than 60 mmHg is generally accepted as an indication for operation, although in subvalvar obstruction, surgery is often recommended at a gradient of 40–50 mmHg because the jet of blood against the valve may, over a period of time, be more damaging than the myocardial hypertrophy.

Principles of Treatment. The relief of all types of left ventricular outflow obstruction is normally by open operation through the aorta. This requires the use of a heart–lung machine to support the circulation and measures to protect the hypertrophied myocardium.

When there is fusion of relatively pliable cusps, these are opened directly, and any secondary muscular hypertrophy should be excised. In calcific aortic stenosis, the valve structure usually cannot be reconstituted; it must be excised and replaced by a tissue or mechanical valve. Subvalvar obstruction is removed by enucleation of the fibromuscular membrane. In cases of supravalvar stenosis, the obstruction is relieved by placement of a pericardial patch in the ascending aorta, from the aortic sinus to beyond the obstructed segment.

Tunnel type obstruction or the hypoplastic annulus both constitute a more difficult problem. One approach is to incise the subaortic septum and open out this area with a Dacron patch, combined with valve replacement (Konno operation). An alternative is complete excision of the aortic root and obstructing subaortic muscle, followed by implantation of a homograft aortic or pulmonary autograft root and reattachment of the coronary arteries (aortic root replacement).

Results. There is a considerable mortality, 15%–20%, for emergency valvotomy in neonates with critical aortic stenosis, but other procedures for the relief of left ventricular outflow obstruction generally can be accomplished with a mortality of 1%–2%. Valvotomy in childhood must be considered a palliative operation, however, for more than three-quarters of the survivors will eventually require further surgery. Subaortic obstruction occasionally recurs, and operation is sometimes complicated by heart block or injury to the mitral valve. It is uncommon for supra-aortic lesions to require reoperation.

Coarctation of the Aorta

By strict definition, coarctation of the aorta is a narrowing or occlusion of the aorta in proximity to the ligamentum or ductus arteriosus. However severe the narrowing, the vessel remains in continuity, which differentiates this condition from interruption of the aortic arch. By convention, any stricture beyond the ascending aorta is referred to as ‘coarctation’. Thus, narrowings proximal to the left subclavian artery or in the lower thoracic or abdominal aorta may be included, provided a pressure drop occurs across them.

Anatomy. Although earlier classifications distinguished adult and infantile types of coarctation, it is now appreciated that a spectrum of malformations may occur at any age. The classical lesion is a localised, concentric narrowing opposite the ductus arteriosus. Internally, a shelf of abnormal tissue further obstructs or occludes the lumen; the distal aorta may be fed from a patent ductus entering below the coarctation or through collateral vessels. Alternatively, there may be a long segment of hypoplasia beyond the left subclavian artery with or without a coarctation shelf at the level of the ductus, or the coarctation may involve the left subclavian artery. Tubular hypoplasia of the transverse aortic arch or an aberrant right subclavian artery arising below the coarctation may also be found, as well as a variety of associated intracardiac defects.

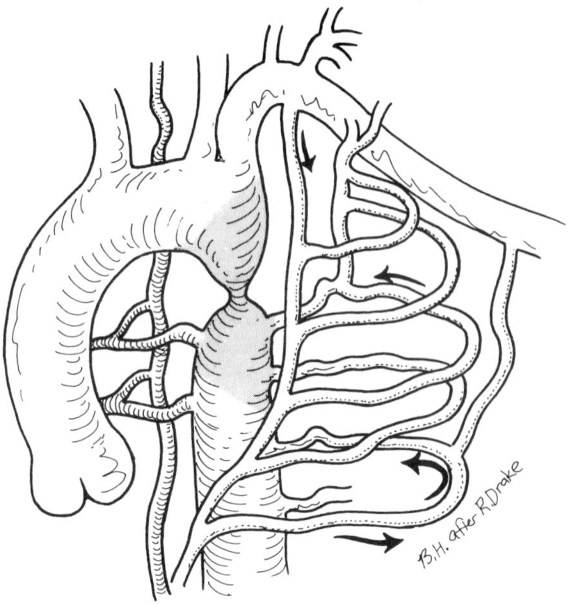

Fig. 6.33. Coarctation of the aorta with collateral vessels feeding the distal circulation (*arrows* show direction of flow into the aorta.

Haemodynamics. The effect of the obstruction is to 'iron out' the systolic fluctuations in blood pressure below the coarctation. This apparently stimulates the kidneys to secrete vasoconstrictor substances which raise the blood pressure. There is thus a high pressure in the vessels of the neck, head and arms with marked systolic fluctuations. In the lower limbs, if collateral development is extensive, there is usually a high diastolic pressure, approaching that in the upper half of the body but without systolic peaks. The high pressure in the proximal aorta is responsible, in some cases, for the rupture of intracranial aneurysms.

In infants, the mechanical effects of the obstruction dominate the picture. A sudden increase in afterload causes ventricular failure, and there is insufficient perfusion of the lower segment, causing loss of blood pressure in the lower limbs. If a persistent ductus enters below the coarctation, unsaturated blood may flow 'right-to-left' into the descending aorta. However, differential cyanosis is rarely apparent clinically, despite a low oxygen saturation in femoral arterial blood samples.

Clinical Features. Coarctication of the aorta may present with sudden collapse and features of ventricular failure as the patent ductus closes in the newborn period. Otherwise, it is unlikely to be diagnosed until the patient is found to have diminished or delayed femoral pulses, or a raised blood pressure, on routine examination. Suggestive symptoms are headache and a tendency to nose bleeds. More dramatic forms of presentation are the result of cerebral haemorrhage, renal failure or bacterial endocarditis. The condition is more common in men than in women.

On examination, older patients are often well-built with strong, bounding pulses in the arms and neck, while the femoral pulses are either absent or markedly diminished in amplitude and delayed in time. Generally, collateral vessels can be seen and felt over the back and round the angles of the scapulae. There may be a thrusting left ventricular type of apex beat, and a systolic murmur can be heard in most instances over the precordium and along the intercostal collateral vessels posteriorly. Flow through the coarctation may also produce a diastolic murmur.

When the features of coarctation are present but the systolic blood pressure in the arms is unduly low, one should suspect associated aortic valve stenosis or the much more rare situation of both subclavian arteries arising distal to the coarctation.

In infants with coarctation, the presentation may be dramatic. Closure of the ductus may cause loss of femoral pulses followed by oliguria, renal failure, metabolic acidosis and left ventricular failure. Conversely, if a ventricular septal defect is associated and the ductus remains open, good femoral pulses may be present even with complete aortic obstruction. This picture is known as preductal coarctation.

Special Investigations. A plain radiograph of the chest confirms the diagnosis by showing the characteristic notching of the lower borders of the ribs that is caused by the enlarged intercostal arteries. This is not seen clearly before 6–8 years of age, but, above this age, the absence of rib notching should cause one to question the diagnosis. In addition, there may be an 'absent' or double aortic knuckle produced by the shadow of the enlarged left subclavian artery and descending aorta beyond the coarctation.

The ECG will show left ventricular hypertrophy in adults, but right ventricular hypertrophy in the newborn.

In infants, the morphology of the aortic arch and coarctation, as well as any associated intracardiac defects, can usually be demonstrated by real-time echocardiography. Cardiac catheterisation is done if there remains a question regarding the arch development or position, or, in older patients, regarding the development of collateral vessels or degree of obstruction.

Differential Diagnosis. Other causes of hypertension must be considered apart from essential hypertension. Steps should be taken to exclude unilateral renal disease (infective or vascular in origin) and also Cushing's syndrome and phaeochromocytoma.

Absent femoral pulses in an adult man may be due to coarctation or terminal aortic occlusion (Leriche's syndrome). In the latter condition, the aortic pulse can be felt clearly in the epigastrium and collateral vessel development will be absent.

Coarctation presenting with bounding neck pulses must be distinguished from persistent ductus arteriosus and aortic regurgitation. In the infant with low cardiac output and generally poor pulses, the possibility of aortic stenosis or interrupted aortic arch must also be considered.

Indications for Operation. The aim is to repair the coarctation before the hypertension is irreversible or complications ensue. This is probably in the first few years of life, and certainly before adolescence. Neonates or infants in cardiac failure demand emergency operation as soon as their condition has been stabilised.

Principles of Treatment. The ideal is to completely relieve the obstruction while, at the same time, conserving growth potential for the future and avoiding complications of aortic clamping during the operation (paraplegia, renal failure, hypertension).

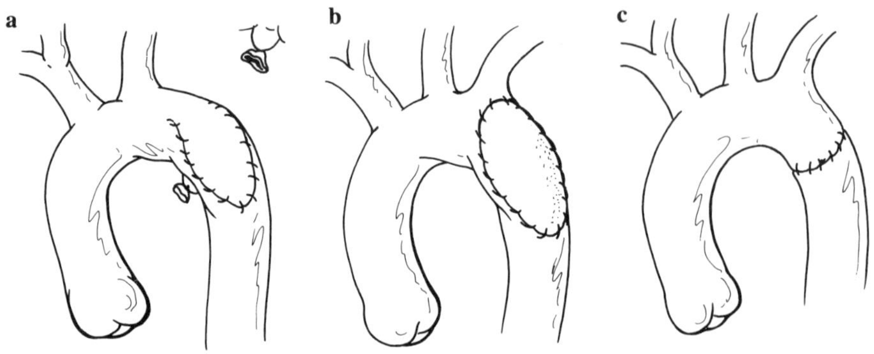

Fig. 6.34. Common operative procedures for coarctation of the aorta: subclavian flap angioplasty (**a**), patch angioplasty (**b**), and resection with end-to-end anastomosis (**c**).

In older patients and infants with suitable anatomy, the coarctation may be excised with end-to-end anastomosis. For long segments of obstruction, it may be necessary to use an onlay patch, while, occasionally, a hypoplastic aorta must be bypassed with a complete prosthetic tube graft. In babies, the subclavian artery is often opened out and turned down as a flap across the coarctation, with the advantage of conserving growth potential.

Perfusion to the lower half of the body is generally adequate if the coarctation is severe and there is good collateral vessel development. In other cases, a degree of protection may be afforded by cooling the patient, but it will sometimes be necessary to maintain circulation to the lower half of the body by means of a shunt or left heart bypass. The duration of aortic clamping should be kept to minumum to avoid anoxic damage to the spinal cord.

Both during and after operation, the blood pressure must be closely monitored to avoid left ventricular failure, haemorrhage and abdominal complications. Most older patients will require pharmacological control of hypertension for several weeks after operation.

Results. Generally, survival is excellent after coarctation repair in children, although some older patients continue to have a degree of hypertension even after satisfactory relief of the obstruction. Mortality among infants also approaches zero, although those with associated intracardiac defects have a lower rate of survival. There is also an incidence of recoarctation, depending upon the age at operation and type of repair. Fortunately, most of these lesions are amenable to balloon dilatation and the need for reoperation is becoming uncommon.

Interrupted Aortic Arch

This is a rare condition in which there is complete separation of two segments of the aortic arch. The distal segment is perfused through a persistent ductus arteriosus. It is usual to have a ventricular septal defect in association.

Anatomy. Based upon the site of interruption, the defects are classified as type A (distal to the left subclavian), type B (between the left common carotid and left subclavian) or type C (between the carotid arteries). Type B is by far the most common. A large patent ductus connects the descending aorta to the pulmonary artery. Usually there is a large ventricular septal defect with displacement of the outlet septum into the subaortic area, but truncus arteriosus, aortopulmonary window, transposition of the great arteries, or single ventricle may also be associated.

Haemodynamics. The right ventricle is at systemic pressure, and perfusion of the lower half of the body depends upon a patent arterial duct. In the presence of a ventricular septal defect, it is not possible to demonstrate a gradient across the left ventricular outflow tract, regardless of the anatomical potential for severe obstruction.

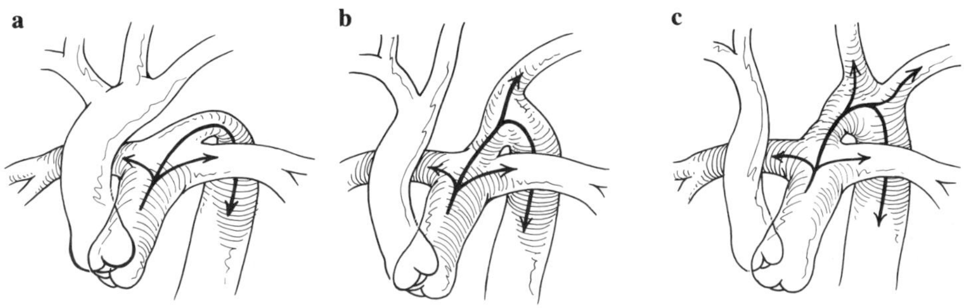

Fig. 6.35. Types of interrupted aortic arch.

Clinical Features. The usual presentation is severe low cardiac output, oliguria and congested lungs with weak or absent pulses in the left arm and both legs. After the ductus is reopened with prostaglandin, a systolic murmur may become apparent.

Special Investigations. The ECG and chest X-ray are non-specific in the newborn and generally will show right ventricular or biventricular hypertrophy and cardiac enlargement with pulmonary congestion, respectively. Real-time echocardiography should visualise the site of the interruption as well as associated intracardiac defects. If a ventricular septal defect is not seen, the diagnosis of aortopulmonary window should be suspected.

Cardiac catheterisation adds insult to metabolic injury in these sick babies and should be reserved for cases with complex associated lesions or in which the side of the descending aorta is in question.

Differential Diagnosis. The only conditions to be excluded are hypoplastic left heart syndrome and coarctation of the aorta, which should be possible by real-time echocardiography. The infant who is septic may present also with circulatory collapse, and sepsis not infrequently complicates interruption of the aortic arch, due to ischaemia of the bowel.

Indications for Operation. Surgical treatment is an emergency and should be undertaken as soon as the infant has been stabilised on prostaglandin and metabolic acidosis has been corrected. Inotropes may also be necessary preoperatively to improve the cardiac output and re-establish urine flow.

Principles of Treatment. Surgery must establish a reliable pathway for blood flow to the lower body segment (arch reconstruction) and control the heart failure and pulmonary overperfusion. In some cases it is possible to join up the two ends of the aorta by direct anastomosis, while in others it is necessary to interpose a tube graft. In a very ill neonate, pulmonary artery banding may be preferable to closure of the ventricular septal defect on cardiopulmonary bypass. However, this requires later removal of the band and septal defect closure, so the present thrust is towards complete correction as a primary procedure.

Results. Both complete primary repair and two-stage correction have achieved a survival of about 70% in this previously lethal condition, and there has recently been some success in treating infants with complex associated lesions (truncus arteriosus, transposition of the great arteries). Some patients require reoperation for subaortic obstruction, and those with a tube graft will probably require replacement of the prosthetic segment when this is outgrown.

Cor Triatriatum

This is an exceedingly rare malformation (less than 0.1% of congenital heart defects) in which a fibromuscular septum partitions the left atrium into two chambers.

Anatomy and Embryology. It is generally thought that there is a failure of absorption of the pulmonary venous confluence into the developing left atrium. This lesion is developmentally midway between total anomalous pulmonary venous connection (where the common pulmonary vein makes no contact with the left atrium) and the normal heart. The pulmonary veins all drain into the upper or proximal chamber, which is separated from the lower or distal chamber by the septum. The lower chamber contains the left atrial appendage and mitral valve. There is usually a small hole connecting the two chambers, and either chamber may communicate with the right atrium through an atrial septal defect. The remainder of the heart is normal.

Haemodynamics. There is near complete obstruction to blood leaving the lungs, and, accordingly, severe pulmonary hypertension.

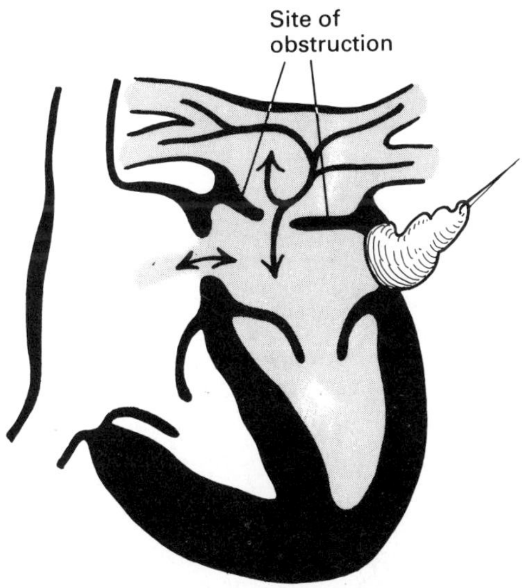

Fig. 6.36. Cor triatriatum with a membrane separating the pulmonary veins from the mitral valve.

Clinical Features. Because there are no murmurs or cyanosis, the diagnosis is frequently overlooked. Patients usually experience breathlessness or cough in the first 2 years, although severe obstruction occasionally leads to low cardiac output in neonates, and older patients with lesser degrees of obstruction may have wheezing and haemoptysis. Signs of pulmonary hypertension are florid, with a right ventricular heave and loud second heart sound.

Special Investigations. The chest X-ray shows pulmonary venous congestion and the pulmonary artery may be enlarged. Right ventricular forces invariably dominate the ECG. The partition between proximal and distal chambers is readily demonstrated by real-time echocardiography, and Doppler studies may show a characteristic diastolic flow pattern across the membrane. While the diagnosis may also be made at cardiac catheterisation, this is unnecessary in most cases and angiography carries the usual risks of contrast injection into a patient with severe pulmonary hypertension.

Differential Diagnosis. Other causes of pulmonary venous obstruction, that is pulmonary vein stenosis, total anomalous pulmonary venous connection, mitral stenosis and supramitral ring, can generally be differentiated by real-time echocardiography.

Indications for Operation. The only treatment is surgical.

Principles of Treatment. Excision of the partitioning membrane on cardio-pulmonary bypass renders the heart anatomically and physiologically normal. If present, the atrial septal defect is closed simultaneously.

Results. Survival is generally excellent (more than 95%) and pulmonary hypertension will regress in most patients. Later deaths are due to occasional cases of irreversible pulmonary vascular disease, and such patients may be candidates for lung or heart–lung transplantation if the pulmonary arterial hypertension does not resolve postoperatively.

Congenital Anomalies of the Mitral Valve

Although only the stenotic lesions will cause cardiac obstruction, anomalies of the mitral valve are conveniently considered together because many cause both stenosis and insufficiency. At one extreme, atresia of the valve produces absent left atrioventricular connection, a rare type of univentricular atrioventricular connection (effectively, a 'single ventricle'). This merges with the hypoplastic left heart syndrome.

Anatomy. Anomalies may occur in the valve leaflets, the chordae, the papillary muscles, or a combination of all three. In addition, infolding of the atrial myocardium above the leaflets may produce an obstructive 'supravalvar ring', or there may be duplication or generalised hypoplasia of the valve. The commonest lesions are an isolated cleft of the aortic leaflet, shortened, fused chordae tethering thickened leaflets to enlarged papillary muscles ('arcuate' or 'hammock' valve), and a single papillary muscle supporting both commissures ('parachute' valve). Dilatation of the mitral ring and elongation of chordae may also result in a prolapsing and regurgitant leaflet.

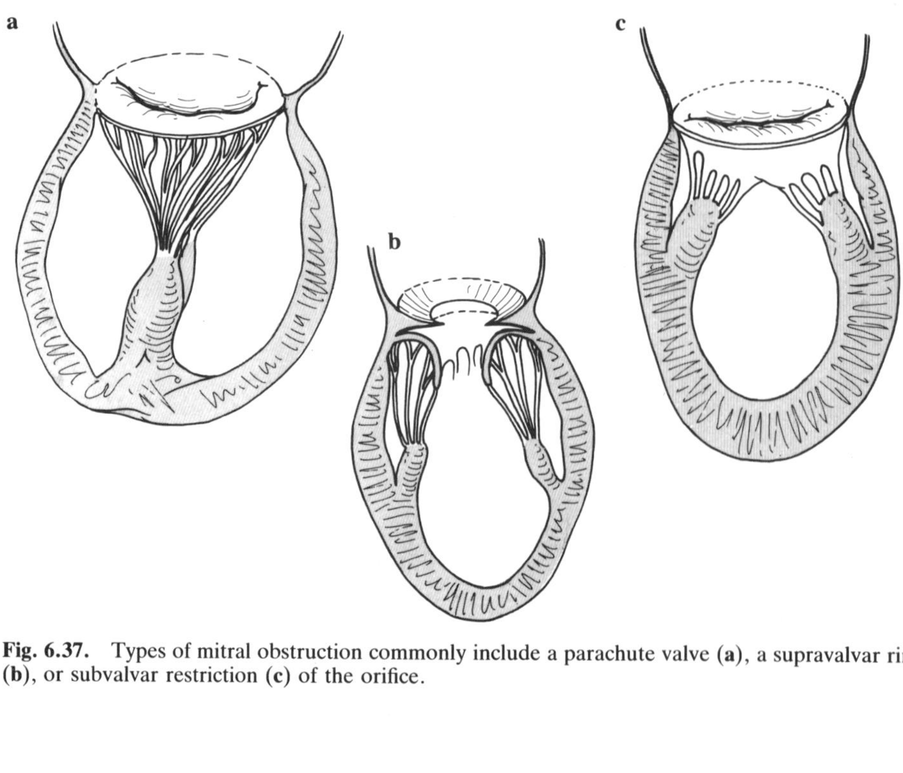

Fig. 6.37. Types of mitral obstruction commonly include a parachute valve (**a**), a supravalvar ring (**b**), or subvalvar restriction (**c**) of the orifice.

Haemodynamics. Obstruction of the mitral valve causes a diastolic pressure gradient between the left atrium and left ventricle, and elevation of left atrial pressure may lead to pulmonary hypertension. With mitral regurgitation, retrograde flow of blood from left ventricle to left atrium may also raise left atrial pressure, but dilatation of the chamber usually accommodates the volume overload and ameliorates pulmonary hypertension. Congenital mitral valve lesions often occur in association with complex anomalies which greatly modify the haemodynamic picture. Thus, increased pulmonary flow through a ventricular septal defect may accentuate mild stenosis, or the presence of an atrial septal defect may off-load the left atrium, obscuring either a stenotic or regurgitant valve.

Clinical Features. The valve lesion is often overshadowed by more complex associated anomalies which also dominate the clinical picture. Elevation of left atrial pressure leads to wheezing, chest infections and, eventually, haemoptysis. In infants, there may be congestive heart failure, sweating and failure to thrive.

The first heart sound may be loud. A pansystolic murmur is heard with mitral incompetence, while a diastolic murmur may be caused either by stenosis or increased flow. Pulmonary hypertension causes a loud second heart sound. There may be crepitations at the lung bases.

Special Investigations. The left atrium tends to be enlarged with a double contour on chest X-ray, and the heart size is also enlarged. Pulmonary venous congestion resembles the oedema or Kerley B-lines seen with other causes of left atrial hypertension. Sinus rhythm is usually present. Right ventricular dominance is more likely with stenotic lesions, and left ventricular with regurgitant ones. If the ECG shows ischaemic changes, the possibility of an anomalous left coronary artery causing ischaemic mitral regurgitation should be considered.

Real-time echocardiography is the investigation of choice and should show the mobility of the leaflets, the number and location of the papillary muscles, and any clefts or prolapse. The degree of stenosis or incompetence can be estimated from Doppler echocardiography.

Cardiac catheterisation may be necessary to document the transvalvar gradient or to investigate associated anomalies. Left ventricular angiography demonstrates any regurgitation and the features of valve morphology.

Differential Diagnosis. The other causes of left atrial enlargement and pulmonary hypertension previously considered must be excluded. It is important also to exclude other problems, such as poor left ventricular function, and to identify associated conditions which may produce a picture of mitral valve disease.

Indications for Operation. These are not always clear-cut and depend to some extent on the associated cardiac lesions. An attempt to relieve stenosis or regurgitation is warranted by pulmonary hypertension, uncontrolled heart failure or pulmonary oedema.

Principles of Treatment. Relief of stenosis may sometimes be achieved by division of a fused commissure or restrictive papillary muscle, while regurgitation may be repaired by annuloplasty or closure of a cleft. However, valve replacement is not infrequently required to achieve satisfactory function, and this depends upon having a sufficiently large annulus to accommodate the prosthesis. When the annulus is severely hypoplastic, the prosthesis may be positioned in the left atrium, but the best option in some cases will be to decompress the left atrium through an atrial septal defect and band the pulmonary artery, with a view to a subsequent Fontan type of procedure.

Results. Mild lesions may cause little incapacity and suffice with medical treatment. Valve repair or replacement carries a mortality of 1%–2% in older children, but this increases sharply to as much as 50% in a critically ill infant. The late results of valve replacement in children remain suboptimal; generally, an effort is made to conserve the valve whenever possible.

Vascular Rings

Anomalies of the great vessels surrounding the trachea and oesophagus in the superior mediastinum have the potential to constrict the airway or the gullet. Other vascular malformations that can cause pressure on the trachea or oesophagus but do not completely encircle them are referred to as 'slings' and are generally considered in the same group of malformations.

Anatomy and Embryology. In the development of the cardiovascular system, six pairs of primitive brachial arches connect the dorsal and ventral aortae. Most vascular rings can be explained in terms of regression or persistence of various parts of this arch system, although it is unlikely that the entire embryonic arch system ever exists at one time in the developing human. The side of the descending aorta is determined independently.

A double aortic arch is formed by the complete persistence of both fourth arches. As such, each arch must give off a carotid and subclavian artery. The arches then join together at the descending aorta. The posterior (right) arch is usually dominant, but either may predominate or have an obstruction within it.

A left aortic arch (the normal situation) results from persistence of the left fourth arch and regression of the right distal to the subclavian artery. The proximal right fourth arch now becomes a branch of the aorta, the innominate artery. If the opposite occurs, it produces a right aortic arch with a left innominate artery, the so-called right aortic arch with mirror-image branching. If the fourth embryonic arch regresses between the subclavian and carotid precursors, the resulting left or right definitive aortic arch will have an aberrant subclavian artery arising as its last branch and passing across the posterior mediastinum behind the oesophagus to reach the arm.

The embryological basis for the pulmonary artery sling is less well understood. In this condition, the left pulmonary artery arises to the right of the trachea and passes between the trachea and oesophagus to reach the left lung. It is probably the only vascular malformation which consistently lies in this position.

A distal or proximal origin of a carotid or innominate artery may cause either vessel to pass obliquely in front of the trachea. The importance of this situation, as regards causing compression of the trachea, is controversial.

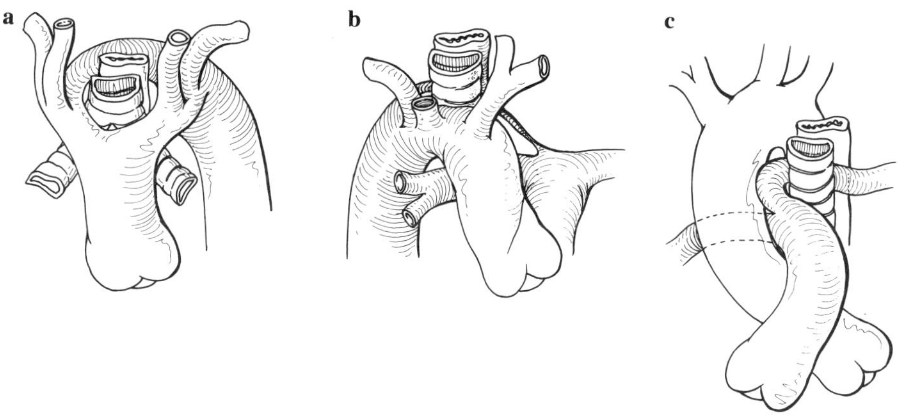

Fig. 6.38. Examples of vascular rings and slings: double aortic arch (**a**), Right aortic arch with left ligamentum (**b**), and pulmonary artery sling (**c**).

Haemodynamics. These are usually normal.

Clinical Features. Stridor, which is both inspiratory and expiratory, is typical of a tight, complete vascular ring. The infant assumes a characteristic position with the head and neck extended to minimise the tracheal compression. When solids are introduced, stridor becomes worse at feeding, and older babies may show signs of dysphagia. With less tight rings, it is possible for the infant to remain asymptomatic.

Special Investigations. Most vascular rings can be identified from their characteristic impressions upon the barium-filled oesophagus. Bronchoscopy and oesophagoscopy permit direct observation of a pulsatile extrinsic compression but add nothing to the preoperative diagnosis and risk trauma that may precipitate complete tracheal blockage. Angiography will give a precise anatomical diagnosis and is most useful for pulmonary artery sling or when it appears that a right thoracotomy may be necessary. It should be recalled, however, that an atretic segment will not be visualised by angiography but may still cause severe compression.

Differential Diagnosis. Much more common causes of stridor, such as respiratory infections and dysphagia, can usually be excluded by a combination of a careful clinical history, a chest X-ray and a barium swallow.

Indications for Operation. Operation is indicated for the relief of symptoms, and is usually necessary for double aortic arch, pulmonary artery sling and right aortic arch with a left ligamentum. Other anomalies must be carefully assessed before recommending surgery.

Principles of Treatment. The compression is relieved by dividing the vascular ring and mobilising the soft tissues around the trachea and oesophagus, at the same time ensuring that important vascular channels are maintained. Thus, in the case of an aberrant pulmonary artery, the left pulmonary artery is resected from the right, passed between the trachea and oesophagus, and reanastomosed to the main pulmonary artery. In a double aortic arch, the smaller arch is divided after a clamping trial to make certain the distal perfusion remains adequate. And, in a right aortic arch with left ligamentum, the ends of the left sided ductus are divided and separated. Usually, the two ends of the divided vascular structure spring widely apart, an indication of the previous tension on the trachea and oesophagus.

Results. Survival is excellent and most patients are completely relieved of their symptoms. In a few cases where the constriction has been severe and prolonged (particularly with the aberrant left pulmonary artery), there may be underlying tracheo- or bronchiomalasia, or strictures in the main bronchi. Some patients eventually 'outgrow' this to a degree, but to the present time only a few have undergone successful surgical relief by implantation of a cartilage graft.

Acyanotic Congenital Heart Lesions: Left-to-Right Shunts

These include atrial and ventricular septal defects, persistent ductus arteriosus, and other communications between the systemic and pulmonary circuits, such as aortopulmonary window, truncus arteriosus and ruptured sinus of Valsalva aneurysm. In general, they place a volume overload on the heart, rather than a pressure load, because a portion of the cardiac output is ineffectively recirculated through the lungs or between the aorta and left ventricle.

Persistent Ductus Arteriosus

This is a persistence of the normal fetal channel lying between the pulmonary artery and the aorta. It usually closes shortly after birth and obliterates to become the ligamentum arteriosum. The duct, if it is present, is by definition patent, so that the use of the term patent ductus is repetitive. Persistent ductus arteriosus is both anatomically and grammatically a more accurate term.

Anatomy. The duct is derived embryologically from the sixth left branchial arch. Medially, the sixth arch forms the pulmonary artery, and the duct, or ligamentum, represents the lateral part of this arch and its connection with the aorta.

At its aortic end, the duct lies almost opposite or just distal to the left subclavian artery, and the recurrent laryngeal nerve winds around its inferior border. The anterior surface of the duct where it joins the pulmonary artery is covered by a short prolongation of the serous pericardial sac. Laterally, where it joins the aorta, there is often a localised dilatation of the aortic wall.

Occasionally, a similar structure is found on the right side, between the innominate artery (or, in the case of right aortic arch, the aorta) and right pulmonary artery.

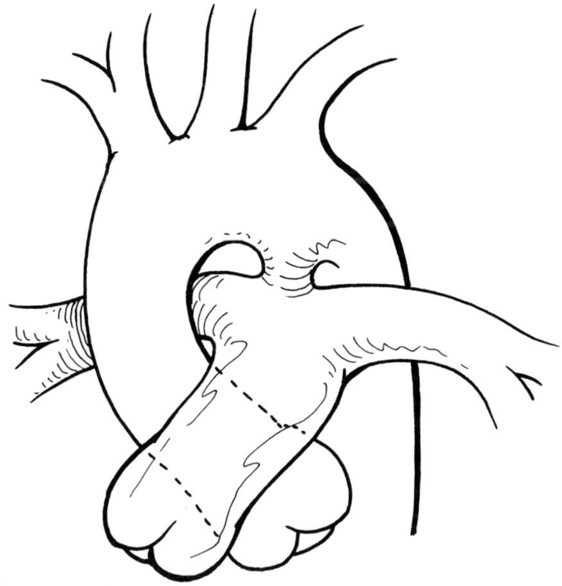

Fig. 6.39. Persistent ductus arteriosus.

Haemodynamics. During fetal life the duct provides a means of bypassing the functionless lungs and it directs blood from the right side of the heart into the descending aorta beyond the head vessels.

At birth, the lungs expand and their vascular resistance subsequently falls. The duct, if it persists, then acts as a fistulous leak from the aorta into the low-resistance pulmonary bed. Eventually, depending upon the size of the duct and the pulmonary vascular resistance, a shunt of blood will be established from the aorta to the lungs and back to the left atrium and left ventricle. Consequently, left ventricular enlargement is expected. Only if the pulmonary resistance remains high or rises again later will right ventricular hypertrophy occur. The aorta, proximal to the duct, carries this heavy blood flow and it is usually of a large diameter, particularly in the region of the aortic knuckle. Persistent ductus, as an isolated lesion, constitutes about 7% of congenital heart malformations.

Clinical Features. The diagnosis of persistent ductus is generally made on routine examination of the heart in children. Symptoms, when present, are those of slight dyspnoea or recurrent 'bronchitis' in cases with very large lung flows. Persistent ductus is, however, a common cause of 'heart failure' in the first weeks or months of life, and may be associated with the development of bronchopulmonary dysplasia in preterm infants. Bacterial endocarditis can be a fatal complication at any age. In the latter stages of the disease, as with any large left-to-right shunt, features of left heart failure may develop or, if pulmonary vascular resistance increases, the flow through the duct may be reversed, with the development of cyanosis or right heart failure.

The pulse is characteristically of large volume and collapsing in quality owing to the continuous leak of blood from the aorta throughout diastole. Arterial pulsation is prominent in the neck vessels. The precordium is overactive, with a left ventricular type of impulse, and a systolic thrill may be felt in the region of the third left interspace. The machinery-like murmur is of a continuous nature with a crescendo in late systole. An increased intensity of the pulmonary component of the second heart sound may be heard in addition to the murmur. At the apex, a rumbling diastolic murmur is often audible as a result of increased blood flow through the normal mitral valve.

In infants, where there is still elevation of pulmonary vascular tone, the flow of blood across the ductus in diastole may be absent or not sufficient to give rise to a murmur. Consequently, an isolated systolic murmur is not unusual in infants and may cause difficulties in distinguishing between this condition and ventricular septal defect. Similarly, in cases associated with increased pulmonary resistance, the pulmonary artery diastolic pressure may approach that in the aorta, with loss of the diastolic component of the murmur. Should the pulmonary artery pressure exceed that in the aorta, there will be a reversed flow of blood from the pulmonary artery into the aorta. This gives rise to differential cyanosis affecting the lower limbs.

Special Investigations. A chest X-ray shows the plethoric lung fields common to all left-to-right shunts and, in older cases, the large aortic knuckle and evidence of left ventricular enlargement. The ECG will confirm the presence of left ventricular dominance.

A combination of the presence of the characteristic murmur, maximal in the third left interspace, together with the chest radiograph is usually all that is required to make the diagnosis, but cardiac catheterisation may be reassuring as the result of the passage of the catheter through the ductus into the aorta. Additional, indirect evidence is obtained by demonstrating an increased oxygen saturation in the pulmonary artery.

While real-time echocardiography may or may not be able to demonstrate the ductus, it is usually possible to detect flow across it with Doppler studies. Retrograde aortography also may be used to delineate the ductus in difficult cases and may be helpful in differentiating it from truncus arteriosus and aortopulmonary window.

Differential Diagnosis. In the differential diagnosis, other forms of left-to-right shunts as well as other causes of a continuous murmur have to be considered, notably septal defects and aortopulmonary window, in addition to less common conditions. Any of these may present with a hyperdynamic precordium and plethoric lung fields on chest X-ray. The prominence of the aortic knuckle in ductus is a useful distinguishing feature.

1. *Atrial septal defect*. Symptoms are unlikely to arise early. The pulse is small to normal in volume, and, although the precordium may be overactive, it is right ventricular in character. The characteristically fixed, wide splitting of the second sound and the ECG should establish the diagnosis. Occasionally in infants a large persistent ductus will be accompanied by an atrial septal defect and the question arises as to which is the dominant lesion. The large flow of blood back to the left atrium tends to 'stretch' the patent foramen ovale, and it will be found in many cases that the atrial defect disappears or becomes insignificant following closure of the ductus.

2. *Ventricular septal defect.* Here the distinction may be difficult or impossible clinically, particularly where a continuous ductus murmur is absent. Also, there may be a pulmonary or aortic insufficiency murmur present in ventricular septal defect which resembles the continuous murmur of ductus.

In ventricular septal defect, the pulse is usually smaller or normal in volume and the thrill is lower (fourth left interspace). In both conditions, there is likely to be an apical mitral diastolic flow murmur. The chest radiography can be helpful in that the aortic knuckle is prominent in ductus and small in ventricular septal defect. Again, the ECG in ventricular septal defect is likely to show biventricular hypertrophy. Real-time echocardiography, particularly with colour-flow mapping should demonstrate either lesion.

Cardiac catheterisation is usually diagnostic, although a ductus with pulmonary regurgitation will show an apparent step-up in oxygen saturation at right ventricular level. The passage of the catheter across the ductus provides incontrovertible evidence of its persistence but this does not exclude the coexistence of the two lesions. For these reasons, both ventricular angiography and aortography may be necessary to establish the presence or absence of a ductus. In difficult cases with pulmonary hypertension, failure of contrast material to pass from the aorta to the pulmonary artery does not necessarily exclude a ductus, because blood flow may be in the opposite direction.

3. *Aortopulmonary window.* This may be impossible to distinguish from a ductus, although the clinical features are more like those of a large ventricular septal defect. A continuous murmur is unlikely to be present unless the aortopulmonary window is small. The diagnosis is not always readily apparent on echocardiography and rests upon the demonstration of a shunt just above the semilunar valves. Passage of a catheter into the aorta above the valves may be helpful, and aortography should confirm the anatomy.

4. *'Pseudo-truncus' or pulmonary atresia* is an important situation to recognise when it is associated with a persistent ductus. Under these conditions the blood flow to the lungs may be entirely dependent upon the ductus, and closure would be fatal. These cases are cyanosed but, with a good flow to the lungs via the ductus, this feature may be minimal. Continuous murmurs may arise also from major aortopulmonary collateral vessels, but these should be loudest in the back of the chest. An important feature to notice on the chest radiograph is the absence of a prominent main pulmonary trunk. In ductus arteriosus, the main pulmonary artery is at least normal and often enlarged.

5. *Ruptured sinus of valsalva aneurysm* into the right atrium or right ventricle gives a collapsing type of pulse and is usually associated with a continuous murmur. A history of sudden onset of cardiac failure is a helpful feature, but the physical signs may again be difficult to distinguish from the ductus. The murmur tends to be louder and a diastolic thrill may be present. Echocardiography may visualise the enlarged sinus, but cardiac catheterisation with aortography is usually necessary to establish the diagnosis and precise anatomy with certainty.

6. *Coronary artery fistula* will produce a continuous murmur but this is usually maximal towards the sternum, and signs of a left-to-right shunt are less impressive. Coronary angiography is necessary to establish the diagnosis.

7. *Pulmonary arteriovenous fistulae* tend to have continuous murmurs which are better heard over the lung fields. Cyanosis is usual but heart failure is less prominent.

Persistent ductus may be responsible for a collapsing pulse and a pronounced arterial pulsation in the suprasternal notch. Other conditions producing this type of neck pulsation are aortic regurgitation and coarctation of the aorta.

In both aortic regurgitation and ductus the pulse is collapsing and the left ventricle is dominant. Also, the to-and-fro murmur may be virtually indistinguishable from a continuous ductus murmur. However, the heart is generally larger and more active in aortic regurgitation and the lung fields are not plethoric. Coarctation is rarely confused with ductus if palpation of the femoral vessels is carried out as a clinical routine.

Indications for Operation. The mortality for closure of uncomplicated ductus should be zero in competent hands, so there is a good case for closure in every patient as soon as the diagnosis is made. In a preterm infant, the ductus is likely to close at term age; if it doesn't, spontaneous closure will have occurred in 90% of patients by 8 months of age and is unlikely after about 1 year. In general, the younger the patient, the more straightforward technically the operation, and complications are less likely to be encountered.

In the adult the duct may be calcified, which adds to the hazards of operation and may be considered sufficient reason to carry out closure as an open operation on cardiopulmonary bypass.

If there is infection or super-added bacterial endocarditis, this should be brought under control if possible before closure is contemplated. When there is an established reversal of flow through the ductus as a result of increased pulmonary resistance, closure is contraindicated.

Principles of Treatment. It is safest to regard the procedure as an operation on the aorta, and a good exposure of this vessel above and below the duct is advisable. As a matter of routine, the arch of the aorta should be identified to avoid ligation in the presence of undiagnosed coarctation or aortic arch interruption.

With a large duct, it is safer to divide and suture the ends in sections to prevent retraction of the cut ends during repair. The use of hypotensive drugs may be beneficial in difficult cases, particularly those with pulmonary hypertension or aneurysm formation. Ligation of the ductus also is effective and probably the technique of choice in young infants, where sutures tend to cut through the friable ductal tissue. It is important, however, to obliterate the entire length of the ductus, possibly incorporating a transfixation suture, if recurrence is to be avoided.

Closure of the persistent ductus with mechanical devices passed by way of the femoral vein is now possible, although the exact indications for nonoperative closure have yet to be established.

Results. Closure of an uncomplicated ductus is probably the most rewarding operation in congenital heart surgery. The patients should all survive and be completely cured, with normal exercise tolerance and life expectancy.

Atrial Septal Defect

This term covers a number of conditions in which there is a communication across the atrial septum. They can be classified as follows:

Fossa ovalis defect, including persistent foramen ovale
Sinus venosus defects
Posterior defect
Inferior vena caval defect
Coronary sinus defect

Partial anomalies of pulmonary venous drainage are included here because the haemodynamic picture is almost identical to atrial septal defect and because there is a frequent association between atrial septal defects and partial anomalous pulmonary venous drainage. The ostium primum defects and common atrium have developmental and clinical features more closely related to complete atrioventricular septal defect (see later) and are accordingly considered with that group of conditions.

Anatomy. The atrial septum has a complex embryological development. The septum primum develops first but with a deficiency below called the ostium primum. A thicker septum secundum then develops on its right side. This has an oval deficiency posteriorly which is floored by the septum primum and forms the fossa ovalis. A small hole (ostium secundum) is present at this stage in the septum primum by virtue of the flap-valve arrangement of the tissues. This valvular foramen ovale is kept open by the high pressure in the right atrium and functions until birth.

A deficiency in the floor of the fossa ovalis constitutes the commonly found ostium secundum or fossa ovalis defect. This is the commonest atrial septal defect encountered clinically and is also one of the commonest congenital heart lesions. It is differentiated from the ostium primum defect by a variable amount of septum being present above the atrioventricular valves. The foramen ovale is probe-patent in about 20% of people, but this is normally of little functional significance. It is sometimes crossed at cardiac catheterisation and then provides good access to the left heart chambers. The patent foramen is not an absence of tissue, in contrast with the fossa ovalis defect, but rather a lack of apposition of the septal flap valve.

The sinus venosus defect lies at the entrance of the superior vena cava into the right atrium. The lower margin is the upper edge of the atrial septum, and the upper margin the posterior or lateral wall of the superior vena cava. There are nearly always some veins from the right lung draining anomalously into the superior vena cava or right atrium in the region of the defect. The embryology is not clear, but the defect is related to the region of the atrium where the sinus venosus and pulmonary veins fuse with the developing common atrium.

A posterior atrial septal defect has no septum at the posterior and inferior margins of the atrium. The right pulmonary veins usually enter in the region of the defect and are thus directed to the right atrium.

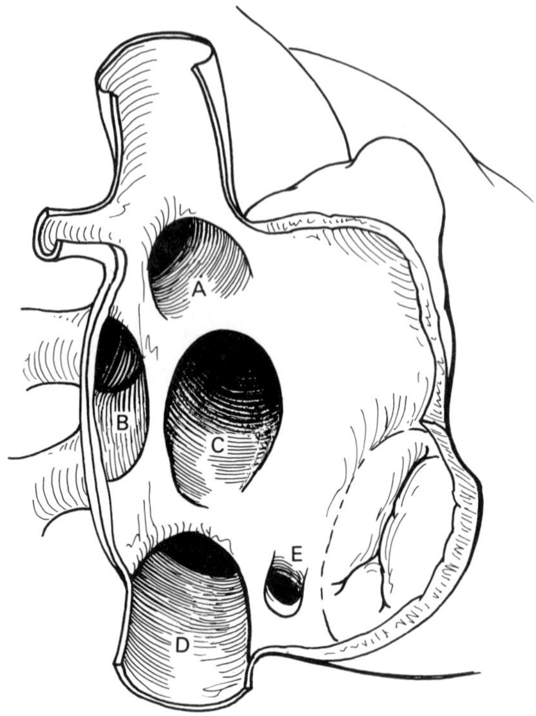

Fig. 6.40. Sites of defects in the atrial septum: A, sinus venosus; B, posterior; C, fossa ovalis; D, inferior vena cava; E, coronary sinus.

The inferior vena caval defect is the counterpart of the sinus venosus defect, having as its lower margin the posterior wall of the inferior vena cava. This must be differentiated from a large fossa ovalis defect, which reaches the inferior vena caval orifice. The inferior vena caval defect will be clearly separated from the fossa ovalis by a portion of septal tissue on its upper margin even if there is a second fossa ovalis defect or a patent foramen ovale. Either defect may be found in association with all the right pulmonary veins draining to the inferior vena cava, called the scimitar syndrome because of its characteristic X-ray appearance.

A coronary sinus defect falls within the spectrum of unroofed coronary sinus syndrome. Because one wall of the coronary sinus is shared with the left atrium, a deficiency will permit blood to flow retrograde through the coronary sinus ostium and into the left atrium or, conversely, from the left atrium through the coronary sinus to the right side of the heart. The unroofing may be partial or complete. A particularly confusing picture may result when a left superior vena cava also drains to the coronary sinus, and the patient is cyanosed with signs of an atrial septal defect.

Haemodynamics. In the uncomplicated atrial septal defect, there will be flow of oxygenated blood from the left atrium into the right atrium. The magnitude of the left-to-right shunt at atrial level is determined by the greater distensibility of the right ventricle. The development of increased pulmonary resistance and hypertrophy of the right ventricle will counteract this distensibility and reduce the shunt.

The right ventricle is usually dominant at birth. Consequently it is relatively inelastic so that a left-to-right shunt is unlikely to be significant in the newborn with an isolated atrial septal defect. As the pulmonary vascular resistance and right ventricular hypertrophy regress, the left-to-right shunt becomes apparent and progressively increases.

The haemodynamics are altered considerably when the patient has pulmonary stenosis, a not uncommon association. The increased diastolic pressure required to fill the hypertrophied right ventricle (which now lacks elastic distensibility) causes a rise in right atrial filling pressure. When this latter pressure rises above that in the left atrium, the shunt may reverse with a flow of blood from right atrium to left atrium. This may also re-open a patent foramen ovale, which is thought to be one mechanism of sudden death from paradoxical embolism, blood clot having formed in the systemic veins and subsequently lodged in a systemic artery.

The left-to-right shunt across the atrial septum is thus variable, even within a given patient at different times. If haemodynamic measurements suggest a very large shunt, however, particularly if it is disproportionate in relation to the size of the defect, anomalous pulmonary venous drainage is likely to be the cause.

Clinical Features. Symptoms are uncommon in childhood but there may be a tendency to frequent chest infections or breathlessness on exertion. Rarely, an infant with atrial septal defect presents with signs of pulmonary hypertension (particularly if Down's syndrome is present) or congestive heart failure. Symptoms usually arise in adult life and take the form of breathlessness and lack of energy.

In spite of the paucity of symptoms during early life, the heart is usually large. The pulse is small to normal in volume and, in young patients, there may be prominent venous pulsations in the neck.

The right ventricle is overactive and imparts a tumultuous quality to the precordial impulse. On auscultation it is usual to hear an ejection type of systolic murmur over the third and fourth left interspaces and sometimes a soft, short diastolic rumbling in the tricuspid valve area. These murmurs are thought to be 'flow' murmurs resulting from an excessive amount of blood passing through normal pulmonary and tricuspid valves. A diagnostic and very characteristic auscultatory feature of atrial septal defect is the wide splitting of the two elements of the second heart sound, both components being of normal intensity. The splitting does not vary with respiration because the increase in venous return to the right heart brought about by inspiration is small in comparison with the amount of blood flowing into the right atrium across the septal defect.

Special Investigations. Chest radiography demonstrates a large heart, the enlargement affecting mainly the right atrium, right ventricle and pulmonary artery. The aorta is small. As in all left-to-right shunts, there is a pleonaemic vascular pattern to the lungs. Occasionally, the chest radiograph suggests the presence of a sinus venosus defect by enlargement of the superior vena cava and displacement of the right superior pulmonary vein upward from the rest of the lung hilum.

The ECG is characteristic for a secundum atrial septal defect, showing the R-S-R[1] pattern of a volume-overloaded right ventricle in the anterior chest leads. A counterclockwise QRS loop and superior axis are more commonly found with atrioventricular septal defects (including a primum atrial septal defect), such that a positive R wave in lead I with a deep S wave in lead III should prompt one to question the diagnosis of a simple atrial defect.

The left-to-right shunt can be quantitated more accurately by radionucleotide angiography than cardiac catheterisation in most patients, and, with demonstration of an atrial defect on real-time echocardiography, this is considered sufficient diagnostic information to undertake operation. When there is doubt about association of other cardiac defects (pulmonary stenosis), or there is a possibility of pulmonary hypertension, or information is needed regarding the pulmonary venous drainage, cardiac catheterisation with angiography is carried out. Catheterisation is also necessary if the patient has a history of cyanosis.

Differential Diagnosis. Other causes of left-to-right shunt, those given under Persistent Ductus Arteriosus, have to be considered. Pulmonary stenosis may also be difficult to distinguish, but in this condition there may be an ejection click and the pulmonary component of the second sound is delayed and soft or inaudible. Usually, it is not possible to differentiate the various types of atrial septal defects clinically.

Indications for Treatment. Atrial septal defects of any type can be closed with a mortality of less than 1%, so the indication for surgical treatment is now regarded to be the presence of a clinically evident defect. This usually corresponds to a left-to-right shunt of more than 1.8 : 1.0.

Principles of Treatment. Closure of the defect should be accomplished without causing obstruction to either systemic or pulmonary venous drainage or causing injury to the conduction system. In all forms, this is best done under direct vision in a 'dry' heart, such that the edges of the defect and the entrance of the pulmonary veins may be seen with certainty.

A typical, small ostium secundum defect may be closed by direct suture. This also applies to the patent foramen ovale and some coronary sinus defects. For large defects or those with a margin involving a venous orifice, closure with a patch is less likely to narrow the orifice or be followed by recurrence.

Results. Provided the defect is securely closed without compromise of systemic or pulmonary venous pathways, the patient should enjoy a normal life.

Ventricular Septal Defect

In this condition, there is a communication between the ventricles. This may be one or many defects, and the defects may be any size. Ventricular septal defects also occur as a component of more complex anomalies, such as Fallot's tetralogy or double outlet right ventricle. It is by far the most frequently diagnosed heart lesion and is found in as many as one-third of heart malformations in children.

Anatomy. The exact embryological basis for all types of septal defects remains uncertain, but at least some are related to the fusion of the components of the ventricular septum or closure of the primitive interventricular foramen. A classification based upon the site of the defect recognises the following types:

1. Membranous or 'perimembranous'
2. Supracristal or 'doubly committed subarterial'
3. Inlet or 'ventricular septal defect of the A-V canal type'
4. Trabecular muscular defect (single)
5. Multiple muscular

The most common of these is the membranous defect, which may extend toward the inlet, trabecular or infundibular portions of the ventricular septum. On its right ventricular aspect, it lies below the crista supraventricularis (that is, the conal or infundibular septum) and usually extends backward for a variable distance toward the medial papillary muscle, beneath the septal cusp of the tricuspid valve. In fact, a good deal of the defect may be obscured by this valve which may assist nature in closing the defect, and contribute to the additional technical problems for the surgeon.

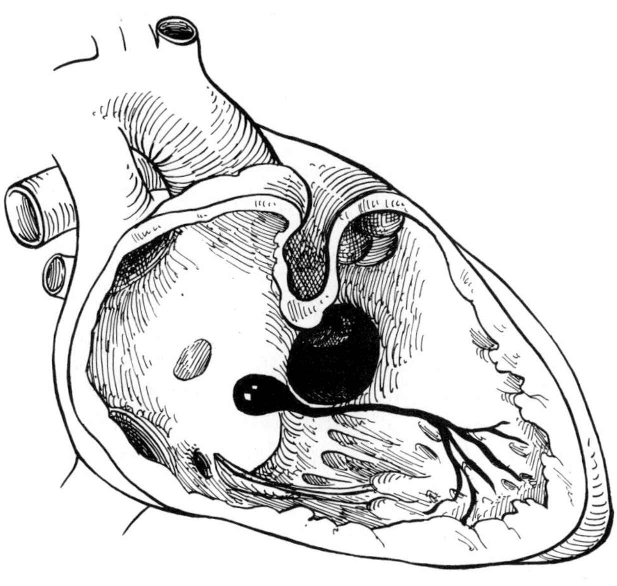

Fig. 6.41. The anatomy of the membranous ventricular septal defect and its relationship to the valves and conducting bundle.

On its left ventricular aspect, this defect is seen to lie in the outflow tract of the ventricle and extends up between the cusps of the aortic valve. The postero-inferior border of the defect is closely related to the main conducting bundle of the heart, and its superior margin is formed by the aortic ring itself.

The supracristal defect lies immediately beneath the aortic and pulmonary valves, being roofed by both. It is remote from the conducting tissue.

An inlet defect extends more posteriorly than a membranous defect and thus has the medial papillary muscle on its anterior aspect. One margin is the septal tricuspid leaflet, but the defect does not usually extend to the aortic valve. The conduction tissue may be displaced posteriorly, as in the A-V canal defects, and thus be related to the posterior half of the defect, or it may pass anteriorly.

When it is single, the trabecular defect often lies in the mid-muscular septum, just beyond the tricuspid valve chordae and papillary muscles. A more distal defect is usually crossed on its right ventricular surface by the large septomarginal trabeculation. While this gives the appearace of two openings in the right ventricle, it is clearly a single, round defect when observed on its left ventricular side. The conduction tissue is not close to either of these ventricular septal defects.

Multiple muscular defects tend to be smaller than a single muscular defect, and they may be located throughout the trabecular septum. This gives the 'Swiss cheese' appearance seen on angiography.

Haemodynamics. Where there is an unrestrictive defect between the two ventricles, blood will be ejected into the great vessel which offers the least resistance. In normal circumstances, the pulmonary vascular bed presents a path of lower resistance than the systemic vascular bed, so that the output of both ventricles will tend to be in the direction of the pulmonary artery.

Were it possible to create a large defect in the ventricular septum of an otherwise normal heart, there would be a catastrophic flooding of the lungs with blood, since the left ventricle would empty most of its contents into this area of low resistance. This shunting of blood would be at the expense of the high resistance systemic vascular bed, and would be incompatible with life. To a lesser degree, this is the situation in an infant who suffers a rapid fall in pulmonary resistance and presents with pulmonary oedema and low cardiac output. If a ventricular septal defect is to be tolerated, there are two alternative mechanisms whereby a systemic circulation is maintained

1. The defect itself when it is small (probably under 5 millimetres in diameter) may act as an obstruction to the passage of blood from the left to the right ventricle. Such a state of affairs is compatible with an almost normal circulation and pulmonary artery pressure. This condition represents the 'maladie de Roger' type of ventricular septal defect, with mild haemodynamic disturbance and a correspondingly benign clinical picture.

2. Alternatively, the ventricular septal defect is large (that is equal or greater than the diameter of the aorta) but an overwhelming left-to-right shunt is prevented by a hindrance to the flow of blood from the right ventricle. This right ventricular impediment tends to counterbalance the stream of blood being ejected through the defect from the left ventricle. It is caused either by some degree of pulmonary stenosis or by an increased pulmonary vascular resistance. This second type of defect with either pulmonary stenosis or pulmonary

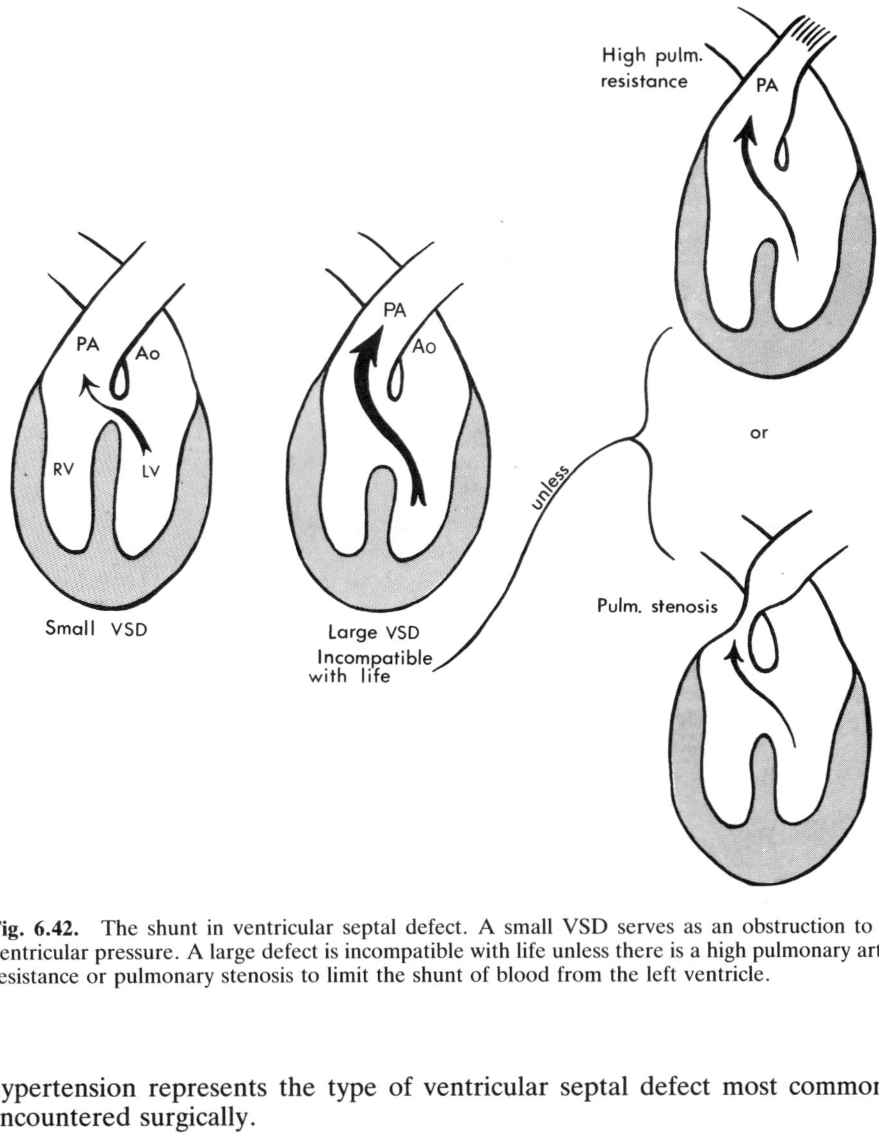

Fig. 6.42. The shunt in ventricular septal defect. A small VSD serves as an obstruction to left ventricular pressure. A large defect is incompatible with life unless there is a high pulmonary artery resistance or pulmonary stenosis to limit the shunt of blood from the left ventricle.

hypertension represents the type of ventricular septal defect most commonly encountered surgically.

It is common to find a *raised pulmonary artery pressure* associated with a ventricular septal defect, and this is closely related to the problem of pulmonary hypertension in general. In ventricular septal defect with a high flow, hyperdynamic pulmonary hypertension will account for some of the increased pulmonary artery pressure and this element will disappear upon closure of the defect. However, changes in the small vessels of the lungs are likely to be an important additional factor. These changes, which vary in severity, include intimal proliferation and hypertrophy of the muscle tissue in the vessel media. In some cases, these changes develop as the result of the ventricular septal defect and thus represent a 'protective' mechanism limiting the shunt. Alternatively, in other cases it seems likely that the histological changes represent a preservation of the high resistance fetal type of lung vessels and that the normal thinning and regression of these vessels does not occur in the face of the large left-to-right shunt. Whatever the mechanism of the changes in the lung vessels, they result in an increased pulmonary vascular resistance, which limits the flow of blood through the septal defect. Without treatment, they will also lead to irreversible pulmonary vascular disease and the Eisenmenger syndrome.

Clinical Features. Before cardiac surgery made possible the closure of ventricular septal defects, the term 'maladie de Roger' served as a convenient label under which to include a large and ill-defined group of conditions associated with a systolic thrill and murmur to the left of the sternum. More careful clinical assessment and the use of accurate diagnostic techniques eliminated most of the other diagnoses from this group, and it became apparent that isolated ventricular septal defects comprised a much smaller number of patients. It also demonstrated that the condition was by no means benign, as was formerly thought.

From a surgical point of view, the condition of a small ventricular septal defect (to which 'maladie de Roger' appropriately refers) with minimal shunting and no disability does not constitute a problem. Although such patients are at risk from bacterial endocarditis, closure of the defect does not prevent this complication. Diagnosis depends on the finding of a thrill and pansystolic murmur maximal to the left of the sternum in an asymptomatic patient with a normal second heart sound, an almost normal lung vasculature and a normal ECG.

In the case of a large ventricular septal defect, symptoms arise mainly from pulmonary congestion. In infants, there may be frank pulmonary oedema and low cardiac output. Extreme tachypnoea, sweating, feeding problems, failure to thrive and recurrent chest infections are all part of the clinical picture. In older age-groups, the stiff lungs result in dyspnoea on exertion, together with recurrent attacks of bronchitis, particularly if there is super-added pulmonary infection. Where pulmonary hypertensive features predominate, the patient tends to be less symptomatic and may present later with cyanosis.

Patients with a large ventricular septal defect are undersized and poorly developed, no doubt as the result of a deficient systemic circulation. Cyanosis is absent unless there is associated pulmonary stenosis or pulmonary vascular resistance approaches systemic levels. In fact, the lips and cheeks are often bright pink, as in other forms of a large left-to-right shunt. Infants with poor cardiac output, however, can present a greyish colour. A prominance of the sternum is a fairly common finding in ventricular septal defect.

The pulse is easily felt, but the jugular venous pressure is not, as a rule, remarkable. The precordium is likely to be tumultuous and reflects the over-activity of the ventricles. The left ventricular apex can often be seen and on palpation it has the hyperdynamic quality of an internal shunt. Right ventricular over-activity may be felt in addition, and a systolic thrill is usually a prominent feature. This is felt most clearly in the fourth left intercostal space. With a muscular defect, its position may be slightly lower. On auscultation a harsh systolic murmur is audible in this area. Classically, the murmur occupies the whole of systole, unlike the ejection murmur of pulmonary and aortic stenosis. This distinction is not always clinically obvious but can usually be confirmed by Doppler echocardiography. Where pulmonary hypertension limits the shunt, the murmur will be correspondingly shorter, and, similarly, the presence of pulmonary stenosis can act as a modifying factor in producing an ejection type of murmur.

At the cardiac apex it is usual to hear a short rumbling mitral murmur which is attributed to excessive blood flow through the mitral valve orifice during diastole.

When there is pulmonary hypertension, the pulmonary component of the second heart sound will be loud, and, as mentioned previously, the systolic murmur may be short. Also, the mitral diastolic flow murmur may be lost.

There may be additional features of pulmonary stenosis, such as a thrill and ejection murmur in the second or third left interspace, and a quiet, widely separated or 'absent' pulmonary component of the second heart sound. Where pulmonary stenosis raises the right ventricular pressure to near systemic level, the condition merges with clinically mild Fallot's tetralogy. Indeed, the term 'acyanotic Fallot' has been coined for this symptom complex.

Special Investigations. The chest radiograph resembles that seen in any left-to-right shunt, namely, plethoric lung fields. The cardiac contour may show a dominant left ventricular silhouette but, with the development of pulmonary hypertension, right ventricular hypertrophy tends to obscure this. A point of importance in distinguishing this condition from persistent ductus is the small aortic knuckle. Where there is associated pulmonary stenosis, the lung fields may be less heavily vascularised than expected, and, where pulmonary hypertension dominates, the lung fields show a large hilar shadow while the outer third of the field is clear.

The ECG shows the features of biventricular hypertrophy, that is, prominent Q and R waves in V_5 and V_6 as evidence of left ventricular hypertrophy as well as prominent right ventricular R waves in V_1 and V_2. Where pulmonary hypertension is considerable, the features of right ventricular hypertrophy, possibly with a strain pattern, will dominate the picture.

Real-time echocardiography can demonstrate most of the larger ventricular septal defects and Doppler echocardiography can estimate the pressure difference across the ventricular septum and thus, indirectly, right ventricular pressure. Cardiac catheterisation is generally needed to ascertain accurate measurements of systemic and pulmonary flows and the pulmonary vascular resistance. The catheter should cross the septal defect into the aorta, which establishes the diagnosis conclusively, but the level of the shunt is not always easy to determine on oxygen saturation studies alone. Owing to blood streaming effects, the catheter may fail to sample a shunt in the right ventricle and may suggest a rise in oxygen saturation in the pulmonary artery instead of the ventricle. Another difficulty is quantitating the shunts at various levels when other defects, such as atrial septal defect or persistent ductus arteriosus, are also present.

Left ventricular angiography demonstrates the position, size and number of defects.

Differential Diagnosis. The small asymptomatic 'maladie de Roger' type of ventricular septal defect presents with a thrill and murmur to the left of the sternum. These cases should be distinguished from isolated pulmonary stenosis, aortic stenosis, persistent ductus arteriosus, coarctation of the aorta and atrial septal defect. Uncomplicated ductus can be distinguished on the murmur alone. Also, the murmurs of aortic and pulmonary stenosis should be of ejection type following upon an ejection click, whereas the ventricular septal defect murmur occupies the whole of systole. Coarctation is diagnosed on the blood pressure and absence of femoral pulsation, and atrial septal defect should be distinguished by the wide fixed splitting of the second heart sound. It is assumed that all the foregoing conditions are in acyanotic patients presenting with a systolic murmur.

Where the clinical disability is marked together with a hyperdynamic heart and congested lung fields, the differential diagnosis depends upon distinguishing between the various forms of left-to-right shunt.

Table 6.1. Differential diagnosis in ventricular septal defect

	Ventricular septal defect	Atrial septal defect	Persistent ductus arteriosus
Clinically	Early symptoms	Later symptoms	Early or late
Ventricles	Right and left	Right	Left
Thrills	4th LIS[a]	Slight or absent	2nd LIS[a]
Murmur	Pansystolic	Ejection systolic	Continuous
X-ray	Small aorta	Small aorta	Big aorta
ECG	Biventricular	Right	Left

[a] LIS, Left intercostal space.

1. *Atrial septal defect* should be eliminated quite easily. It rarely presents early in infancy and the right heart features predominate clinically, electrocardiographically and radiographically.

2. *Persistent ductus* may be difficult to distinguish with certainty if the continuous murmur is absent, as in infants or in the presence of pulmonary hypertension. Also, in cases of ventricular septal defect with pulmonary or aortic regurgitation, this regurgitant murmur may be difficult to distinguish from a continuous murmur. Both ductus and ventricular septal defect show a left ventricular dominance but the pulse in ductus should be of a collapsing quality.

The size of the aortic knuckle on the chest radiograph should be carefully studied, if necessary with the aid of a barium swallow. In ductus the aortic knuckle is large, while in ventricular septal defect it is small. Also the ECG in ductus is likely to be predominantly left ventricular while it is usual to have a biventricular picture in ventricular septal defect. The presence of pulmonary hypertension in either condition will increase the right ventricular contribution. Aortography is the most reliable method of demonstrating or excluding a ductus in a difficult case.

3. *Aortopulmonary window* can be extremely difficult to differentiate from ventricular septal defect on clinical examination. A continuous murmur is not usual and the two conditions may be clinically indistinguishable. Echocardiography, however, should visualise the ventricular septal defect, and sometimes it is also possible to demonstrate an aortopulmonary window with certainty. The cardiac catheter may cross from pulmonary artery to aorta at a

level just beyond the pulmonary valve, but, where doubt remains, angiography will be necessary to establish the anatomy.

4. *Truncus arteriosus*. Here again the picture may be indistinguishable from ventricular septal defect or aortopulmonary window. Even the cardiac catheter is not infallible, and echocardiography may be more precise in establishing the diagnosis. Although, in theory, these patients should be cyanosed from the mixing of blood within the ventricles, the large pulmonary shunt makes the degree of desaturation such that it may not be clinically detectable. The chest radiograph may be helpful in demonstrating a deep pulmonary bay, together with plethoric lung fields.

5. *Atrioventricular septal defects*. In some of these defects, the ventricular component may dominate the clinical picture, making differentiation from isolated ventricular septal defect difficult. The ECG should be helpful, while real-time echocardiography clearly demonstrates atrioventricular valves at the same level and the loss of an atrioventricular septum in these cases.

Indications for Operation. Many ventricular septal defects, indeed the vast majority, will close spontaneously. Nevertheless, some will lead to death from congestive heart failure in infancy or irreversible pulmonary vascular disease, a regrettable and completely avoidable complication. Thus, the clinician must select those cases which will not close by themselves and which will cause disability.

In infants, regardless of the size of the defect, symptoms rarely occur before the natural regression of the pulmonary resistance at 6 weeks of age. If the baby is 'in trouble' before this, it is nearly always as the result of an associated lesion, coarctation being the most common.

After about 6 weeks, some infants will develop a massive left-to-right shunt with uncontrollable heart failure and low cardiac output. Surgery is urgently needed in such patients. A more common picture is failure to thrive despite maximal medical treatment, and surgery is also clearly needed in this group if they are to survive beyond a few months.

In some patients symptoms will be mild, due to elevation of pulmonary vascular resistance, and this is the group who are likely to subsequently develop irreversible changes in the lungs.

The association of a large persistent ductus arteriosus and ventricular septal defect is a particularly lethal combination. Studies of lung biopsies have shown that changes in the pulmonary vessels are nearly always reversible up to about 1 year of age and this correlates with clinical experience. Thus, any infant with significant pulmonary hypertension should be operated upon by about 9 months of age in order to abolish the risk of established pulmonary vascular disease.

In patients who have a large defect without severe congestive failure or elevation of pulmonary arterial resistance, the decision to recommend operation depends upon the magnitude of the shunt and evidence of spontaneous closure of the defect. If the shunt is large ($Q_p/Q_s > 2:1$) and there is no evidence that the defect is closing, elective repair is generally done at between 1 and 3 years of age. Some 80% of ventricular septal defects close during the first year and there is usually some sign of tricuspid valve tissue around the defect if this is likely to happen in the remainder. If tricuspid valve tissue is beginning to occlude the hole, further observation is justified and does not constitute a risk to the patient.

Other indications for operation are the onset of aortic incompetence and recurrent or uncontrollable endocarditis. In the former, the ventricular septal defect may be either membranous or subarterial. A cusp of the aortic valve prolapses into the defect and often gives the false impression of a small defect, such that right ventricular pressure is low and there is a modest left-to-right shunt. Progression of the aortic incompetence is the rule, however, and may be arrested by closure of the ventricular septal defect. Cases of endocarditis may have large vegetations on the tricuspid valve. When medical treatment has failed to control the infection, closure of the ventricular septal defect and removal of vegetations is carried out.

Where the ventricular septal defect is part of Eisenmenger's syndrome, closure is contraindicated as it may actually accelerate the pulmonary vascular disease. Such patients should be evaluated for possible lung or heart–lung transplantation.

Principles of Treatment. The aim of treatment is to achieve secure closure of the defect without injury to the cardiac valves or the conduction tissue. Occasionally this can be done by direct suture, but a patch is generally preferable. Any pulmonary stenosis or muscular hypertrophy of the infundibulum, or a persistent ductus, are dealt with at the same time. Accurate closure necessitates support of the circulation with cardiopulmonary bypass or, in very small infants, deep hypothermia and total circulatory arrest.

The relation of the conduction tissue to the postero-inferior rim of the membranous defect must be kept in mind in planning the repair. Complete heart block, should it occur, necessitates the implantation of a permanent pacing system.

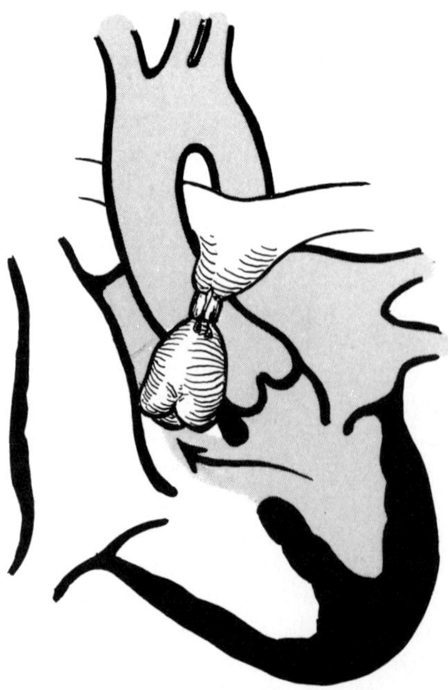

Fig. 6.43. Banding of the pulmonary artery in ventricular septal defect.

An alternative to complete closure is banding of the pulmonary artery, which creates an artifical pulmonary stenosis. This is rarely done as the subsequent removal of the band and closure of the defect carry greater risk and less likelihood of satisfactory result than primary closure, even in very small infants. However, it can be performed where there are no facilities for cardiopulmonary bypass and may then be life-saving.

Results. An uncomplicated ventricular septal defect can be closed with a risk that approaches zero at any age by an experienced surgical team, and this should provide the patient with a normal exercise tolerance and, probably, normal life expectancy. The outlook may be altered by the presence of multiple defects, elevated pulmonary vascular resistance or aortic regurgitation. All patients who have undergone closure of a ventricular septal defect remain at risk from bacterial endocarditis and accordingly require antibiotic prophylaxis.

Atrioventricular Septal Defects
(Endocardial cushion defects; atrioventricular canal malformations)

This group of malformations share a deficiency of tissue at the atrioventricular junction. As a result, there may be an interatrial defect, an interventricular defect and/or abnormalities of the atrioventricular valves.

Anatomy. The underlying abnormality is a defect in the atrioventricular septum. The tricuspid valve normally inserts at a lower level than the mitral valve, such that a portion of the septum comes to lie between the left ventricle and the right atrium. When this is absent, the two valves are at the same level, and instead of being wedged between them, the aorta is displaced anteriorly. Displacement of the aorta causes the outlet portion of the ventricular septum to be longer than the inlet portion, which is responsible for the characteristic 'goose-neck' appearance seen on the left ventricular angiogram in this malformation. The common atrioventricular junction may be partitioned into a left and a right orifice (as seen in a 'partial' or 'ostium primum' defect) but the valve leaflets are quite different from normal mitral and tricuspid valves. Alternatively, the common orifice may be undivided, with a single, large valve opening into both ventricles. This is the usual situation in a 'complete' defect.

Usually, there is an atrial septal defect of variable size immediately above the valve, the so-called ostium primum atrial septal defect. Rarely, there is a complete absence of atrial septum, in which case the malformation is called a 'common atrium'. The left atrioventricular (mitral) valve usually has a gap between its anterior and posterior leaflets in both conditions. The separation, or 'cleft', may reach the ventricular septum, in which case it said to be complete, as opposed to a partial or incomplete cleft. There may also be a deficiency in the right atrioventricular (tricuspid) valve.

In the complete form, the valve leaflets are not partitioned into a right and left side by attachment of the ventricular septum but rather float above a ventricular septal defect. This again may vary in size from a few millimetres to the entire length of the ventricular septum. The conduction system must pass more posteriorly because of the defect, and this gives rise to a counterclockwise or superior QRS axis commonly seen on the ECG.

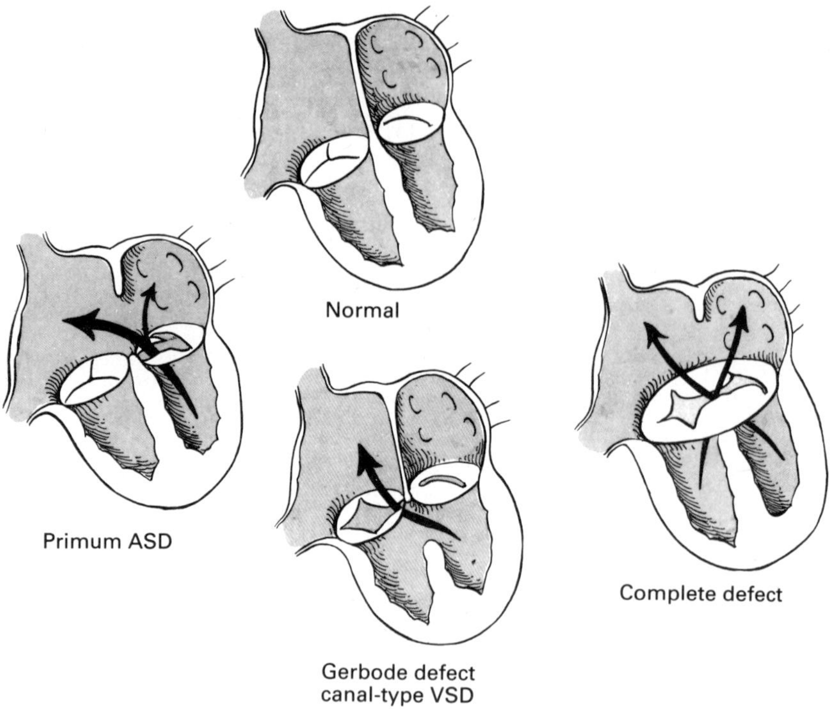

Fig. 6.44. Types of atrioventricular septal defects (left-to-right): partial (ostium primum ASD), VSD of AV canal type, and complete. Valve regurgitation suggested by arrows.

Intermediate defects (in which there is a fibrous tongue of tissue partitioning the common valve) and associated malformations such as Fallot's tetralogy also occur rarely. Atrioventricular septal defects may be part of more complex malformations, such as single ventricle or isomeric hearts.

Formerly, it was held that part of the mitral and tricuspid valves as well as the adjacent septum developed from the primitive endocardial cushions, and hence the name 'endocardial cushion defects' for this group of lesions. However, it is now appreciated that the endocardial cushion make only a small contribution and the developmental basis of the defect must involve several components.

Haemodynamics. The partial defect has the basic left-to-right shunt of an atrial septal defect with or without additional left atrioventricular valve regurgitation. In the complete form, the haemodynamics are generally dominated by the ventricular septal defect. Thus, there may be a large left-to-right shunt with pulmonary hypertension and a tendency to develop pulmonary vascular disease. Other important factors are the relative size of the two ventricles, the presence of obstruction to left ventricular outflow, and incompetence of the common atrioventricular valve.

Clinical Features. The complete forms tend to present early with an enlarged heart and symptoms of a large pulmonary flow, as seen in ventricular septal defect. In less florid cases the symptoms and signs are almost indistinguishable from those of ostium secundum atrial septal defect, but, when it is present, the apical systolic murmur of mitral regurgitation is suggestive of an atrioventricular septal defect.

Special Investigations. The chest X-ray may be virtually normal in mild cases, but cardiac enlargement and pulmonary plethora are more common. When the left atrium is greatly enlarged, a double shadow may be apparent.

The ECG is most useful, a superior or counterclockwise axis being typical of atrioventricular septal defects. This produces a deep S wave in leads I and II.

Of all malformations, real-time and Doppler echocardiography probably make the greatest contribution to diagnosis in this group. In addition to visualising the common valve or two valves at the same level, it is possible to demonstrate the size of the interatrial and interventricular communications, the size of each ventricle and regurgitation through the valve leaflets.

Cardiac catheterisation permits quantification of shunts and resistances, while angiography will outline the size of the ventricular chambers and any incompetence of the valves. The catheter may cross the atrial septum just above the atrioventricular valves and it is more likely to enter the left ventricle than in a secundum defect.

Differential Diagnosis. Other forms of left-to-right shunt must be considered, but, in practice the diagnosis resolves into distinguishing this condition from a straightforward atrial or ventricular septal defect.

Indications for Operation. As in other septal defects, surgery is done to prevent heart failure or the development of pulmonary vascular disease. The complete form generally requires operation in the first year of life, while partial defects are repaired electively, usually around 3–4 years or whenever the diagnosis is made. Probably left atrioventricular valve incompetence should be regarded as a reason for operation, as this causes the valve leaflets to become progressively thickened and deformed.

Principles of Treatment. The goal is to achieve competent left and right atrioventricular valves and secure closure of the septal defects without causing damage to the conduction system or narrowing of the left ventricular outflow tract. There are several techniques by which this may be done, and great controversy regarding their relative merits. In general, the atrial septal defect is closed with a patch of pericardium, and it may be necessary to approximate the two edges of the 'cleft' to obtain a competent left atrioventricular valve. The ventricular septal defect is also closed with a patch, usually of cloth material, taking care to avoid stitches in the area of the conduction tissue.

In theory, pulmonary artery banding is also an option for infants with the complete form of the defect. But in practice infants with a competent atrioventricular valve do equally well with complete primary correction. When the valve is incompetent, pulmonary artery banding intensifies the regurgitation.

A small number of patients will have extreme dominance of one ventricle over the other. For either right or left ventricular dominance, the mortality of repair becomes prohibitive. While pulmonary artery banding will protect the lungs, most patients have Down's syndrome and would not be considered for transplantation. At present, a solution to this problem is subsequent bidirectional cavopulmonary or Glenn anastomosis with a view to an ultimate Fontan-type circulation.

Results. For the partial defect, surgery is usually successful, with approximately 99% survival. Some patients require reoperation for subsequent repair or replacement of a leaking left atrioventricular valve. With favourable anatomy and some patient selection, the complete form can be repaired with a mortality of between 5% and 15%.

Aortopulmonary Window

In this condition, there is a hole between the proximal aorta and the pulmonary artery, distal to their respective valves.

Anatomy. This lesion arises as a defect in the spiral septum dividing the ascending aorta and pulmonary artery. Usually, the communication is just above

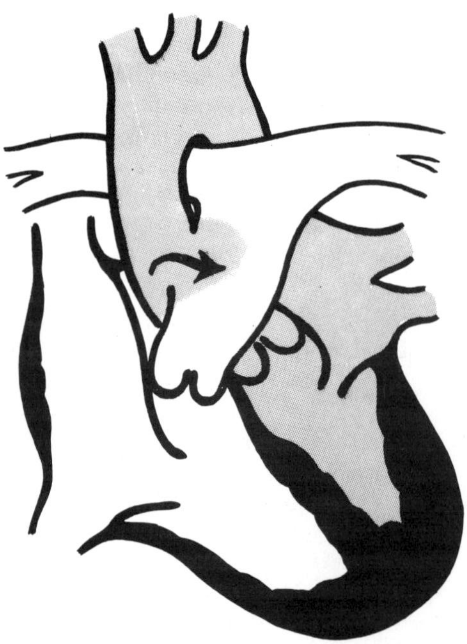

Fig. 6.45. An aortopulmonary window.

the valve sinuses, but it may be more distal, connecting the posterior aorta to the anterior right pulmonary artery. The whole septum may be deficient but the aortic and pulmonary valve rings are both present and separate, in contrast with truncus arteriosus. As suggested by the term 'window', there is no length to the connection, in contrast with persistent ductus. Associated anomalies are not uncommon, including coarctation of the aorta, interrupted aortic arch or origin of the right pulmonary artery from the aorta.

Haemodynamics. The haemodynamics are basically similar to a very large persistent ductus, although the proximity of the lesion means that the pulmonary arteries receive the full force of left ventricular ejection. There is a left-to-right shunt from aorta to pulmonary artery with increased flow through the lungs. The left atrium and left ventricle are enlarged. The ascending aorta is dilated, but the arch and descending aorta distal to the site of the shunt are small. If the defect is large, the clinical picture is complicated by pulmonary hypertension early on, and Eisenmenger's syndrome may develop.

Clinical Features. Patients with aortopulmonary defect present with features common to other large left-to-right shunts. They are subject to respiratory infections, dyspnoea and tiredness. There may be failure to thrive or retardation of growth among infants and young children.

The physical signs depend on the size of the communication and degree of left-to-right shunt. A small defect may be indistinguishable from a small ductus with a continuous murmur. When the defect is larger, the pulse is collapsing, the left ventricular impulse is hyperdynamic and the right ventricle may also be palpable. A continuous murmur is unusual in large communications because aortic and pulmonary arterial pressure equalise, but there is sometimes a diastolic flow murmur across the mitral valve at the apex. Signs of pulmonary hypertension may be dominant. The right ventricle is then powerful, a systolic murmur may be less obvious, and a pulmonary ejection click and loud pulmonary second sound are heard. There may also be a long early diastolic murmur of pulmonary regurgitation. When pulmonary hypertension is severe, clubbing of the fingers and central cyanosis appears.

Special Investigations. The ECG shows either pure left ventricular enlargement or combined right and left ventricular forces as seen in ventricular septal defect. The chest radiograph demonstrates lung plethora and cardiac enlargement. The ascending aorta and pulmonary artery are dilated, but the aortic knuckle is small.

Echocardiography will show the presence of aortic and pulmonary valves, but visualisation of the window itself may be difficult, particularly if it is small and positioned distally. Cardiac catheterisation indicates a shunt at pulmonary artery level and the catheter may pass from the pulmonary artery into the ascending aorta. Sometimes, with a larger or distal window, it appears to pass into the descending aorta in a position similar to that of a ductus. Aortography is the best investigation for the diagnosis of this condition accurately and will show rapid passage of contrast into the pulmonary arteries above the valve. The origin of the coronary arteries, which may be to the pulmonary side of the defect, and the pulmonary arterial branches should also be seen.

Differential Diagnosis. The main problem is to differentiate aortopulmonary window from persistent ductus arteriosus, ventricular septal defect with aortic incompetence, ruptured sinus of Valsalva and truncus arteriosus. This is difficult clinically, and aortography is usually required. The aortic knuckle is large in ductus, and passage of a catheter into the ascending aorta from the pulmonary artery may help to differentiate the two conditions. When severe pulmonary hypertension is present, truncus arteriosus may be particularly difficult to differentiate. In the latter, there is usually a shunt at ventricular level, the second sound is single and the origin of the pulmonary arteries may be unusually high with a deep pulmonary bay or absent main pulmonary trunk on the chest X-ray. Echocardiography and ventricular angiography will, however, demonstrate the presence of separate pulmonary and aortic outflow tracts in aortopulmonary window.

Indications for Operation. All patients in whom there is not already irreversible pulmonary vascular disease should undergo closure of an aortopulmonary window to prevent congestive heart failure, pulmonary vascular disease and endocarditis.

Principles of Treatment. Because there is no length to the connection, simple ligation, even of small aortopulmonary windows, does not reliably obliterate the communication. Separation of the two trunks is done with the support of the heart–lung bypass machine. In small windows this may be accomplished by detaching the aorta and pulmonary artery, while in those which are large or involve the valve sinuses a patch is sewn across the defect, usually through the pulmonary artery. Care is taken to leave the coronary artery ostia in free communication with the aorta. The window must be occluded at the start of bypass prior to cross-clamping of the aorta in order to prevent run-off into the lungs and distension of the heart.

Results. Operation leaves a normal cardiovascular system, and both early and late results are excellent if pulmonary vascular disease has not become established preoperatively.

Sinus of Valsalva Fistula

The right aortic sinus or the adjoining portion of the noncoronary sinus may have an area of weakness which allows a 'blow-out', producing an aneurysm of the sinus of Valsalva. When this ruptures into the heart, a fistula results. Oriental races are more commonly affected.

Anatomy. A lack of elastic and muscular elements in the aortic wall just above the attachment of the valve cusp results in an area of weakness which progressively distends. The right and non-coronary sinuses are most commonly involved, but aneurysms and fistulae have been seen in the left coronary sinus also. The aneurysm generally ruptures into the right ventricle or right atrium, characteristically with a 'wind-sock' projection into the cardiac chamber. Rarely, it communicates with the left ventricle. The length of the fistulous tract may be a

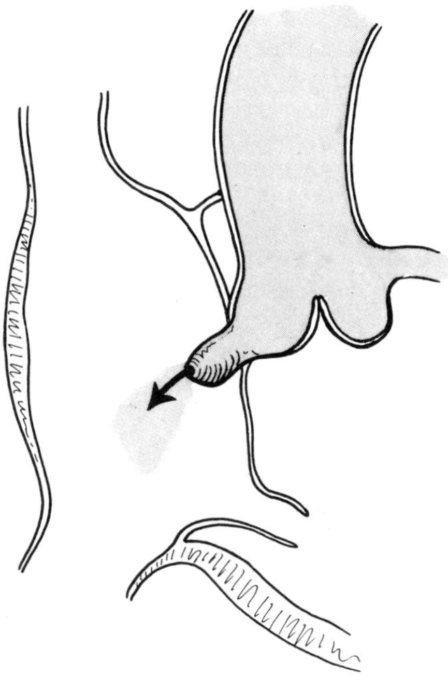

Fig. 6.46. Sinus of Valsalva fistula to the right atrium.

function of age, as the communication appears to be more direct when it is present at birth.

Haemodynamics. These will depend upon the chamber into which the fistula empties. There is a large left-to-right shunt if the communication is with the right atrium or right ventricle. Ventricular septal defect and valvar aortic incompetence are not infrequently associated with a sinus of valsalva fistula, in which case there may be additional volume overloading of the right or left ventricle, respectively.

Clinical Features. About half the cases present with mild symptoms of heart failure or an asymptomatic murmur. The other half experience a dramatic, sudden precordial pain followed by breathlessness and a loud murmur that may be audible without the aid of a stethoscope. This episode relates to actual rupture of the aneurysm with formation of a large fistula.

The murmur may be loud and continuous. It is often accompanied by a thrill and heard best to the right of the sternum. When only a diastolic murmur is heard, the fistula is either into a hypertensive right ventricle or the left ventricle.

The pulse tends to be collapsing and, in a right atrial fistula, there may be signs of right heart failure with an elevated venous pressure and pulsatile liver.

Special Investigations. Although pulmonary plethora may be present, the chest X-ray tends to be non-specific. The degree of cardiac enlargement reflects the size of the shunt, while the right atrium may be disproportionately big if the fistula enters this chamber.

Left ventricular or biventricular hypertrophy is seen on the ECG. Conduction disturbances may be produced by a lesion in proximity to the atrioventricular node, particularly with fistulae into the right ventricle and septum.

Echocardiography will confirm the clinical diagnosis, while cardiac catheterisation with angiography should establish the course of the fistula as well as the presence of any associated lesions.

Differential Diagnosis. The clinical history and physical findings are frequently sufficiently distinctive to make the diagnosis. Other lesions that cause continuous murmurs need to be considered, such as persistent ductus, coronary artery fistula and ventricular septal defect with aortic regurgitation. In some cases, these lesions may coexist. The more rare aortico-left ventricular tunnel tends to lay at right angles to the aorta, a feature which can be recognised in echocardiographic studies.

Indications for Operation. When present at birth, the fistula may be small and cause few symptoms. Rupture of an aneurysm usually occurs in the third or fourth decade, and most of these patients die of heart failure during the next 5 years. Both groups suffer a significant incidence of bacterial endocarditis and progressive aortic incompetence. Accordingly, closure is recommended in all cases.

Principles of Treatment. Closure of any fistula from its high pressure side is logical, and the sinus of Valsalva usually is repaired by suturing a patch into its aortic opening. The aortic valve is repaired if necessary, and other associated defects treated on their own merits. If the distal end of the wind-sock is approached in the right atrium, its proximity to the conduction tissue should be respected.

Results. Despite the high mortality that occurred in the initial phases of surgery for this lesion, it is now common to carry out successful repair, with a mortality approaching zero. Late complications are generally related to the presence of aortic valve incompetence.

Aortico-Left Ventricular Tunnel

This extremely rare condition is mentioned in order to differentiate it from sinus of Valsalva fistula. While both may produce a fistula between the aorta and the left ventricle, the aortic orifice of the tunnel is found more distally, beyond the sinus of Valsalva and represents a detachment of the base of the cusp. It presents as a characteristic cherry-like swelling at the base of the right coronary sinus and is invariably present at birth. Aortic flow into the left ventricle is considerable, and death from heart failure is usual during the first months of life in untreated cases. The right coronary artery may arise from the tunnel, which is the justification for some regarding this as a variant of coronary artery fistula. The diagnosis of aortico-left ventricular tunnel should be considered in all cases of apparent aortic regurgitation in young infants, since primary valve regurgitation in this age-group is uncommon. Closure of both ends of the tunnel is achieved through the cherry-like swelling and aims to prevent later development of aortic regurgitation or a left ventricular aneurysm.

'Gerbode' Defect

This term is used to refer to a group of situations in which there is shunting of blood from the left ventricle to the right atrium. Historically, when atrial septal defects were closed without the aid of cardiopulmonary bypass, it became apparent that a shunt that came from the left ventricle to the right atrium carried a very high surgical mortality. Thus, much interest centred upon diagnosing the condition preoperatively. It is now appreciated that three embryologically and anatomically distinct types of malformation may produce a communication and hence a shunt between the left ventricle and right atrium.

The most common situation is a membranous ventricular septal defect in association with one of a variety of tricuspid valve anomalies. These may range from an exaggerated commissure between septal and anterior tricuspid leaflets to a frank Ebstein's malformation.

The second group of conditions in which left ventricular to right atrial shunting is by no means uncommon are the atrioventricular septal defects. Here the 'cleft' in the valve or a deficiency of tissue overlies the left ventricle, permitting regurgitation of blood through the atrial septal defect into the right atrium. These two types are called 'infra-annular', because the malformation lies below the level of the tricuspid valve annulus.

The 'supra-annular' lesion is extremely rare. This is an isolated communication directly from the left ventricle, through the atrioventricular septum, into the right atrium. Unlike the other two, the ventricular septum is intact beneath the tricuspid valve.

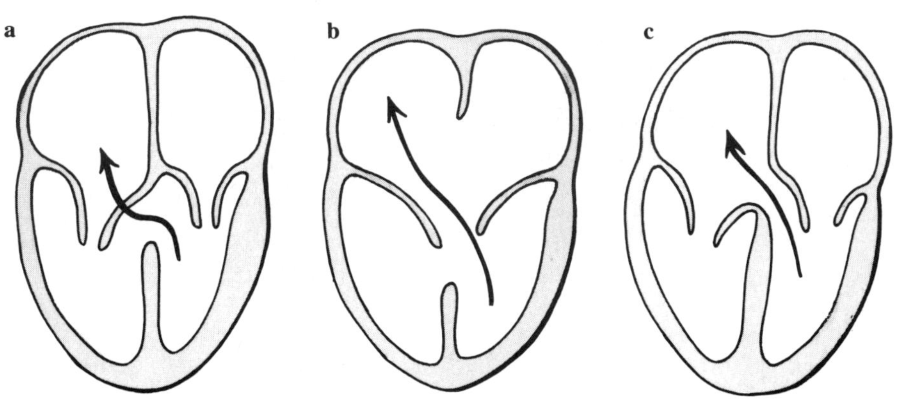

Fig. 6.47. Lesions that permit a left ventricular-to-right atrial shunt. VSD with abnormal tricuspid valve (**a**); atrioventricular septal defect (**b**); supra-annular defect (**c**).

Lesions Which may be Cyanotic or Acyanotic

The malformations in this group generally have a common mixing chamber, but, because of the variability in morphology, patients may either be cyanosed or not, depending upon streaming and shunting of blood within the heart or the amount of pulmonary blood flow. A given patient may also change from acyanotic to cyanotic during the evolution of the cardiac lesions.

Truncus Arteriosus (Common arterial trunk)

In this condition, there is a single great artery arising from the heart: this vessel gives off branches to the coronary, pulmonary and systemic circulations in the anterior mediastinum. A defect in the ventricular septum is also part of truncus arteriosus.

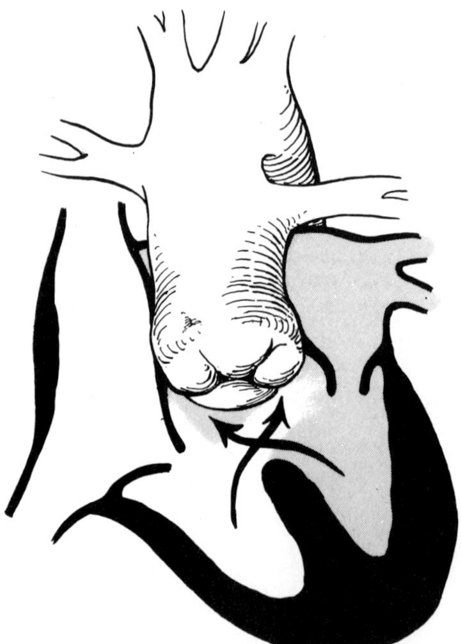

Fig. 6.48. Truncus arteriosus.

Anatomy. There is probably a failure of septation of the primitive truncus arteriosus, such that the pulmonary arteries arise from the common trunk as remnants of the sixth branchial arch. Hence, the alternative names for this condition: 'persistent truncus arteriosus', 'common aorticopulmonary trunk'.

Based upon the origin of the pulmonary arteries, truncus arteriosus is subdivided into three types. In type I, a short branch arises from the leftward side of the aorta and divides into right and left pulmonary arteries. Each branch arises from a separate orifice, but they are still close together in type II, while in type III, the orifices are widely separated. The so-called Type IV or 'pseudotruncus' is now recognised to be a variant of pulmonary atresia with ventricular septal defect in which collateral vessels to the lung are given off from the descending aorta.

The single arterial outlet ('truncus') usually arises from the left ventricle but may sit astride the ventricular septal defect or come off the right ventricle. Its valve has three or four cusps, and a degree of dysplasia giving rise to stenosis or regurgitation is not uncommon.

A ventricular septal defect is invariably present. Usually it has a muscular rim and lies immediately beneath the truncal valve. Less commonly, the defect extends to the tricuspid valve and then has relations with the conduction tissue as found in other membranous ventricular septal defects (see Ventricular Septal Defect).

Haemodynamics. Mixing of blood occurs at ventricular level across the ventricular septal defect, so that the peripheral arterial blood is desaturated. However, there is such a heavy blood flow from the aorta directly into the lung fields that the clinical picture is virtually one of a large left-to-right shunt and the desaturation of the blood is largely obscured. When there is severe stenosis or incompetence of the truncal valve, the equivalent of left and right ventricular outflow obstruction or combined aortic and pulmonary regurgitation are superimposed.

Clinical Features. These patients are not markedly cyanosed, unless the pulmonary vascular resistance is high. They present with features common to all cases of a large left-to-right shunt. Signs favouring a diagnosis of truncus arteriosus are a clear second heart sound arising from the common valve and the absence of a prominent main pulmonary artery on the chest radiograph. In fact, the combination of a sabot-shaped heart with plethoric lung fields and high pulmonary arteries should always raise the question of truncus arteriosus, particularly if there is a right-sided aortic arch. Other defects with a large left-to-right shunt and prominent lung markings are usually assciated with a prominent pulmonary artery shadow.

Special Investigations. The chest X-ray has been mentioned above. The ECG features are non-specific. Real-time echocardiography can demonstrate the single arterial trunk; in small infants, usually the pulmonary artery origins can also be seen. The ventricular septal defect is said to be so consistent in truncus arteriosus that further investigations are unnecessary. Cardiac catheterisation and, particularly angiography, not infrequently tip the haemodynamic balance in an already compromised ventricular myocardium. Their potential value must be carefully balanced against the possibility of precipitating massive pulmonary congestion and low cardiac output with consequent elevation of operative risks. If there is a possibility of associated defects, it is probably best to carry out catheterisation early, before the pulmonary vascular resistance falls and the myocardium suffers from a low diastolic perfusion pressure, rather than waiting for clinical deterioration.

Differential Diagnosis. Clinically, this condition may resemble aortopulmonary window, pulmonary atresia with ventricular septal defect and massive collateral flow, and older patients with ventricular septal defect and aortic incompetence. Real-time echocardiography is invaluable for differentiating between them, particularly in the sick infant.

Indications for Operation. Patients with truncus arteriosus do not improve, and half will die of congestive heart failure in the first month of life. The remainder will acquire severe pulmonary vascular disease, usually during childhood. Operation, even though it carries considerable risk, should be advised for almost any patient who does not have advanced pulmonary vascular changes.

Principles of Treatment. The pulmonary arteries are separated from the aorta and connected to the right ventricle by means of a valved extracardiac conduit. Closure of the ventricular septal defect and the defect in the truncus produced by detachment of the pulmonary arteries completes the repair. An alternative is to reduce run-off to the lungs by banding each pulmonary artery, but this makes the subsequent correction more complicated and carries much the same risk as complete primary correction.

Results. Survival of 80%–90% has now been achieved for truncus arteriosus in some centres, although repair in the first weeks or in the presence of severe truncal valve incompetence may carry a much greater mortality. Interestingly, however, some centres have demonstrated improved survival by elective operation in the neonatal period, before malnourishment, infection, and pulmonary damage have set in. Survivors generally outgrow the right ventricle-to-pulmonary artery conduit in a few years, and occasionally repair or replacement of the truncal valve also becomes necessary later in life.

Corrected Transposition
(Atrioventricular discordance with ventriculoarterial discordance)

Congenitally corrected transposition of the great vessels is a malformation in which transposition of the great arteries (ventriculoarterial discordance) is physiologically rectified by the concurrent presence of atrioventricular discordance.

Anatomy. The morphological right atrium is connected to the morphological left ventricle, which gives off the pulmonary artery, and the morphological left atrium is connected to the morphological right ventricle, giving off the aorta. The atrioventricular valves follow the ventricular morphology; thus, the systemic ventricle has a 'tricuspid' valve, and the pulmonary ventricle, a 'mitral' valve. Abnormalities of cardiac position are common in this malformation, including dextrocardia, situs inversus and 'upstairs-downstairs' ventricles. The conduction tissue usually connects with an anterior node.

Although corrected transposition may exist without other cardiac abnormalities, it is the rule to have one or more associated defects. These included ventricular septal defect, left ventricular outflow obstruction (pulmonary stenosis), atrial septal defect or left atrioventricular valve malformations. In addition, the elongated course of the conduction tissue predisposes to fibrosis, and spontaneous complete heart block is not uncommon.

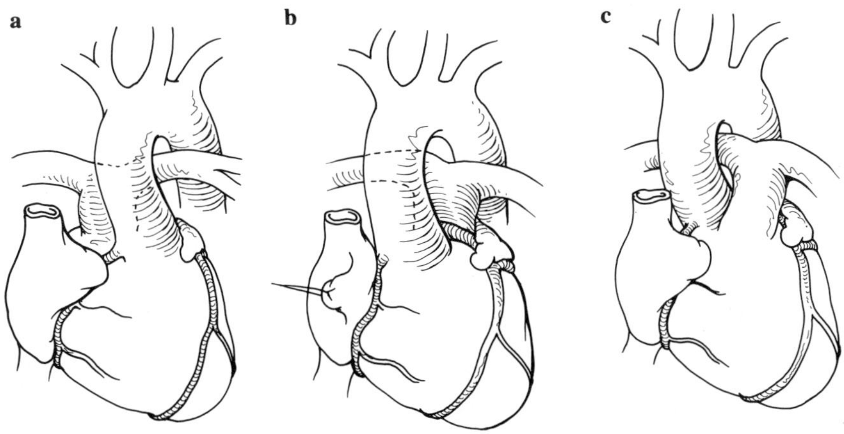

Fig. 6.49. Normal heart (**c**) compared with the great vessels in simple transposition (**b**) and corrected transposition (**a**).

Haemodynamics. In uncomplicated cases, venous return from the body enters the right atrium and flows across the morphological mitral valve ('right atrioventricular valve') into the left ventricle. It is then pumped to the pulmonary artery, and oxygenated blood returns to the left atrium to pass across the morphological tricuspid valve ('left atrioventricular valve') and into the right ventricle. From here it is pumped to the aorta. The systemic and pulmonary circulations are thus in series, and haemodynamics are physiologically correct, although the systemic circulation is supported by a morphological right ventricle.

The left atrioventricular valve, being designed for the low pressure pulmonary circulation, tends to suffer in the systemic circulation and also may be intrinsically abnormal (similar to an Ebstein's malformation). It is not uncommon for left atrioventricular valve incompetence to develop which is equivalent to mitral regurgitation in a normally connected heart.

Ventricular septal defects occur frequently and usually are large. It is not unusual for there to be a degree of pulmonary stenosis, which may be valvar, subvalvar or due to the abnormally positioned left ventricular outflow tract. It is the relative contributions of these two lesions which determines the prevailing haemodynamic state. Severe pulmonary stenosis will produce right-to-left shunting with decreased pulmonary blood flow and arterial desaturation, while a large ventricular septal defect in the absence of pulmonary stenosis results in left-to-right shunting.

Clinical Features. In the absence of associated lesions, patients may remain asymptomatic, an abnormal heart shadow being found on the chest radiograph. Infants may present with a large left-to-right shunt and heart failure or cyanosis, although it is uncommon for either to be severe before one year of age. Occasionally, the presentation is a slow heartbeat due to complete heart block.

The murmurs and other physical signs tend to reflect associated lesions. The anteriorly placed aorta may give rise to an unusually loud second heart sound, which should not be confused with the accentuated pulmonary component in pulmonary hypertension.

Special Investigations. Conduction defects are common, and the ECG may show first or second degree heart block, complete atrioventricular dissociation or Wolff–Parkinson–White syndrome. The chest X-ray shows the left sided ascending aorta, but this can be seen also in other complex congenital anomalies.

On echocardiography, this is one condition which produces atrioventricular valves at the same level, and it is possible also to demonstrate discordance between the atrioventricular connections and the ventriculoarterial connections. The definitive morphological and haemodynamic diagnoses are provided by cardiac catheterisation with cineangiography.

Differential Diagnosis. Corrected transposition with a large ventricular septal defect may be difficult to differentiate from a univentricular heart, even after complete invasive studies; indeed, this may be more a question of definition than diagnosis in some cases. Simple or complex transposition can usually be excluded by echocardiography, but when there are positional anomalies, this may be difficult.

Indications for Operation. When pulmonary stenosis and ventricular septal defect are present with corrected transposition, operation is undertaken to relieve hypoxia in the first instance, and to correct the circulation subsequently. The indications for closure of a ventricular septal defect or left atrioventricular valve replacement are similar to those in patients without corrected transposition. Bradycardia accompanied by syncope or heart failure may necessitate cardiac pacing, while tachyarrythmias from associated Wolff–Parkinson–White syndrome are treated pharmacologically or by ablation of the accessory conducting pathways.

Principles of Treatment. The positional abnormalities of the great vessels and cardiac chambers may complicate access to what would be a surgically straightforward undertaking in other circumstances. Also, the position of the conduction tissue limits the use of some techniques.

Thus, closure of a ventricular septal defect in a heart with atrioventricular discordance by placement of a patch within the pulmonary ventricle usually causes heart block because the conduction system (in the morphological left ventricle) lies beneath the suture line. Modifications must be used to place the patch in the systemic (morphological right) ventricle, but this, in turn, may be complicated by limited access (the usual right ventricular incision being undesirable in the systemic pumping chamber) or injury to the systemic atrioventricular valve. While closure of a ventricular septal defect in this condition is possible during infancy, these problems may favour pulmonary artery banding to protect the lungs early in life and subsequent secondary repair at 2–3 years of age.

Similarly, direct relief of pulmonary stenosis is rarely possible, due to the posterior position of the pulmonary artery and proximity of the conduction tissue. Patients who require augmentation of pulmonary blood flow are generally managed by systemic pulmonary artery anastomosis early in life and placement of a valved extracardiac conduit between the left ventricle and pulmonary arteries at about 6 years of age.

Left atrioventricular valve incompetence generally necessitates valve replacement because the morphological tricuspid valve does not lend itself to repair on the high pressure side of the heart. When a pacemaker is needed, it may be necessary to affix leads to the surface of the heart for an 'epicardial' system. This is because the smooth-walled left ventricle which would be accessible for placement of a lead through the venous system, may not permit secure fixation. In response to some of the problems which occur with a systemic right ventricle and the left atrioventricular valve, a more aggressive surgical approach has been advocated recently. This involves combining atrial redirection (Mustard or Senning operation) with either tunnelling of the morphologic left ventricle to the aorta and a right-ventricle-to-pulmonary artery conduit or an arterial switch procedure (see Transposition). In the end, the left ventricle and mitral valve support the systemic circulation.

Results. In general, the risks of a repair in cases with atrioventricular discordance are higher than in normally connected hearts, and early mortality is about 10%. There is also a continued late mortality, such that only about 60%–70% of patients remain alive 10 years after operation.

Double Outlet Right Ventricle

This is a type of connection between the heart and the great arteries in which one great vessel and at least half of the other arise from the morphological right ventricle. As such, it includes an extensive spectrum of cardiac defects, including those with two functional pumping chambers, single ventricle and isomeric hearts.

Anatomy. From the surgeon's point of view, the important features are the size and location of the ventricular septal defect, the position of the great vessels and the relationship between the great vessels and the ventricular septal defect.

The great vessels may be positioned side-by-side, anterior–posterior or in a more or less normal relationship. The aorta may be anterior, to the left or posterior to the pulmonary artery, and either one or both great vessels may be supported by a complete muscular conus.

A ventricular septal defect is nearly always present. This is said to be 'restrictive' if its size is small and there is a pressure gradient across it. The defect may be in proximity to the aorta ('subaortic'), the pulmonary artery ('subpulmonary'), both great arteries ('doubly committed') or neither ('noncommitted'). It may be classified also according to the usual morphological criteria as membranous, muscular, and so forth, independent of the origin of the great vessels.

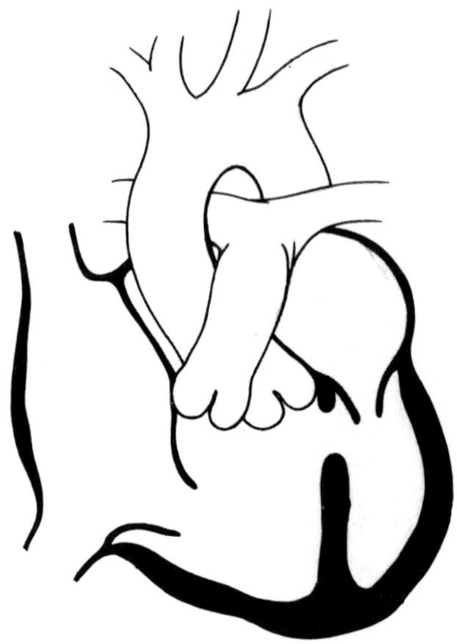

Fig. 6.50. Double outlet right ventricle.

Haemodynamics. The haemodynamic picture depends upon streaming of blood within the heart as well as the prevailing left-to-right or right-to-left shunts. When the ventricular septal defect is restrictive, the left ventricle builds up pressure to discharge its contents into the right ventricle, as this is its only outlet. Left ventricular pressure may exceed the systemic pressure in this situation, and left atrial pressure may be elevated as a result. When there is a large ventricular septal defect, pressures on the left and right side will be equal, and the ratio of systemic and pulmonary flow will depend upon their respective resistances or obstructions, including such factors as aortic coarctation and pulmonary stenosis. The determinants of oxygen saturation, however, may be more complex. Streaming of systemic venous return into the pulmonary artery, in cases with subpulmonary ventricular septal defect, may cause severe hypoxia even though overall flow to the lungs is increased.

Clinical Features. The presentation will reflect the amount of pulmonary blood flow, which in turn depends upon the underlying morphology. When pulmonary stenosis is present, the clinical course may resemble that of Fallot's tetralogy, while a large ventricular septal defect without restrictions of pulmonary blood flow causes heart failure with a large left-to-right shunt. Both heart failure and cyanosis tend to be present when the ventricular septal defect is subpulmonary, and these patients tend to have 'transposition' physiology.

Special Investigations. While the chest X-ray and ECG may give clues to the diagnosis, detailed investigation with real-time echocardiography and cardiac catheterisation is usually necessary to establish the exact diagnosis. In borderline cases, it may still be difficult to distinguish double outlet right ventricle from Fallot's tetralogy, transposition of the great vessels with ventricular septal defect and a large ventricular septal defect.

Differential Diagnosis. This includes almost any cardiac malformation, given the spectrum of intracardiac anatomy which may be associated with double outlet right ventricle.

Indications for Operation. These follow the general guidelines of the closely related cardiac malformations. Thus, in double outlet right ventricle, normally related great vessels and pulmonary stenosis, the clinical situation is very similar to Fallot's tetralogy, and treatment may be needed for severe or increasing cyanosis. Congestive heart failure and increased pulmonary arterial pressure will be the reason for operation in patients with large ventricular septal defect and unprotected lungs, while those with transposition physiology may require improved mixing to relieve hypoxia.

Principles of Treatment. In general, the ideal surgical solution is to route the blood from the left ventricle into the systemic circulation, while providing an unobstructed pathway for flow from the right ventricle into the pulmonary arteries. With normally related great vessels, this may simply involve an intracardiac tunnel between a subaortic ventricular septal defect and the aorta. However, with anterior–posterior great vessels and a subpulmonary ventricular septal defect, the Dacron patch would leave the left ventricle connected to the pulmonary artery and it would then be necessary to also 'switch' the great vessels or perform an interatrial redirection of blood flow to separate the circulations. Restrictive and noncommitted ventricular septal defects tend to pose the more complex surgical problems. Occasionally, a satisfactory two-ventricle repair is not possible, and a Fontan type of procedure is carried out.

Results. These depend upon the type of malformation and, in some cases, the type of operation carried out. For the ventricular septal defect end of the spectrum, creation of an intraventricular tunnel carries a mortality of less than 5%. Repair of the Fallot-like lesions also has a low operative risk. In more complex anomalies, such as the Taussig–Bing heart, there is a 15%–25% mortality. Occasional reoperation may be needed to relieve obstruction within an intraventricular tunnel or to replace an extracardiac conduit.

Double Outlet Left Ventricle

This is an extremely rare and complex malformation in which both great arteries arise from the left ventricle. The right ventricle may be underdeveloped, but the left ventricle is always well formed. Surgical repair is possible by closure of the ventricular septal defect and connecting the right ventricle to the pulmonary arteries by means of a valved extracardiac conduit, or in some cases, by a Fontan type operation.

Single Ventricle
(Univentricular atrioventricular connection; univentricular heart)

The definition of a 'single ventricle' remains controversial, as does its proper nomenclature. The concept of a single ventricle is that the heart possesses one

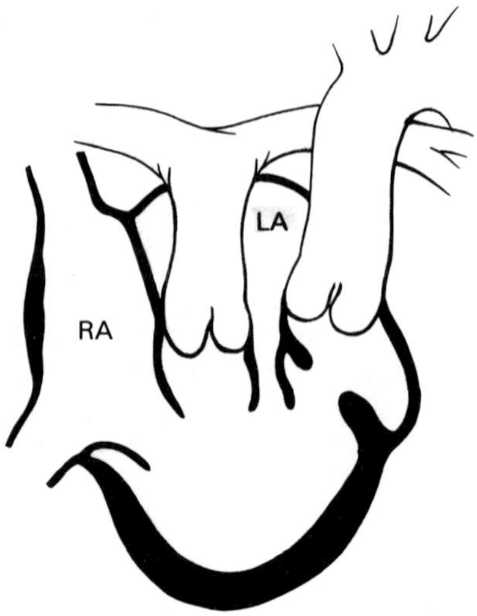

Fig. 6.51. In the most common type of single ventricle, the pulmonary artery arises from the main (left) ventricular chamber, and the aorta from a small outlet chamber.

effective pumping chamber. One atrioventricular valve and most of another are committed to this chamber. In fact, a second, smaller chamber is usually present.

Anatomy. Hearts that have 'single ventricle' tend to have other complex features, and sequential chamber analysis is useful for their description.

Based upon the trabecular pattern of the dominant chamber, the ventricle is said to be left, right or indeterminate (the so-called 'primitive' ventricle). The smaller chamber is of the opposite morphology and may give off one or more great arteries. Thus, the ventriculoarterial connection can be concordant, discordant or double outlet. When the small chamber is of right ventricular morphology, it tends to be found on the front of the heart. Those of left ventricular morphology are usually posterior.

In the most common type of univentricular atrioventricular connection, left and right atria are connected to a morphological left ventricle by way of mitral and tricuspid valves. The dominant left ventricle gives off the pulmonary artery directly, and there may or may not be associated pulmonary stenosis. The smaller, morphological right ventricle is on the left anterior aspect of the heart and connected to the left ventricle through a ventricular septal defect or 'outlet foramen'. This small chamber gives off the aorta, such that there is ventriculoarterial discordance. Narrowing of the ventricular septal defect or heavy trabeculations within the right ventricular outlet chamber will produce the equivalent of left ventricular outflow obstruction or subaortic stenosis in a normally connected heart.

Haemodynamics. The prevailing haemodynamic picture will be determined largely by the presence of pulmonary or aortic stenosis. Some patients will have excessive pulmonary blood flow and pulmonary hypertension, while others will have the extreme of pulmonary atresia and depend upon a persistent ductus arteriosus for perfusion of the lungs. Within the heart, there may be favourable streaming of systemic and pulmonary venous return to the pulmonary artery and aorta, respectively, such that oxygen saturations are nearly normal. Conversely, unfavourable streaming causes a picture similar to simple transposition of the great arteries, with severe arterial desaturation. The presence of stenosis or incompetence of one or the other atrioventricular valve (or a common atrioventricular valve) or coarctation of the aorta may further complicate the haemodynamic picture.

Clinical Features. As can be inferred from the haemodynamics, this ranges from cases that resemble a large ventricular septal defect, to those that present with severe cyanosis. Occasionally the haemodynamics are balanced, and such patients may reach the fifth or sixth decade without complaints of cardiac disease.

Special Investigations. Echocardiography is usually necessary to make a diagnosis of single ventricle, while cardiac catheterisation with angiography is required for precise definition of morphology and haemodynamics.

Differential Diagnosis. The conditions most likely to be confused with single ventricle are Fallot's tetralogy, which resembles the Holmes heart, and corrected transposition with a large ventricular septal defect.

Indications for Operation. Few patients with single ventricle will survive childhood without operation. Surgery is undertaken to control pulmonary blood flow, relieve congestive heart failure, encourage development of the pulmonary arteries, improve systemic oxygenation or to relieve obstruction to systemic blood flow.

Principles of Treatment. Cases of single ventricle, should, in theory, be correctable by either septation of the main chamber or a Fontan type of operation, and management should be planned with one of these options as the eventual goal.

Partititioning of the dominant ventricle can be done only if the two atrioventricular valves are separate and the chamber is large enough to be divided into two portions. In general, this will be in patients who have had excessive pulmonary blood flow. A Fontan type of repair gives both ventricles to the systemic circulation, and systemic venous blood is conveyed directly to the pulmonary arteries. In order for this to be successful, there must be good development of the pulmonary arteries with a low vascular resistance, competent atrioventricular valve mechanisms and good ventricular function. In general, patients with reduced pulmonary blood flow are better candidates for the Fontan operation. It may be necessary to carry out pulmonary artery banding or systemic pulmonary anastomoses to relieve symptoms early in life or to prepare the circulation for one or the other of these procedures.

Results. The septation operation can, under ideal circumstances, be accomplished with a hospital mortality of around 10%, and exercise tolerance is generally good, although not normal, for these patients. About half will acquire heart block as the result of the operation and need a permanent pacemaker.

There is still, to date, a significant late mortality and incidence of reoperation following septation, with about 50%–60% survival 5 years after operation.

The early mortality for the Fontan type of repair in single ventricle has thus far been 20%–30% in most centres, but late deaths appear to be rather less common, with about 80%–90% surviving another 3 years. Very late results are not yet available for this procedure, but exercise tolerance appears to be maintained in most survivors.

Congenital Anomalies of the Coronary Arteries

It is sometimes forgotten that 'coronary artery disease' may occur in the infant and young child. Although it does not always result in the classical adult picture of ischaemic myocardium, these anomalies still cause severe cardiac disability or complicate the repair of other congenital malformations. They are thus outlined briefly below.

Anomalous Origin of the Left Coronary Artery from the Pulmonary Artery

In this condition, the left coronary is given off from the pulmonary artery. The high pulmonary vascular resistance at birth maintains antegrade perfusion,

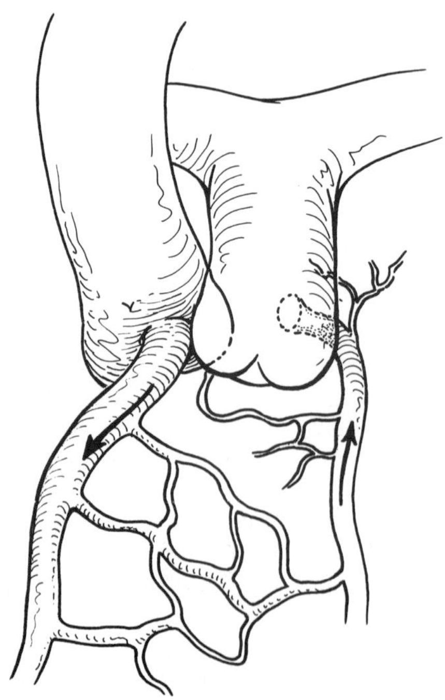

Fig. 6.52. Anomalous origin of the left coronary artery from the pulmonary artery.

albeit with desaturated blood. As pulmonary resistance falls, flow reverses and the left coronary may steal blood by shunting from the myocardium into the pulmonary artery. Survival probably depends upon the development of collateral vessels. Myocardial infarction is not uncommon, but murmurs are generally not present until the onset of ischaemic mitral regurgitation. Thus diagnosis is often delayed.

Surgery is probably best directed toward the re-establishment of a two-coronary artery system, although obliteration of the coronary steal by ligation of the anomalous vessel in older patients with well-developed collateral vessels may be beneficial. The anomalous left coronary artery may either be excised from the pulmonary artery and transferred to the empty aortic sinus, or aortic blood may be tunnelled to it through a small aortopulmonary connection. Despite extensive impairment of left ventricular function, survival of 80%–90% has been achieved, and there appears to be potential for myocardial recovery in young infants. Occasionally, mitral valve replacement is also necessary.

Coronary Artery Fistula

A communication between a coronary artery and one of the cardiac chambers or the coronary sinus produce a continuous murmur and may lead to symptoms of congestive heart failure. Bacterial endocarditis may also occur in relation to the turbulent blood flow. Occasionally the coronary artery proximal to the fistula reaches aneurysmal proportions, and multiple fistulae may also occur.

Closure is usually undertaken with the support of cardiopulmonary bypass, although small communications at the termination of the coronary may be closed by ligation. Early survival and late results are generally excellent.

Single Sinus Origin and Single Coronary Artery

These rare anomalies are usually incidental findings in hearts with normally connected great vessels, although a left coronary artery arising from the right sinus may be compressed by aortic dilatation during exercise and lead to left ventricular ischaemia in an otherwise healthy young person.

Single sinus origin is not uncommon in cases of transposed great arteries with ventricular septal defect. Its importance lies in the fact that direct transfer of the coronary as part of the arterial switch operation will cause kinking of the coronary vessel. Several techniques have been described to deal effectively with this problem.

Origin of the Left Anterior Descending Coronary from the Right Coronary Artery

When this variation is found in association with Fallot's tetralogy, it will limit the use of a transannular patch and the site of a ventriculotomy. In some cases, it becomes necessary to use a valved extracardiac conduit.

Further Reading

Jordan SC, Scott O. Heart disease in paediatrics, 3rd edn. Butterworths, London, 1989
Lock JE, Keane JF, Fellows KE. The use of catheter intervention procedures for congenital heart disease. J Am Coll Cardiol 1986; 7: 1420–1423
Stark J, deLeval M (eds). Surgery for congenital heart defects. Grune & Stratton, London, 1983

Chapter 7

Acquired Valvular Heart Disease

Included under this heading are inflammatory and degenerative conditions involving the cardiac valves. Similar lesions involving the myocardium and pericardium are considered in subsequent chapters, while traumatic lesions of the valves are included in the section on cardiac trauma.

By far the most common of the inflammatory lesions in most parts of the world is rheumatic carditis. This affects the endocardium, myocardium and pericardium, but it is surgically important chiefly as a result of the valve (endocardial) lesions. The mitral valve is most often affected, with the aortic next in frequency, followed by the tricuspid and pulmonary valves, in that order.

Other less common inflammatory lesions like tuberculosis may involve the pericardium and give rise to constrictive pericarditis, while syphilis may result in dilatation of the aortic valve ring and stenosis of the coronary artery ostia.

Mitral Valve Disease

Mitral Stenosis

Acquired obstructive lesions of the mitral valve are virtually all of rheumatic aetiology. Even though prompt treatment of streptococcal infections has decreased the incidence of rheumatic fever in some parts of the world, rheumatic mitral valve disease is by no means uncommon and may also cause considerable disability in children and young adults.

Pathology. During the healing phase of rheumatic valvitis it is likely that the valve commissures become adherent initially at the point of insertion of the papillary muscles; this was first described by Brock. Adherence at this point leaves a central pathway approximately 1.25×0.50 cm in diameter, and through this orifice the left atrial blood must flow to reach the left ventricle.

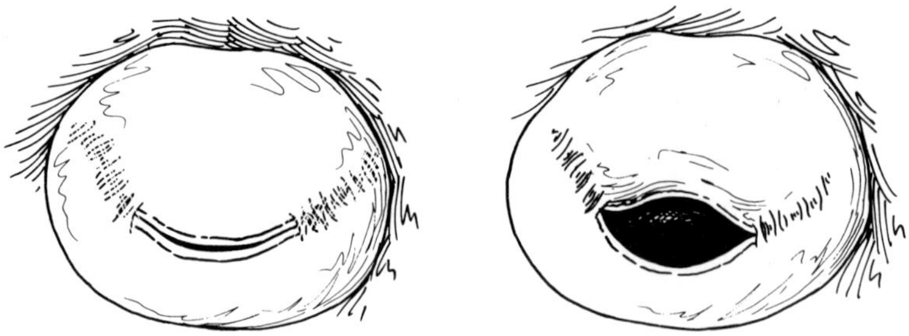

Fig. 7.1. Stenosis of the mitral valve.

Depending upon the severity of the inflammatory process, there will be a greater or lesser degree of scarring of the valve and, consequently, there may be gross thickening of the cusps, areas of calcification or loss of valve substance. Moreover, the valve ring and adjacent atrium may be involved in the scarring and an important feature which bears on the success of conservative surgery is the degree of thickening. The chordae may form an almost solid and funnel-shaped scar, resulting in a rigid, secondary subvalvar orifice. These rigid valves are unable to close in systole, so there will often be a mixture of stenosis and regurgitation. Valve orifices greater than 1 cm^2 probably do not give rise to severe symptoms of obstruction and cases coming to operation usually have valve openings smaller than this.

Haemodynamics. As a result of the narrow mitral orifice, there will be an obstruction to the passage of blood from the left atrium to left ventricle during diastole. The right ventricle overcomes this obstruction quite easily by increasing

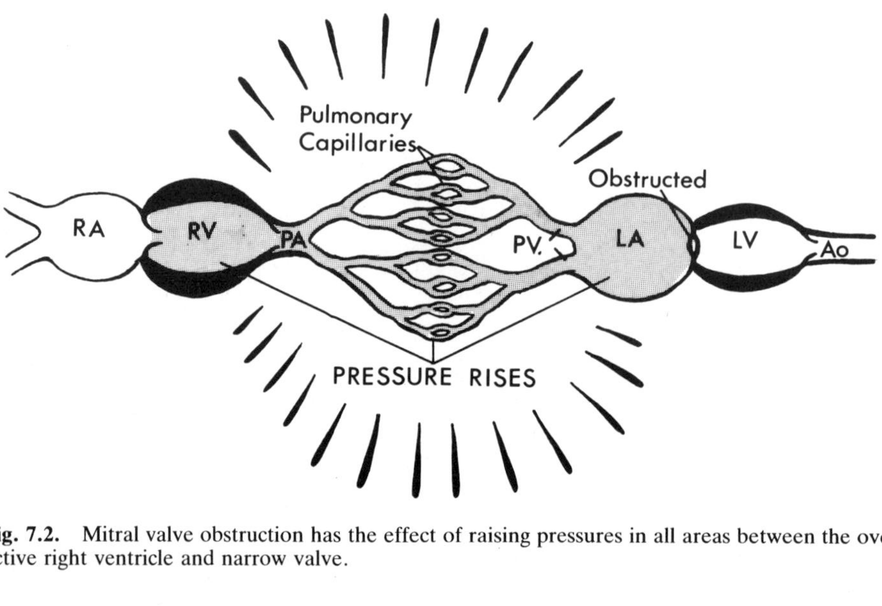

Fig. 7.2. Mitral valve obstruction has the effect of raising pressures in all areas between the over-active right ventricle and narrow valve.

its force of contraction and, consequently, the pressure gradient across the mitral valve. This results in a rise in left atrial pressure.

In addition, the pressure in the pulmonary vascular bed intervening between the overactive right ventricle and the obstructed left atrium will rise. As a result, the lungs become stiff and the patient must do more work to ventilate the lungs. In other words, he becomes conscious of his breathing, which means that he is dyspnoeic.

In some cases, possibly as a result of reflexes from the pulmonary veins or arterioles, the pulmonary capillaries are 'protected' against a sudden rise of pressure which would precipitate pulmonary oedema. This protection is brought about by an increased resistance in the pulmonary arterioles proximal to the vulnerable lung capillaries, a form of pulmonary hypertension. As a result of the increase in the pulmonary vascular resistance, the right ventricle must work against this additional obstruction; ultimately, this results in right ventricular failure manifested by distended peripheral veins, engorged liver, peripheral oedema, and ascites.

Frank pulmonary oedema, when it occurs, is a result of fluid passing from the pulmonary capillaries into the pulmonary interstitial space and alveoli. The hydrostatic and colloid osmotic pressures acting on the alveolar capillary membrane have been summarised by Fishman's modification of Starling's law, as follows:

$$F = \mathrm{k}(P_c - p_c - P_{if} + p_{if}),$$

where F is fluid flux across the alveolar capillary membrane; k is a permeability factor of the alveolar capillary membrane; P_c and P_{if} are the hydrostatic pressure within the capillaries and pulmonary interstitial space, respectively; and p_c and p_{if} are plasma colloid osmotic pressure and colloid osmotic pressure within the pulmonary interstitial space, respectively.

This equation is applicable to all forms of cardiac pulmonary oedema.

A serious complication of rheumatic mitral valve disease is the onset of atrial fibrillation and this may often herald the onset of symptoms. This, together with enlargement of the left atrium, predisposes to the formation of clots, which are likely to be disseminated as cerebral and peripheral emboli. Bacterial endocarditis is a further hazard.

Clinical Features. The disease is more common in women and a clear history of rheumatic fever is not invariable. Symptoms do not, as a rule, come on until early adult life and may be precipitated by an illness or pregnancy. In many instances they date from the onset of atrial fibrillation.

Typically, there is progressive dyspnoea on effort, at first only with unusual exertion, but later restricting day-to-day activities. With the dyspnoea comes cough, a history of winter 'bronchitis' and haemoptysis. These episodes may vary from an occasional streak of blood associated with the bronchitic episodes to copious bright red 'pulmonary apoplexy'. Infarction of the lung is another cause of haemoptysis, but the most ominous form is the pink, frothy sputum of frank pulmonary oedema. There may be recurrent episodes of paroxysmal nocturnal dypsnoea or, more dramatically, the disease may be ushered in with bacterial endocarditis or with embolic occlusion of the cerebral or peripheral arteries.

On examination, these patients are usually thin and have a slightly cyanotic or ruddy 'mitral' facies. They are often orthopnoeic and cannot comfortably lie flat upon the examination couch. The pulse is small in volume and the hands are cold, reflecting the low cardiac output. Engorged neck veins may reveal evidence of right heart failure. There may be an *a* wave of pulmonary hypertension or a systolic venous pulsation from functional tricuspid regurgitation. The apex beat has a tapping quality, and a diastolic thrill can frequently be felt. In addition, one can sometimes feel the closing shock of the mitral valve, that is, a palpable first heart sound. To the left of the sternum an over-active right ventricle is often palpable.

On auscultation, a loud first sound is audible at the apex. The normal second sound is closely followed by a sharp opening snap and a low-pitched rumbling diastolic murmur, which may continue into the first sound with presystolic accentuation. At the base of the heart, there may be an easily heard pulmonary component of the second sound, dependent for its intensity upon the degree of pulmonary hypertension.

The opening snap is thought to indicate the presence of pliable valve cusps. It is lost in some cases with mitral incompetence and where the valve is calcified or rigid.

Special Investigations. The radiograph of the heart shows a small aorta with an enlarged pulmonary artery, a right ventricular contour and small left ventricle. The hypertrophied dense left atrial shadow can usually be seen through the superimposed cardiac shadow. Rarely, evidence of calcification in the mitral valve area may be seen. The lung fields are moderately congested and may show Kerley B-lines in the costophrenic angles. Where recurrent haemoptyses have occurred, haemosiderosis of the lung fields may be prominent.

The ECG can be diagnostic, showing a widened and double-peaked P-mitrale. There may also be evidence of moderate right ventricular hypertrophy. In the presence of left ventricular hypertrophy, one should consider the possibility of associated or dominant mitral regurgitation, aortic valve disease, or systemic hypertension.

M-Mode echocardiography shows thickened leaflets with impaired mobility and left atrial enlargement. The severity of the stenosis is reflected by flatness of the E-F slope, and the degree of fibrosis and calcification by the density of the echoes from the mitral valve. Real-time echocardiography demonstrates leaflet movement and any calcification, while an estimate of the gradient across the valve can be made from Doppler echocardiography.

In difficult cases, cardiac catheterisation may supply additional information regarding the diastolic left atrial-to-left ventricular gradient and degree of pulmonary hypertension, but this investigation is used more often in the assessment of mixed mitral stenosis and regurgitation. Patients of more than 40 years of age may have associated coronary artery disease, which should also be investigated preoperatively.

Differential Diagnosis. An important condition to distinguish from mitral stenosis is atrial septal defect. Both lesions are more common in women and are likely to cause symptoms at about 30–40 years of age. The chest radiograph and ECG can be remarkably similar, as can some of the physical signs. A soft and widely spaced opening snap may be confused with the wide, fixed second sound of atrial septal defect. Also, in atrial septal defect, there may be a short tricuspid diastolic murmur not unlike a mitral stenotic rumble. With careful attention to clinical signs and the X-ray, and with the aid of echocardiography, it should rarely be necessary to have to recourse to catheterisation to make the distinction.

Other causes of a mitral diastolic 'flow' murmur are persistent ductus arteriosus and ventricular septal defect. Both have left ventricular dominance, and the other distinguishing features are usually clear.

A myxoma within the left atrium may mimic mitral stenosis very closely. Indeed, prior to the advent of echocardiography, a number of cases were discovered at operation for presumed mitral stenosis. The tumour is very soft and friable, such that a history of systemic emboli, particularly in the absence of atrial fibrillation, should suggest the possibility of myxoma. The diagnosis is usually clear on real-time echocardiography.

A pedunculated ball-valve thrombus in the left atrium may also give rise to typical features of mitral stenosis, but the sign may be variable and impaction of the thrombus in the mitral valve can give rise to syncopal attacks.

Cor triatriatum can present a picture indistinguishable from mitral stenosis, but without the associated findings on the ECG or chest radiograph. A correct preoperative diagnosis is usually possible, again, with the aid of real-time echocardiography. Supravalvar mitral ring, however, may not be appreciated until visualised directly at operation.

Where mitral stenosis is associated with marked pulmonary hypertension, the characteristic auscultatory features tend to be obscured and are replaced by those of pulmonary hypertension. That is, the long mitral diastolic murmur is reduced in length or lost while the right ventricle becomes dominant and the pulmonary element of the second sound is accentuated. Also, the raised pressure on the right side of the heart is likely to be associated with the development of functional tricuspid, and possibly pulmonary, regurgitation. The systolic murmur of the former condition may then be confused with mitral regurgitation, and the significance of the mitral valve lesion is further masked. Furthermore, the pulmonary regurgitant murmur is often confused with the murmur of aortic regurgitation and an otherwise deserving case of severe stenosis may be rejected for surgery on the grounds of free mitral and aortic regurgitation. Fortunately, improved diagnostic techniques, as well as the surgeon's capacity to manage double valve disease with the aid of cardiopulmonary bypass, make this occurrence unlikely.

Mitral regurgitation occurring as an isolated phenomenon should not be confused with mitral stenosis, although both may have a diastolic murmur. Unfortunately, when the two conditions are present as a mixed mitral valve lesion, difficulty arises in deciding the relative severity of each. A loud first sound and clear, sharp opening snap favours dominant stenosis even in the presence of a systolic murmur. On the other hand, a loud systolic murmur, soft first sound and easily heard third heart sound favour a diagnosis of mitral regurgitation. Tricuspid systolic murmurs are likely to cause confusion, but they are loudest on inspiration and are not as a rule conducted towards the axilla. Mitral regurgitation is more common in male patients, particularly with a history of severe, repeated rheumatic affections. Again, a large heart, particularly an aneurysmal left atrium, favours mitral regurgitation, while severe pulmonary hypertension is more usual in mitral stenosis.

Indications for Operation. The indication for operation is the presence of mitral stenosis causing symptoms, a resting diastolic gradient of 10 mmHg across the valve being considered to be objective haemodynamic evidence of significant obstruction.

It is generally acknowledged that the presence of active rheumatic fever is a contraindication to surgery, although in very rare instances it may be necessary to perform mitral valvotomy in order to aid a heart labouring under a second attack of rheumatic fever.

Intractable pulmonary oedema may occasionally make emergency mitral valvotomy obligatory and, similarly, pregnancy in the presence of mitral stenosis may be an indication for operation in the interests of both the mother and the child. Ideally, however, planned operaton should be carried out prior to pregnancy.

Atrial fibrillation is certainly not a contraindication, and most cases are fibrillating when they come to operation. A history of embolic episodes is an added indication for operation; in the presence of an acute systemic embolus, it may be expedient to do a valvotomy and remove the emboli at the same time.

The involvement of other heart valves, particularly the association of mitral and aortic stenosis, is no bar to operation, since both lesions can be treated. Similarly, coronary artery disease in the presence of mitral stenosis can also be treated at the same time.

Age is not in itself a contraindication to relief of mitral valve obstruction. Where the valve is critically stenosed and giving rise to symptoms, surgical relief should be considered whatever the age of the patient, although older patients may have to accept a higher operative risk.

Principles of Treatment. The surgical management of mitral stenosis has demonstrated the value of good preoperative condition, and several factors may help to bring the patient to surgery in the best possible circumstances. This is particularly important for far-advanced cases, which fortunately have become uncommon.

Gross pulmonary hypertension, with its associated poor systemic output, predisposes to peripheral deep vein thrombosis and pulmonary embolism. In these cases, anticoagulants can be helpful while awaiting operation. Anticoagulation may also be beneficial in patients who require bed rest and loss of fluid preoperatively, to avoid clot formation in the left atrium. Digitalisation is useful in those not already receiving the drug. This ensures that postoperative arrythmias, particularly atrial fibrillation, will be immediately under control if they should arise. In patients liable to pulmonary oedema, precautions are taken to prevent undue anxiety and a sedative is given when the day of operation is at hand. The orthopnoeic patient is not laid flat while awaiting anaesthesia.

The object of surgical treatment is not only to enlarge the mitral orifice, but also to restore its function. An enlarged but rigid orifice will provide only a temporary remission of symptoms and 're-stenosis' is almost inevitable. Given the options of closed valvotomy, open valvotomy under direct vision and valve replacement, it should be possible to achieve this objective in virtually all patients.

Anatomically, the mitral valve has a crescent orifice which is almost 4 cm long in adults. The anteromedial or aortic cusp is more mobile and functionally more important. The posterolateral cusp acts as an opposing baffle. The papillary muscles are inserted via the chordae tendinae into the lateral and medial commissures. Brock has emphasised the importance of opening the valve beyond the points of insertion of the tendons; this is important if one is to restore the normal hinge-like action of the valve.

If the valve is suitable for commissurotomy, i.e. there is a good opening snap and no evidence of calcification, a choice must first be made between closed dilatation through the left ventricular apex, or with a balloon passed across the atrial septum, and an open operation on cardiopulmonary bypass. While the latter allows more precise control and mobilisation of fused chordae beneath the valve, it should not be forgotten that closed dilatation often achieves an excellent result and can thus offer treatment where facilities for cardiopulmonary bypass are not available.

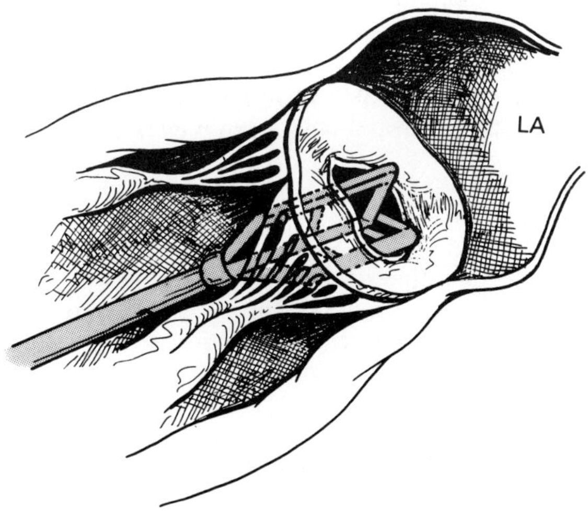

Fig. 7.3. Transventricular 'closed' mitral valvotomy with an expanding dilator.

A calcified valve may not be salvageable, and in such cases open operation is mandatory. An attempt may be made at commissurotomy under direct vision, but if this does not achieve a competent and mobile valve, the leaflets are excised and replaced with an artificial valve. The valve may be a mechanical device, in which case anticoagulation is necessary to stop clot forming on the valve, or a preserved pig or pericardial valve.

When the patient is in atrial fibrillation, or when there has been a history of systemic emboli, the left atrial appendage is obliterated to reduce the risk of blood clots forming within it postoperatively.

After operation, all the peripheral pulses should be felt while the patient is still on the operating table. Emboli, if present, should be removed immediately.

A complication occurring usually at 10–14 days but in some instances a few weeks or months postoperatively, is a condition called 'pleuropericarditis', also known as the post-commissurotomy or post-pericardiotomy syndrome. It is characterised by the features of pericarditis, often with recurrent attacks of pleurisy and effusion. The syndrome is suggested when the patient feels unwell, perhaps with substernal pain which may be referred to the back, or even the back and sides of the neck. There is sometimes a dry irritable cough with some elevation of temperature, tachycardia and a friction rub over the precordium. There may also be raised neck veins and an enlarged cardiac shadow on the chest X-ray if there is fluid accumulation in the pericardial space. There is no evidence that the condition represents a further attack of rheumatic fever, and it may in fact result from homologous blood transfusion. Symptoms may recur for weeks or months postoperatively. If fluid causes cardiac compression, it should be aspirated without delay.

Results. Survival following mitral valvotomy is excellent, as is that for mitral valve replacement in this condition. Low cardiac output in patients with advanced disease occasionally leads to failure of other organs, from which the patient cannot rally.

Although commissurotomy is haemodynamically effective, most patients eventually develop re-stenosis and require further surgery. Biological valves also need to be replaced at around 7–10 years postoperatively in a number of patients: those with mechanical prostheses may suffer thromboembolic or haemorrhagic complications. All patients remain at risk of endocarditis.

Mitral Regurgitation

Incompetence of the mitral valve may be rheumatic in origin or it may follow bacterial endocarditis or instrumental mitral valvotomy. An increasingly common cause is mitral valve prolapse. Infarction of a papillary muscle from coronary artery disease also produces mitral regurgitation; this is considered in Chapter 8.

Pathology. In rheumatic cases, there may be rigidity, deficiency or binding-down of the valve leaflets which prevents their accurate closure in systole. Alternatively, there may be dilatation of the mitral valve ring such that the otherwise essentially normal leaflets do not oppose. In these circumstances, the disease is self-perpetuating in that regurgitation causes a large left ventricle

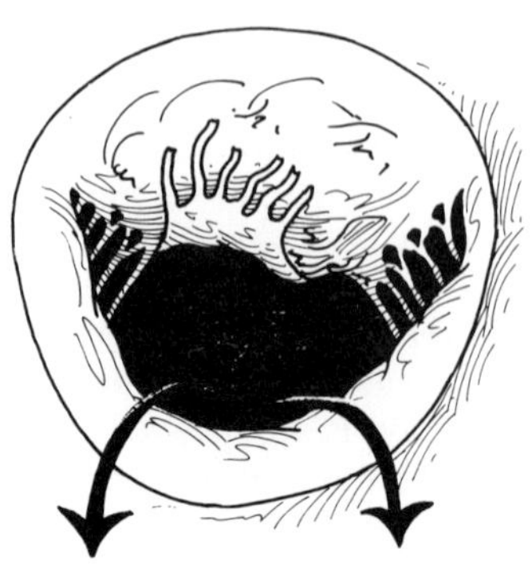

Fig. 7.4. Mitral incompetence due to ruptured chordae.

which, in turn, further enlarges the mitral ring. Rupture of the chordae — those in the posterior leaflet are particularly prone to this — may result in acute onset of mitral regurgitation.

Mitral valve prolapse, or the 'floppy valve' syndrome results from myxomatous degeneration of the chordae and leaflets, although there may be an underlying congenital deformity of the valve. Part of the valve collagen may be replaced by mucopolysaccharides; this causes the leaflets to become thickened and prolapse into the left atrium. The chordae eventually elongate and rupture, increasing the regurgitation through a flail segment of the leaflet. Changes occur earlier in patients with Marfan's syndrome.

Mitral regurgitation in isolation is only rarely caused by infective endocarditis destroying a leaflet. It is more common to find regurgitation through a damaged anterior leaflet, where infection has spread from the aortic valve.

Haemodynamics. The cardiac output is maintained by an increased left ventricular stroke volume which compensates for the retrograde loss of left ventricular output into the left atrium. The left ventricle is consequently large and dilated as in aortic regurgitation. The left atrium is also enlarged, which tends to modulate the increase in left atrial pressure. Pulmonary hypertension is thus less marked than in obstructive lesions of the mitral valve.

Clinical Features. Rheumatic mitral incompetence is more common in men and this may be due to the greater incidence of calcification and rigidity of the valve. Myxomatous degeneration, is contrast, tends to occur slightly more frequently in women.

The pulse is usually rapid and flicking in character but small in volume. There is usually enlargement of the heart, and a hyperdynamic left ventricular type of impulse can be felt at the apex. A systolic thrill is felt exceptionally but may be more common with ruptured chordae. It is characteristic to hear a blowing pansystolic murmur immediately following a normal first heart sound. The murmur is conducted from the apex laterally towards the axilla, unless the regurgitation is directed through a the posterior leaflet towards the base of the heart. A ventricular filling sound or third heart sound may also be heard. A mid-systolic click is typical of the floppy valve.

Although it is not difficult to make a diagnosis of mitral regurgitation clinically, it is often difficult to assess its degree and to decide upon the relative importance of stenosis and regurgitation where the two lesions co-exist.

Special Investigations. The ECG confirms the presence of left ventricle preponderance; the chest radiograph usually shows a considerably enlarged or aneurysmal left atrium. Pulmonary congestion may be present in acute regurgitation.

The echocardiogram may visualise prolapsing leaflets, while Doppler echocardiography, particularly with colour-flow mapping, will demonstrate the position and the degree of regurgitation.

Cardiac catheterisation adds little to the clinical diagnosis but will permit direct measurement of the left atrial *v* wave, and this will be accentuated in mitral regurgitation of acute onset. Left ventricular angiography will show regurgitation of dye from the ventricle into the atrium.

Differential Diagnosis. The only cardiac lesions likely to be confused with mitral regurgitation on clinical examination are tricuspid regurgitation and aortic stenosis. The pansystolic murmur of tricuspid regurgitation tends to be loudest along the right sternal border and accompanied by large venous pulsation. When mitral regurgitation directs the jet of blood towards the roof of the atrium, it may be conducted into the neck, similar to aortic stenosis. Invasive studies or echocardiography may be necessary to differentiate the two lesions.

Indications for Operation. It is difficult to define precise indications for operation because the progression of symptoms in mitral regurgitation is quite variable and mild-to-moderate incompetence of the valve may cause florid clinical signs with little disability. Pulmonary hypertension is certainly an indication for operation, as are severe symptoms. Probably more than moderate enlargement of the left ventricle also justifies operation, as does uncontrolled bacterial endocarditis.

Principles of Treatment. Open operation is necessary to determine the precise cause of the regurgitation. Various techniques have been described for mitral valve annuloplasty or cusp repair to restore competence of the valve. Where the leaflets are grossly disorganised and/or rigid, particularly with heavy calcification, it is necessary to excise the valve and replace it with a prosthesis.

Results. For either repair or replacement of an incompetent mitral valve the early mortality ranges from 0 to about 6%, depending upon the preoperative condition of the patient and underlying pathology.

Aortic Valve Disease

Aortic Stenosis

Isolated aortic stenosis in young patients is obviously congenital in origin, and this lesion has already been discussed (Chap. 6). Where the disease is diagnosed in middle-age, the aetiology is less certain. A congenitally bicuspid valve may have undergone extensive calcification by this time, obscuring the underlying architecture.

Alternatively, aortic stenosis may be rheumatic in origin. Involvement of the aortic valve in rheumatic fever is common but it is almost invariably associated with mitral valve disease. The problem then is to define the relative importance of each lesion when they coexist. The presence of mitral stenosis masks some of the features of aortic stenosis by reducing the blood flow through the aortic valve and thereby limiting cardiac output as well as the patient's activities.

Pathology. The rheumatic valve has preservation of the normal three-cusp architecture, but each commissure becomes fused by the inflammatory process. The cusps themselves are thickened and stiff. Some calcification is not unusual, but this is rarely as extensive as seen in the congenitally bicuspid valve. The rheumatic valve is fairly easily differentiated from 'senile' aortic stenosis in which the cusps are thickened by deposits of calcium and atheroma at their bases but not fused. This lesion tends to occur late in life.

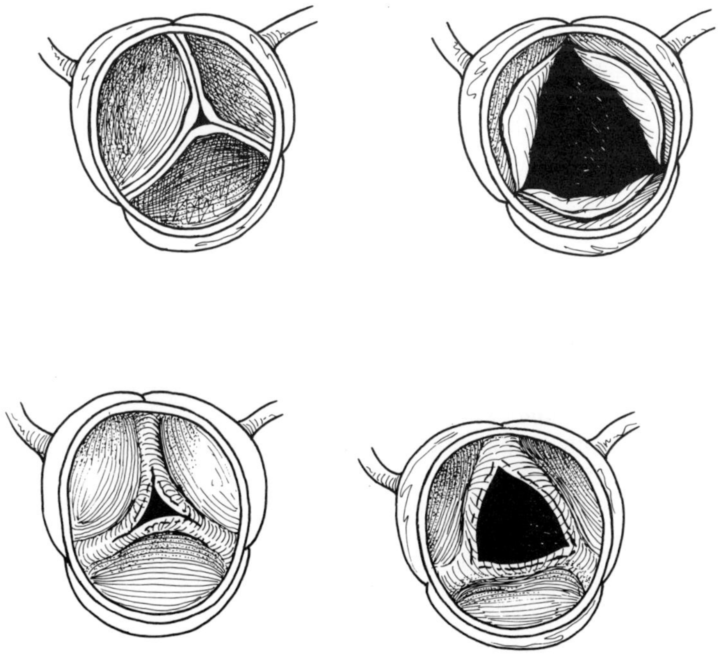

Fig. 7.5. Opening of the normal aortic valve (*top*) contrasted with one in which the commissures have fused (*bottom*).

Haemodynamics. The obstructed left ventricle builds up pressure to maintain cardiac output, and this causes massive muscular hypertrophy. Gradients across the valve often exceed 100 mmHg. Eventually the muscle fails, causing left ventricular dilatation and elevation of end-diastolic pressure. At this point, the gradient may decline as the result of low cardiac output, and the patient suffers elevation of pulmonary venous and arterial pressure.

Clinical Features. Many patients with aortic stenosis appear deceptively healthy despite classical symptoms of exertional angina, dyspnoea or syncope. The presence of aortic stenosis can often be suspected from the nature of the pulse, which should have a small volume, a slow rise and a sustained quality. Also, a left ventricular thrust at the apex and signs of left ventricular hypertrophy on the ECG in a case of mitral stenosis raise the possibility of aortic valve disease. Other causes of these findings are mitral regurgitation and systemic hypertension. Confirmatory evidence of valvar aortic stenosis is the presence of a systolic thrill over the aortic root and an ejection systolic murmur conducted into the neck vessels. The second sound at the base may be 'single' due to the rigidity of the diseased valve leaflets. Pulmonary congestion is present in advanced cases.

Special Investigations. The chest radiograph may show a post-stenotic bulge of the ascending aorta. Valve calcification may also be present, although this is neither as common nor as extensive as in isolated, congenital aortic stenosis. The ECG nearly always shows evidence of left ventricular hypertrophy, and there may be a 'strain pattern' of T wave inversion in the left ventricular leads.

The stenotic valve can usually be demonstrated on echocardiography. Cardiac catheterisation is undertaken to assess the severity of the obstruction if this is in doubt. In patients older than about 40 years of age, coronary angiography is also carried out, as associated coronary disease may contribute to the patient's angina.

Differential Diagnosis. As mentioned previously, a localised jet of mitral regurgitation may imitate the murmur and thrill of aortic stenosis. Other, rare, causes of left ventricular outflow obstruction must be kept in mind, such as an accessory mitral valve leaflet or abnormal insertion of the anterior mitral leaflet across the outflow tract.

Indications for Operation. Relief of the obstruction should be carried out before the myocardium becomes severely damaged. A gradient of 60–70 mmHg is usually significant; but in the presence of associated mitral stenosis an aortic valve gradient of 40 mmHg can be important. Also, angina or syncope, and left ventricular changes in the ECG, all point to the severity of the obstruction.

Principles of Treatment. When the valve cusps remain pliable and the basic architecture is preserved, it may occasionally be possible to divide the fused commissures and achieve a functional valve. More often, valve replacement is necessary, and this can be done with a mechanical or biological prosthesis or with a homograft or pulmonary autograft valve. Percutaneous balloon valvuloplasty has recently been used to dilate non-calcified, fused commissures in patients not considered fit for routine operation, and this procedure may accomplish relief of the obstruction.

Results. The relief of aortic stenosis may produce a dramatic improvement in cardiac output with a gratifying remission of symptoms. Surgical mortality is low (about 2%–3%) and dependent primarily upon preoperative left ventricular function. There is, however, a significant late mortality, about 85% of patients being alive 5 years after aortic valve replacement. This is again due, in part, to impaired ventricular function, and serves to emphasise the desirability of early diagnosis and treatment.

Aortic Regurgitation

Aortic regurgitation refers to dominant or isolated regurgitation at the aortic valve. Aortic diastolic murmurs are common in association with rheumatic mitral valve disease, but the lesion is often trivial. A number of conditions may cause aortic regurgitation.

Pathology. Free aortic regurgitation presenting as an isolated lesion must always raise a suspicion of syphilitic aortitis, but this is now rare. Aortitis may complicate systemic diseases such as ankylosing spondylitis or rheumatoid arthritis, causing dilatation of the aorta and secondary valvar incompetence. Dilatation of the ring and ascending aorta is typical of Marfan's syndrome, where it is called 'annulo-aortic ectasia', and is also found as a degenerative arteriosclerotic process. In these cases, the valve leaflets tend to be normal or mildly thickened and deformed. Even though the leaflets appear normal, however, aortic regurgitation may be severe. The competence and strength of the thin aortic leaflets are dependent upon their length and close apposition in diastole. The coapting surfaces press closely against one another, cancelling out the distraction forces applied to them. A minor degree of shortening or displacement of one or more cusps upsets this delicate balance and allows free regurgitation.

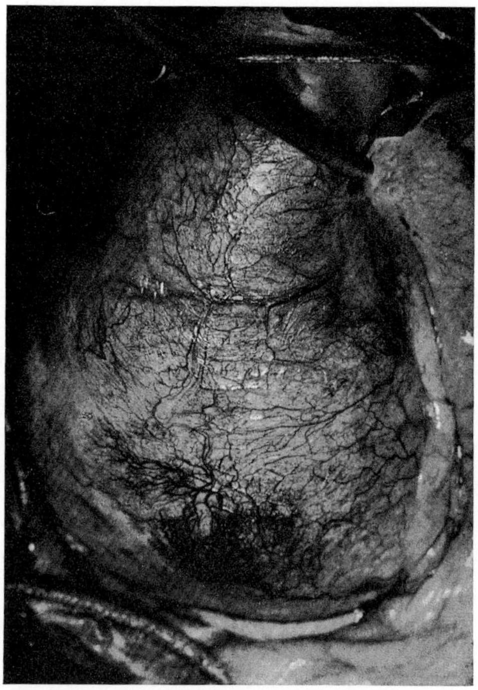

Fig. 7.6. The aneurysmal type of aortic root in Marfan's disease with aortic regurgitation.

Other acquired lesions causing aortic regurgitation include rheumatic valve disease, where the leaflets retract due to scarring in the healing process, and bacterial endocarditis, which causes destruction of a cusp. Here the mechanism of regurgitation involves loss of leaflet substance or cusp rupture. Since the advent of valve replacement, prosthetic degeneration or dysfunction or paravalvar leaks have also become important causes of aortic regurgitation.

Haemodynamics. Depending upon the degree of regurgitation, the left ventricle dilates in order to eject an increased stroke volume. This is to compensate for the volume of blood returning from the aorta to the left ventricle during diastole.

The end-diastolic pressure is raised, and this is reflected in an elevated left atrial and pulmonary venous pressure.

Clinical Features. The pulse volume is large and has a collapsing quality, the 'water-hammer' pulse. This is due to rapid ejection of blood, which may produce a peak systolic pressure in excess of 200 mmHg, followed by rapid run-off into both the systemic vascular bed and the left ventricle. This is particularly noticeable in the neck, where dynamic pulsation of the carotid arteries may cause rhythmic movements of the ear lobes. The diastolic blood pressure is usually very low or unrecordable in severe aortic regurgitation.

Free regurgitation gives rise to an enlarged, hyperdynamic heart, and the characteristic immediate diastolic murmur is high-pitched, decrescendo and best heard along the left of the sternum. There may be an accompanying rumbling mitral diastolic murmur at the apex (Austin Flint murmur), possibly due to the regurgitant aortic stream displacing the aortic leaflet of the mitral valve in diastole. If the cardiac output is impaired, the signs of aortic incompetence will be less florid, and, indeed, the murmurs may disappear altogether.

Other clinical features may point to the aetiology of the aortic regurgitation. The presence of mitral stenosis or incompetence suggests rheumatic fever, while a high arched palate, long spidery fingers and poor vision may suggest Marfan's syndrome.

Special Investigations. The chest radiograph often shows a very large aortic shadow with marked enlargement of the left ventricle. It is sometimes described as an ox heart (cor bovinum). The left ventricular hypertrophy is reflected in the ECG. In long-standing cases, there may also be a P mitrale.

A quantitative assessment of the degree of regurgitation is difficult to obtain, but injection of contrast into the ascending aorta during cardiac catheterisation permits an estimation of the amount of reflux into the left ventricle. This will also demonstrate the morphology of the aortic sinuses and ascending aorta. Similar information is available from echocardiography. Coronary angiography is also done routinely in older patients.

Differential Diagnosis. Persistent ductus arteriosus can mimic aortic regurgitation very closely both haemodynamically and on clinical examination. The pulse is collapsing in both conditions, but the murmur of ductus should be continuous in character and heard best below the left clavicle. Also, the lungs are usually plethoric.

Coarctation of the aorta may present a similar picture on superficial examination because of the bounding neck and arm pulses. Nevertheless, the absence of femoral pulses, the proximal hypertension and the typical radiological picture, should make the diagnosis clear. However, the two conditions may coexist.

Ruptured aneurysm of a sinus of Valsalva into the right atrium or right ventricle may be indistinguishable from aortic regurgitation. The onset may be more sudden when the aneurysm ruptures, producing overloading of the right heart and a raised venous pressure. The murmur may be more continuous in nature, due to the absence of a valve in the fistulous connection. Cardiac catheterisation is usually necessary to make the diagnosis with certainty. It shows a rise in saturation in the right heart chambers, while aortography demonstrates the anatomy.

Indications for Operation. Minor degrees of aortic regurgitation are well tolerated for long periods, but a progressively enlarging heart is a sign that the compensating mechanisms are failing. Also, crippling angina or the onset of cardiac failure may demand surgical relief. Cases of severe regurgitation are liable to sudden arrythmia and a fatal outcome.

Principles of Treatment. Surgical treatment is guided by the pathology. Where the regurgitation is caused by a localised defect in the valve as a result of trauma or bacterial endocarditis, this may sometimes be repaired with pericardium or prosthetic material. Where the valve is totally disorganised and destroyed, it has to be excised and replaced by an artificial prosthesis, a heterograft, an autograft or a homograft.

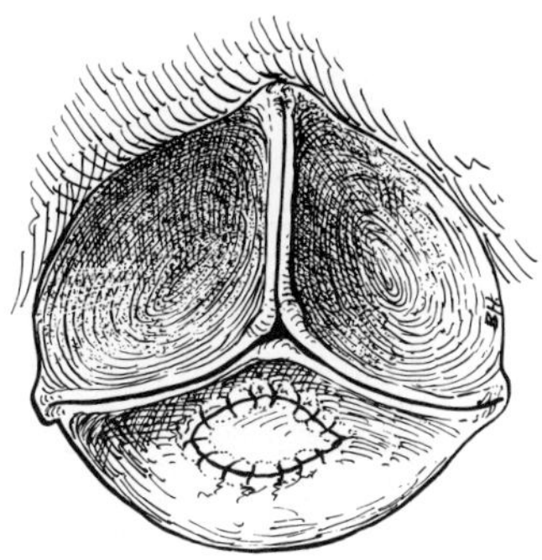

Fig. 7.7. Illustration of a possible repair method with pericardium for aortic regurgitation due to localised destruction of a valve leaflet.

In Marfan's syndrome, the valve and ascending aorta may have to be replaced. This may also be necessary if endocarditis has destroyed the valve cusps and spread to the supporting aortic ring and septum. The timing of

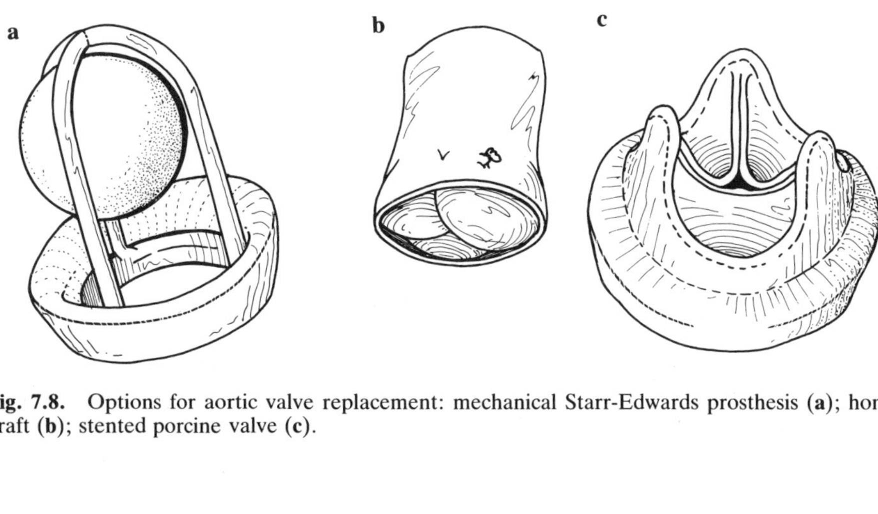

Fig. 7.8. Options for aortic valve replacement: mechanical Starr-Edwards prosthesis (**a**); homograft (**b**); stented porcine valve (**c**).

operation for aortic regurgitation due to bacterial endocarditis may be difficult. The general tendency is to defer operation too long, in the hope of first curing the infection or controlling the cardiac failure by medical therapy. While this is the ideal, it is not always possible, and many deaths from active endocarditis could be prevented by earlier surgical referral and treatment. While not wishing to operate unnecessarily in an infected field or to deprive the patient of a reasonable trial of medical treatment, it is a good policy to advise early operation if there is evidence of ongoing infection, repeated systemic emboli or heart failure which cannot be controlled.

Results. Both early and late survival is very good, and the symptoms should be completely relieved if the myocardium has not become decompensated prior to operation.

Tricuspid Valve Disease

Symptoms emanating from the tricuspid or the pulmonary valve in isolation are extremely rare. Usually they are 'functional' in origin; that is, they represent regurgitation in rheumatic valve disease, occurring as a result of the development of pulmonary hypertension, or flow gradients due to an intracardiac shunt.

Rheumatic involvement of the tricuspid valve itself does occur but nearly always in association with mitral and aortic lesions. It produces stenosis, and less commonly regurgitation which should be considered in patients with rheumatic heart disease and features of pronounced right heart failure (ankle oedema and ascites). The symptoms of dyspnoea or orthopnoea may not be severe, since the lungs are 'protected' by the proximal obstruction at the tricuspid valve. As in congenital tricuspid atresia, there will be an enlarged liver and a prominent *a* wave if the patient is in sinus rhythm. A tricuspid diastolic murmur may be audible. This is differentiated from the mitral diastolic murmur by enhancement on inspiration, although this feature may be subtle.

Stenosis of the tricuspid valve also occurs in carcinoid syndrome. The fusion of leaflets, with shortening and thickening of the chordae, tends to cause incompetence of the valve at the same time.

Isolated incompetence may result from tricuspid valve endocarditis, a disease which is virtually limited to intravenous drug abusers. Incompetence of the valve produces characteristic pulsations in the neck veins and systolic pulsation of the liver. A pansystolic murmur is present and often loudest, with inspiratory accentuation, to the right of the sternum.

The chest X-ray tends to show right atrial enlargement. Tall, peaked P waves are characteristic on the ECG. Echocardiography, particularly with colour Doppler, is useful to show thickening of the leaflets and the degree of stenosis or regurgitation across the valve. A gradient of 4 mmHg at cardiac catheterisation represents significant stenosis.

It is occasionally possible to perform a valvotomy for stenosis, but even under direct vision this often results in severe incompetence. Usually, it is necessary to replace the valve with a prosthesis.

Tricuspid incompetence can often be dealt with by one or another annuloplasty technique. Often, the decision regarding treatment will have to be made at operation, after palpation of the valve has allowed an assessment of its function.

It is difficult to estimate the results of tricuspid valve surgery because other associated lesions tend to dominate the clinical picture. Early and late mortality range from 0 to about 30% in various series. There is also a small incidence of complete heart block developing after tricuspid valve replacement.

Pulmonary Valve Disease

Fusion of the valve cusps may occur in carcinoid syndrome or rheumatic valve disease, in which case the other features of the disease predominate. Cardiac catheterisation is usually necessary to make the diagnosis, although refinements in echocardiography approach the same level of accuracy for measurement of gradients. Pulmonary regurgitation is usually secondary to pulmonary hypertension, but occasionally infective endocarditis involves the cusps or vessels beyond the valve.

Pulmonary stenosis should be amenable to valvotomy, as the basic architecture of the valve tends to be preserved. When there is severe and sustained elevation of pulmonary arterial pressure, causing pulmonary regurgitation, a competent valve in the pulmonary position may benefit right ventricular function. This is usually accomplished by orthotopic pulmonary valve replacement using a prosthetic or homograft valve.

Prosthetic Valve Disease

With the long-term survival of patients who have undergone successful replacement of one or more cardiac valves, there is now considerable information regarding the late performance and complications of various prosthetic devices. Valve replacement does not 'cure' the patient of cardiac disease but rather exchanges the disability of the diseased native valve for a different group of problems. Some of these problems may be peculiar to a certain type of prosthetic valve, while others relate to the underlying cardiac disease or valve replacement in general.

Valve Failure. All tissue or biological valves, with the possible exception of the pulmonary autograft, eventually suffer wear-and-tear producing stenosis or incompetence or both. In gluteraldehyde-preserved bioprostheses, this becomes evident about 7 years after implantation. Valve dysfunction progresses slowly, permitting elective replacement of the prosthesis in most cases.

Structural failure of the mechanical prosthesis is less common but more sudden and catastrophic. It may be due to fracture of one of the components, which then allows the movable ball or disc to escape into the circulation and produces massive incompetence of the prosthesis. Mechanical devices may also become obstructive as the result of tissue ingrowth or clot formation. This process is usually slower and allows time for diagnosis and treatment.

Thromboembolism. The presence of non-human material in the circulation promotes clot formation, and the clots are then released into the systemic or, less commonly, the pulmonary circulation. The risk of thromboembolic complications is low for tissue valves but much greater with mechanical devices. Anticoagulation is thus routine after implantation of most mechanical prostheses, and also if the patient is in atrial fibrillation.

Paravalvar Leak. When the implanted valve incorporates a ring to anchor sutures between the heart and the prosthesis, it is possible for leakage to develop between the sewing ring and the native valve annulus. This is usually a technical problem related to poor quality of the tissues available for support of the prosthesis, but it may occur also with infection.

Endocarditis. Blood flow through any prosthetic valve has an element of turbulance, and inert or non-biological surfaces are exposed constantly to any organisms within the patient's circulation. It is thus not surprising that infection may involve a prosthetic valve almost as readily as an abnormal native valve. The haemodynamic consequences, however, are often much more serious.

Infection of a biological prosthesis tends to produce marked systemic symptoms (pyrexia, systemic emboli, renal impairment), soon followed by severe incompetence of the valve due to leaflet destruction. While a mechanical prosthesis may continue to function normally in the face of infective endocarditis, haemodynamic deterioration usually indicates the onset of a paravalvar leak due to destruction of the annulus. In both cases, the infection tends to spread into adjacent tissues with abscess formation.

The mortality for this condition exceeds 50%, even with antibiotic therapy, and there should be a very low threshold for reoperation to remove the infected prosthesis and any other infected material. Aggressive surgical therapy, using a homograft valve whenever possible, has reduced the overall mortality to around 20% in recent series.

Further Reading

Davies MJ. Pathology of cardiac valves. Butterworth, London, 1980

Edmunds LH Jr, Clark RE, Cohen LH, et al. Guidelines for reporting morbidity and mortality after cardiac valvar operations. Ann Thorac Surg 1988; 40: 257–259

O'Rourke RA, Crawford MH. Editorial: Timing of valve replacement in patients with chronic aortic regurgitation. Circulation 1980; 61: 493–495

Perloff JK. Evolving concepts of mitral valve prolapses. N Engl J Med 1982; 307: 369–370

Roberts WC. The silver anniversary of cardiac valve replacement (editorial). Am J Cardiol 1985; 56:503–506

Ross DN. Homograft replacement of the aortic valve. Lancet 1972; i: 487–491

Ross DN. Biologic valves. Their performance and prospects. Circulation 1982; 45: 1259–1272

Chapter 8

Ischaemic Heart Disease

In this chapter, acquired ischaemic heart disease refers to atherosclerotic coronary artery disease and its sequelae. Other causes of cardiac ischaemia – connective tissue disorders, coronary embolism and various types of arteritis – together comprise less than 1% of cases. The overwhelming magnitude of the problem becomes apparent when it is appreciated that ischaemic heart disease is one of the most common causes of death in the populations of industrialised nations. In some countries, it accounts for one-third to one-half of all deaths. Moreover, the disease tends to affect patients around 50–60 years of age, causing disability during the prime of life.

Anatomy

The two main coronary arteries lie in the atrioventricular grooves and circle the base of the heart like a crown (or corona, hence coronary). The right coronary artery arises from the aorta anteriorly and turns downwards and to the right in the right atrioventricular groove. It gives off a conus branch, ventricular branches, and the acute marginal artery. This latter vessel runs along the margin between the anterior and inferior surfaces of the right ventricle. The right coronary then continues in the back of the atrioventricular groove and gives off further branches. The largest of these is the posterior descending artery, which lies in the posterior interventricular groove. The most distal extremity of this branch anastomoses with the left anterior descending artery. The main right coronary artery may continue onwards for a variable distance, giving off further ventricular or posterolateral arteries. It terminates by anastomosing with the distal left or circumflex coronary artery.

In most people the posterior descending artery arises from the right coronary, and this common circulatory pattern is called 'right dominant'. In the remainder, the posterior descending artery comes from the left coronary. In such cases of 'left dominance', the right coronary artery is usually quite small.

The left coronary artery arises from the anterior or left-hand sinus of the aorta and runs behind the pulmonary artery. It gives off its major anterior descending branch and continues in the atrioventricular groove as the circumflex artery until it reaches the posterior interventricular groove. Here it anastomoses with the distal right coronary artery. Branches of the circumflex coronary pass from the atrioventricular groove towards the apex of the heart. These so-called 'marginal' branches supply the lateral and posterior walls of the left ventricle. As with the right coronary artery there is a great deal of variation.

The left anterior descending coronary, which may be considered the first major branch of the left coronary, runs towards the apex along the anterior interventricular groove. It gives off a number of important septal branches, which pass downward, as well as diagonal branches running to the lateral wall of the heart from its left side. Occasionally, the highest diagonal artery arises in a 'trifurcation' at the junction of the left anterior descending artery and the circumflex. It is then called the intermediate coronary or ramus intermedialis. In a coronary arteriogram, the left anterior descending artery can usually be identified as the vessel that extends to the apex of the heart and gives off septal branches.

Pathology

Ischaemic heart disease is generally regarded as the clinical manifestation of advanced atherosclerotic narrowing in the coronary arteries, although recently it has become apparent that spasm or lesser degrees of obstruction may also result in impaired myocardial function. There are probably several major mechanisms by which obstruction may come about.

One possibility is that a coronary artery embolism, arising from mural thrombus in the left atrium or left ventricle, occludes a branch of the coronary artery. The healing of this lesion includes infiltration of lipids into the arterial

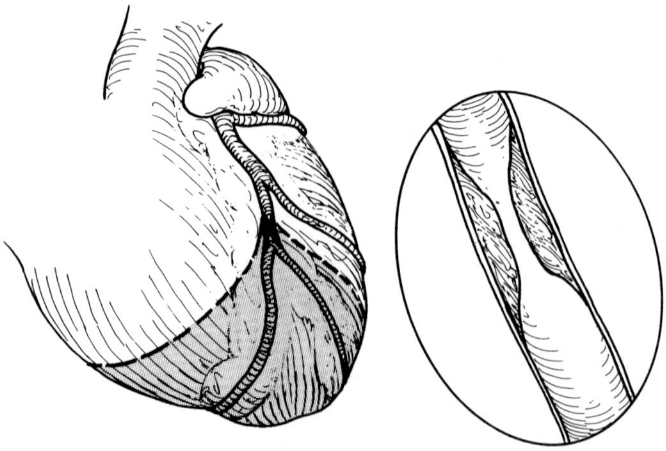

Fig. 8.1. Myocardial infarction resulting from critical narrowing of the coronary artery. The area affected by loss of blood supply is *shaded*.

wall, which sets the stage for further damage to the intima and formation of arteriosclerotic plaques.

The other major theory, that of primary endothelial damage, holds that the endothelium of a muscular artery suffers injury that induces platelet aggregation and subsequent migration of smooth muscle cells into the intima. The 'injury' may be an underlying biochemical or metabolic abnormality predisposing the patient to atheroma formation.

The end result of either process is the formation of an elevated, white fibrous plaque within the lumen of the vessel, the 'atheroma'. Of its own accord, atheroma causes little disability in this form. However, progressive thickening, sometimes with superimposed ulceration, haemorrhage, thrombosis or calcification, produces further narrowing of the lumen. Probably at about 70% narrowing, there is a critical reduction of blood flow.

If the narrowing develops gradually, many patients will, for reasons not entirely understood, generate a collateral flow of blood from other coronary branches to the myocardium distal to the obstruction. On the other hand, if sudden thrombosis or haemorrhage around a previously small plaque causes abrupt cessation of blood flow, the dependent area of cardiac muscle has little chance of survival.

The narrowing process tends to affect multiple vessels, and when one artery is completely occluded, the other two will nearly always have some areas of stenosis. Plaques tend to form at the sites of major coronary artery branches and in the more proximal distribution of the vessels. It is still unpredictable precisely what cardiac damage will result from a given picture of coronary arteriosclerosis.

Another cause of myocardial ischaemia is spasm of the coronary artery. Human coronary arteries have been shown to possess both alpha and beta adrenergic receptors as well as reactivity to peptides and chemical substances. While the exact role of contraction and relaxation in regulation of coronary blood flow is uncertain, the occurrence of severe ischaemia as the result of reversible spasm has been well documented.

Inadequate blood flow to the cardiac muscle results in the death of muscle cells or 'myocardial infarction'. This is a 'heart attack' in lay terms. While some areas may be salvaged by early reperfusion, the dead tissue usually heals by fibrosis and scarring. In some cases, this will produce streaks of fibrous tissue intermingled with active myocardium, while in others, the scar will be 'full-thickness' without myocardial cells. The latter may be the precursor of a ventricular aneurysm. If the infarcted area involves the inferior surface of the heart, it may affect a papillary muscle of the mitral valve. Usually, it is the posteromedial papillary muscle which is involved. In milder cases, this may result in reversible ischaemic mitral regurgitation, but severe damage causes complete disruption of the tip of the papillary muscle with florid mitral incompetence. This is found in about 2% of the patients who die after myocardial infarction.

The other complications of myocardial infarction are also acute or chronic manifestations of muscle death in a critical area of the heart. Rupture of the free wall of the heart (*cardiac rupture*) or the ventricular septum (*postinfarction ventricular septal defect*) tend to occur between 7 and 14 days after the acute ischaemic episode. Cardiac rupture is estimated to be about ten times more frequent than septal rupture, but is diagnosed far less commonly during life. The frequency of cardiac rupture – found in as many as one-quarter of patients who die after myocardial infarction – may be due to the greater frequency of ischaemia involving the free wall of the heart as well as the larger pressure difference between the ventricle and the pericardial space. Both cardiac and septal rupture occur in association with hypertension after myocardial infarction, which, paradoxically, augers favourably for the recovery of the rest of the myocardium.

An *aneurysm of the left ventricle* is an area of full-thickness fibrous scar which moves paradoxically – that is, expands during ventricular contraction. It occurs most commonly in the territory of an occluded anterior descending coronary and thus involves the anterior wall and apex of the left ventricle. Aneurysms become apparent several weeks or months after the infarction and may become lined with clot or calcification.

After myocardial infarction *arrythmias* are not uncommon. An ischaemic region involving the conduction fibres may fail to conduct the heartbeat altogether, as in complete heart block after an inferior infarction. The conduction defect may or may not revert to normal with healing. Ventricular arrythmias result from irritable areas of the myocardium, probably in regions of salvageable but damaged heart cells. In the acute phase, this may produce isolated ventricular ectopics of little consequence, or runs of sustained ventricular tachycardia with severe haemodynamic embarrassment. Following the production of scar tissue, circular types of conduction may become established between the normal and fibrous areas of the myocardium and cause prolonged ventricular tachycardia. Arrythmias may also be associated with left ventricular aneurysms.

Although a complication of myocardial infarction, *cardiogenic shock* is a haemodynamic situation rather than a single anatomical or pathological lesion. It may result from any of the above complications, as well as from widespread myocardial damage without specific structural disruption of the heart. Generally, more than half of the left ventricular muscle mass is damaged, and the infarction nearly always involves the septal and anterior regions.

A number of so-called 'risk factors', have been found in association with the development of arteriosclerotic coronary artery disease. These include such things as elevated lipids, hypertension, diabetes, male sex, older age, a family history of ischaemic heart disease, cigarette smoking and the use of oral contraceptives. The mechanisms by which they influence the development of coronary artery disease is uncertain.

Haemodynamics

These may be grossly normal or there may be extensively impaired ventricular function. Moreover, ventricular function may alter during episodes of ischaemia.

Recently, it has been suggested that biochemical and ultrastructural changes which have functional implications for the left ventricle occur when there are either brief periods of severe ischaemia ('stunned myocardium') or chronic mild ischaemia ('hibernating myocardium') which are not severe enough to cause outright cellular death. These haemodynamic alterations may also be important in the ventricular dysfunction seen after open heart surgery.

Several tests are used to evaluate overall left ventricular function, including an estimation of the ejection fraction of the left ventricle on cine angiogram, echocardiogram or radioisotope scan, measurement of cardiac output and quantification of pulmonary artery and left ventricular end-diastolic pressure at cardiac catheterisation. These investigations may be repeated during exercise in order to unmask haemodynamic abnormalities when there is borderline myocardial blood flow.

Following myocardial infarction, a large area of scar may show paradoxical pulsation and result in an overall reduction in cardiac output. When the left ventricle contracts, this area distends outward because it contains no muscle fibres to shorten with the rest of the heart. Blood pumped in and out of a true aneurysm thus adds nothing to cardiac output. Such patients usually have an elevated end-diastolic pressure, reflecting left ventricular failure.

Mitral incompetence as the result of papillary muscle dysfunction will produce an elevated left atrial pressure and volume overload of the left ventricle. In severe cases, this may also produce an elevated pulmonary artery pressure and low cardiac output.

Rupture of the ventricular septum generally results in a very large left-to-right shunt in the context of recovery from an acute myocardial infarction. This causes pulmonary oedema due to flooding of the lungs and, usually cardiogenic shock as the result of low systemic output.

External cardiac rupture following myocardial infarction usually results in acute haemopericardium and cardiac tamponade. The pressure of fluid within the pericardial sac impairs venous filling of the heart. There is sudden elevation of right atrial pressure, bradycardia, and profound shock from low cardiac output. Most patients die very rapidly, but occasionally the rupture is contained by the pericardium, and the haemodynamic picture evolves into that of a pseudoaneurysm or chronic tamponade.

The most extreme haemodynamic deviation is cardiogenic shock. As the result of 'pump failure', there is an elevated left atrial pressure and a very high end-diastolic pressure in the left ventricle. Cardiac output is reduced and there is severe systemic hypotension, such that perfusion of vital organs is inadequate. This leads to metabolic acidosis and decreased urine flow, which further impair cardiorespiratory function. Usually this picture corresponds to a massive myocardial infarction, often with perforation of the heart or septum or with severe mitral regurgitation. The prognosis is extremely poor.

Clinical Features

There is no clear-cut correlation between the clinical presentation of coronary artery disease and the morphologic changes, nor is the clinical course entirely predictable from the mode of presentation. However, several 'syndromes' are now well recognised as manifestations of arterioscelerotic coronary artery narrowing.

The classical symptom of myocardial ischaemia is chest pain precipitated by exertion and relieved by rest. The pain is often described as a tightness or sensation of pressure in the mid-chest region, radiating to the lower jaw or to the left arm. The patient himself may not recognise the sensation as a pain so much as a squeezing or burning discomfort. The characteristic feature is that the sensation comes with circumstances of increased myocardial oxygen requirements which, as the result of inadequate coronary blood flow, cannot be met. These include exercise, meals, cold weather, emotional stress, increased systemic blood pressure and high altitude. The pain generally subsides after a few minutes' rest. There may be associated breathlessness if left ventricular function is impaired by the ischaemic episode. Physical examination is usually unremarkable, although a fourth heart sound may become audible and there may be elevation of the systemic blood pressure during an attack. If these symptoms are more or less unchanging in severity or frequency, the patient is said to have *chronic stable angina pectoris*. An unusual type of angina, which tends to occur at rest, is the so-called Prinzmetal's variant angina. This is thought to be caused by coronary artery spasm, and, paradoxically, is sometimes relieved by exercise.

Chest pain occuring at rest or during sleep, or increasing in intensity or duration, becomes *unstable* (crescendo) *angina*. This may be due to coronary artery spasm or other precipitating factors such as anaemia or arrhythmias. But most commonly it is due to critical obstruction of the vessel. The patient is therefore at a considerable risk of suffering a myocardial infarction or developing ventricular arrhythmias.

The cause of *acute myocardial infarction* is the actual death of cardiac muscle cells deprived of oxygen supply. This may occur in circumstances other than atherosclerotic coronary artery disease, such as septic shock or massive haemorrhage, or even a long period of aortic cross-clamping during cardiac surgery. It may be preceded by chronic or unstable angina, or myocardial infarction itself may be the initial presentation of coronary artery disease.

Pain is usually the dominant complaint, and, as in angina pectoris, may be described as a tightness or crushing sensation in the mid-chest. However, it may radiate more widely and is usually more severe and prolonged than anginal pain. Not uncommonly, the patient feels nauseated, light-headed and generally weak. There may be syncope due to systemic hypotension, signs of low cardiac output such as cold peripheries, and a weak, fast pulse or frank pulmonary oedema. Systemic signs, such as fever and tachycardia, tend to follow the acute event by 1–2 days. Occasionally, in perhaps 10% of cases, myocardial infarction occurs with symptoms so mild that they are not recognised by the patient. The infarction is then said to be 'silent' and is diagnosed retrospectively on the ECG or because the patient presents with complications. This is more likely in association with diabetes mellitus.

A smaller group of patients seek medical attention for symptoms of congestive heart failure or arrythmias. Complete heart block may produce sudden loss of consciousness or 'Stokes–Adams attacks' as the initial and isolated manifestation of coronary artery disease, or there may be self-limited episodes of ventricular fibrillation. Sudden death is the unfortunate presentation in about a quarter of patients with ischaemic heart disease, presumably due to ventricular fibrillation.

Special Investigations

The ECG is the principal investigation and will show ST or T wave abnormalities in the presence of ischaemia or Q waves when there has been actual infarction. When the ECG is normal at rest, the presence of coronary artery disease may be unmasked by an exercise test. In this examination, the patient performs an increasing amount of work on a treadmill or exercise cycle until the development of chest pain or changes of ischaemia on the ECG. A positive exercise test – that is, one in which the patient experiences angina and there are ST changes on the ECG – is suggestive of coronary artery disease but must be interpreted in conjunction with other investigations. Arrythmias may also be seen on the ECG.

The chest X-ray is often normal, even in the presence of extensive coronary atheroma. When the cardiac shadow is enlarged, one should consider the possibility of left ventricular failure or previous systemic hypertension. A bulge on the margin of the heart may indicate a ventricular aneurysm, and organised clot within this may become calcified. Pulmonary venous congestion or pulmonary oedema raise the possibilities of severely impaired left ventricular function, ischaemic mitral valve regurgitation or a post-infarction ventricular septal defect.

A number of non-invasive techniques have been applied to the investigation of coronary artery disease. Radioisotope scanning with thallium will show areas of unperfused myocardium as ‘cold spots’ where the isotope has not reached the heart muscle. This test may also be carried out before and after exercise. Radioisotope studies may also demonstrate areas of poor contraction and what proportion of blood is pumped by the ventricle with each cardiac contraction (the ejection fraction).

An estimate of left ventricular function may also be gained from real-time echocardiography, which may give additional information about mitral valve function, rupture of the ventricular septum or the presence of a pericardial effusion.

The most conclusive investigations, however, are left ventricular cine angiography and coronary angiography carried out at cardiac catheterisation. The injection of contrast material into each coronary artery ostium should visualise the coronary arterial system as well as any areas of narrowing or obstruction and collateral development. Left ventricular angiography permits an estimate of the ejection fraction, ventricular dilatation and areas of impaired contraction. The presence of mitral regurgitation or a ventricular septal defect also will be apparent.

Differential Diagnosis

A variety of disorders may cause chest pain, and most of these can be differentiated by a good clinical history. However, it should not be overlooked that any of these disorders can occur also in a patient with arteriosclerotic coronary artery disease, and some patients who present with ‘sudden death’ have been previously diagnosed as having chest pain of another aetiology.

Gastrointestinal problems such as hiatus hernia, cholycystitis or peptic ulcer disease often cause epigastric pain or lower chest pain. Usually symptoms are related to eating or position, and the diagnosis can be made on barium studies or endoscopy.

Musculoskeletal disorders not infrequently cause sharp or aching pain in the chest and shoulders or arms. The pain caused by degenerative disc disease is usually caused by movements of the neck or back and accompanied by sensory changes. Similarly, joint pains from inflammatory or degenerative lesions of the shoulder come on with movement of the arm or shoulder. The 'Tietze's syndrome' is due to inflammation of the costosternal junctions and results in localised tenderness as well as anterior chest pain.

Severe mitral stenosis with pulmonary hypertension or chronic pulmonary disease may cause a type of chest pain which is very similar in character to angina and which is accompanied by ST depression on the ECG. However, there will usually be clear signs of valvular heart disease or right ventricular hypertrophy. Other cardiovascular causes of chest pain include pulmonary embolism, acute aortic dissection and pericarditis. These conditions tend to produce severe discomfort unrelated to effort. Pulmonary embolism may be accompanied by haemoptysis and pleuritic pain on one side of the chest. In acute aortic dissection, the pain has a tearing nature and may go directly through to the patient's back. The pain of pericarditis is relieved by leaning forward, but it should not be forgotten that pericardial inflammation may also accompany myocardial infarction. A typical friction rub is generally apparent on examination.

The possibility of a psychological aetiology for chest pain should be remembered also. These patients usually characterise their discomfort as being sharp or stabbing or a prolonged dull aching sensation. Their symptoms may be precipitated by exertion and exacerbated by anxiety and fatigue, but they do not necessarily obtain relief from rest. Headaches and generalised fatigue are commonly associated.

Indications for Operation

The role of surgery in the treatment of ischaemic heart disease is continually being refined in the light of early and late results, advances in pharmacological therapy, new therapeutic procedures (such as balloon angioplasty) and modification of natural history by the recognition and neutralisation of 'risk factors'. At the same time, developments in surgical technique, support devices (see Chap. 5) and heart transplantation have extended the possibility of treatment to many cases that formerly would have been considered hopeless. Thus the indications for operation are likely to undergo continued evolution and modification.

In patients with chronic, stable angina, pain may be adequately controlled by beta-blockers, vasodilators and/or calcium blocking agents, and the indications for operation are then the angiographic demonstration of lesions of the types known to be associated with a high probability of sudden death or myocardial infarction. These include left main stem stenosis, proximal stenosis of all three major coronary branches, or triple vessel disease with evidence of impaired left ventricular function. In cases with single or double vessel disease, percutaneous transluminal angioplasty may be advised as the initial treatment, although associated ventricular dysfunction tends to favour surgical therapy.

Unstable angina is an indication for intensified medical treatment, as it is frequently a precursor of frank myocardial infarction. If angina is not rapidly controlled, urgent operation is indicated, although angioplasty may again be considered an alternative.

There is growing evidence that re-establishment of blood flow soon after the onset of acute myocardial infarction – that is, within about 4–8 hours after the onset of chest pain – may limit the amount of muscle death and decrease the incidence of complications. In many cases, this can be achieved acutely by the administration of agents to dissolve blood clots (thrombolytic agents), with demonstrable improvement in survival. Surgical revascularisation of the myocardium or balloon angioplasty may be required as an emergency if thrombolytic agents are ineffective or the vessel blocks again. Thus, acute myocardial infarction is becoming an indication for operation, whereas previously it was considered an absolute contraindication.

Surgery is also required to deal with the sequelae of myocardial infarction, including repair of post-infarction ventricular septal defect, replacement or repair of an incompetent mitral valve, or resection of a ventricular aneurysm. Ventricular arrythmias may be amenable to surgical ablation or treatment with an implantable defibrillator, and insertion of an intra-aortic balloon or insertion of left or right ventricular assist devices may be indicated to treat cardiogenic shock acutely or as a bridge to cardiac transplantation. For patients with severely damaged myocardium, transplantation of the heart may offer the only possible chance of survival.

An increasingly frequent indication for operation is recurrence of symptoms due to blockage of bypass grafts or progression of arteriosclerotic disease in the native vessels. This tends to occur about 8–10 years after the initial myocardial revascularisation.

Principles of Treatment

The aims of surgery for ischaemic heart disease are to alleviate the distress of angina pectoris, prevent sudden death, prevent or limit myocardial infarction and to improve cardiac function by repair of structural defects. In general, this involves bringing a new source of blood to the myocardium, with or without additional procedures.

The most common method of bypassing coronary arterial stenoses is with a reversed segment of the long saphenous vein, removed from the patient's leg, anastomosed between the ascending aorta and the coronary artery ('coronary artery bypass graft' – CABG). In some circumstances the vein is attached in turn to several obstructed arteries as a 'sequential' graft, while in others it carries blood to a single vessel. It remains controversial whether every single obstructed branch should receive a new blood supply ('complete revascularisation') or whether only the major obstructed vessels need be grafted, leaving the collateral development to carry increased blood flow to the smaller branches. In general, at least two and sometimes as many as six or seven distal anastomoses will be constructed at operation.

The internal mammary artery, when it is of sufficient size and has been freed from the chest wall without injury, provides an excellent alternative source of

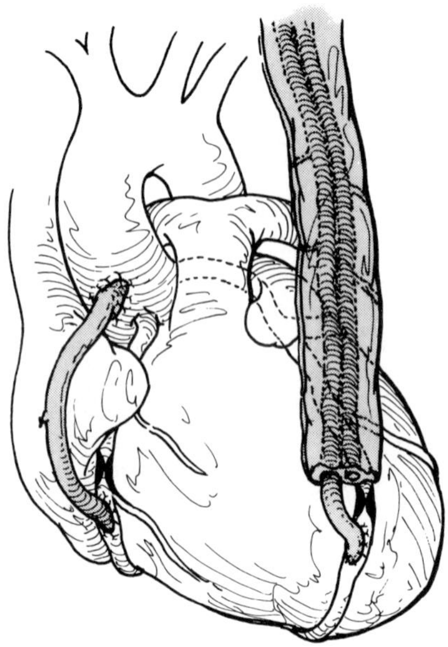

Fig. 8.2. Saphenous graft to the right coronary artery and left internal mammary artery anastomosis (IMA) to the distal left anterior descending artery.

blood flow for the coronary circulation. On the left side, it is generally anastomosed to the left anterior descending coronary artery or its diagonal branch, while on the right side (used less frequently) it may be used on the right coronary. Both graft patency and patient survival are improved by use of the internal mammary artery graft.

Where a large infarct has healed by fibrous replacement of the myocardium and, paradoxically, the aneurysmal area pulsates, its removal may both benefit cardiac output and help to alleviate ventricular arrythmias. The aneurysmal area is excised and the edges of the left ventricle are sutured together. The fibrous sac may be filled with clot, and care must be exercised to prevent its dislodgement into the systemic circulation while the heart is still ejecting. Revascularisation may or may not be required. It is frequently proximal blockage of the left anterior descending artery without significant disease in the other coronaries which leads to the formation of a left ventricular aneurysm, and the territory supplied by this vessel may be completely removed during excision of the fibrotic tissue.

Ischaemic mitral regurgitation may be due to infarction or rupture of a papillary muscle, or it may be secondary to generalised left ventricular dilatation. In some cases, it is possible to achieve a competent valve by performing an annuloplasty. As a less satisfactory alternative, the valve is excised and replaced with a prosthesis. Coronary bypass grafting is virtually always necessary at the same time.

When myocardial infarction is complicated by a ventricular septal defect, the patient will often develop severe low cardiac output. Formerly, surgery was deferred for about 4–6 weeks in order to allow some fibrosis and healing of the muscle. To do this, the patient usually required circulatory assistance, either

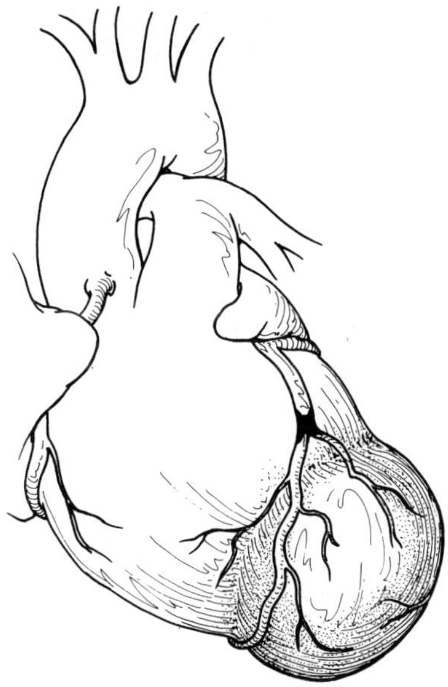

Fig. 8.3. Left ventricular aneurysm due to blockage of the anterior descending coronary artery.

with an intra-aortic balloon pump or a ventricular assist device. Closure of the ventricular septal defect and myocardial revascularisation were then carried out electively, albeit on a selected population of patients, many having died in cardiogenic shock prior to this time. Nowadays, surgery is best done in the acute phase of infarction, closing the defect through the site of infarction. The ventricular muscle is generally of very poor quality at this time and needs to be supported with material like Teflon felt. There is currently some interest in development of a clam-shell type of device which possibly could be positioned by cardiac catheter to close the ventricular septal defect without open heart surgery.

Rupture of the heart demands emergency intervention as soon as the diagnosis is made. Aspiration of blood from the pericardium, inotropic support and volume replacement may 'buy' enough time to transfer the patient to the operating theatre. Usually, it is possible to close the ventriculotomy with large bites of suture reinforced with Teflon felt. In general, patients who survive the acute catastrophe have a favourable outlook because the remainder of the myocardium is often preserved (indeed, it generated sufficient force to 'blow-out' the necrotic area).

The management of ischaemic ventricular arrythmias may be either pharmacological or surgical. Surgical techniques involve electrophysiological mapping and ablation of dysrhythmic foci by freezing or incision of the muscle. Implantation of a pacemaker or an automatic defibrillator may be indicated in some cases.

Cardiogenic shock results from 'pump failure' either due to massive 'global' ischaemia of the myocardium or secondary to acute ventricular septal defect or ischaemic mitral regurgitation. The patient will be hypotensive, mentally clouded, pale, sweaty, with a tachycardia and with little or no urine output. The breathing is rapid and with congestive features. Immediate resuscitation includes admission to an intensive care ward, and often intubation and positive pressure ventilation to reduce pulmonary oedema.

Arterial, venous and pulmonary catheter lines are inserted and pressures and urine output are charted. Electrolytes and metabolic acidosis need correction, and supporting drugs such as dopamine, phosphodiesterase inhibitors, and vasodilators are used to off-load the failing ventricle and support the cardiac output. Diuretics may help to reduce the pulmonary oedema.

The patient may improve; if not, balloon pump counterpulsation should be started through a femoral artery. Coronary angiography may be carried out if the patients condition is stable. Persistent shock in spite of resuscitative measures and balloon pumping carries a grim prognosis, with over 80% mortality.

An alternative is to put the patient on bypass, primarily with a view to decompressing the heart and carrying out emergency revascularisation in the hope of salvaging myocardium, if the infarct occurred within the preceding 4–6 hours. Beyond this time revascularisation is likely to exacerbate the injury (reperfusion syndrome) by increasing the metabolic demands on an ischaemic myocardium.

Although myocardial 'protection' or 'preservation' is fundamental to any type of cardiac surgery it assumes even greater importance when operating upon patients with arteriosclerotic coronary artery disease. Indeed, most of the modern techniques of myocardial preservation and knowledge about ischaemic injury – applicable to other areas of cardiac surgery – have evolved in the context of managing patients with ischaemic heart disease. The vulnerable or previously compromised myocardium may have little reserve, particularly in the presence of severely obstructed coronary vessels. Periods of hypotension should be avoided during anaesthesia and preparation for cardiopulmonary bypass, as should severe hypertension which increases systemic afterload and may cause sub-endocardial ischaemia.

Our current thinking in the management of cardiogenic shock is to decompress the left ventricle to remove its work-load and perfuse the coronary arteries with warm oxygenated blood with potassium to arrest all heart action. Metabolic substrate factors can be added to this blood. This technique is reputed to reverse the ischaemic damage, after which revascularisation can be effective. Should the patient fail to wean from bypass after revascularisation and the correction of any mechanical lesions, the next step would be establishment of long-term ventricular assistance to await myocardial recovery or transplantation.

Several methods have proved satisfactory for arresting myocardial metabolism during periods of aortic cross-clamping, despite the theoretical difficulty of delivering cardioplegic solution beyond stenosed segments. Solutions of blood or crystalloid 'cardioplegia' may be given into the aortic root or retrograde up the coronary sinus, followed by additional infusions through the graft as each distal anastomosis is completed. A variety of cardioplegic solutions are now available with various components to enhance myocardial energy stores and prevent ischaemic injury. Probably the most important elements of cardioplegia are *cold* (which reduces the metabolic requirements of the tissues) and *potassium* (which arrests the heart in a relaxed state). Infusion of warm cardioplegia prior to unclamping the aorta may ameliorate reperfusion injury also. Topical cooling of the heart by irrigation of the pericardial cavity with cold fluid is often a useful addition to cardioplegic techniques.

An alternative in elective coronary artery surgery is to use moderate hypothermia with brief periods of intermittent aortic cross-clamping and ventricular fibrillation for each distal anastomosis. The heart is then defibrillated and allowed to beat spontaneously while the proximal anastomosis is attached to the aorta. This method has the advantage of progressively reperfusing each part of the heart as the grafts are completed, as well as avoiding cardiac distension and oedema. It does, however, demand the technical efficiency to limit the periods of aortic cross-clamping to about 8 minutes each.

Results

Survival for coronary artery bypass surgery in patients with at least fair ventricular function approaches 100%, and remains in excess of 90% 5 years after operation. Initially, about 80% will be completely relieved of angina, and most patients will also have improved exercise tolerance as the result of improved left ventricular function.

The vein grafts tend to have a late closure rate of somewhere between 3% and 5% per year during the first 5 years, so that about 75%–80% are patent 5 years after implantation and 50%–60% at 10 years. Internal mammary artery grafts, however, have a 90% patency rate 10 years postoperatively.

Resection of a ventricular aneurysm has about a 5% early mortality but usually produces considerable haemodynamic improvement, with relief of cardiac failure postoperatively. Other procedures, such as repair of cardiac rupture or ventricular septal defect with revascularisation, carry a greater risk but are still of benefit to a considerable number of patients who would otherwise die of acute myocardial infarction.

Further Reading

Buckberg GD. Studies of controlled reperfusion after ischaemia. J Thorac Cardiovasc Surg 1986; 92: 483–487

Gibson DG, Greenbaum RA, Pridie RB, Yacoub MH. Correction of left ventricular asynchrony by coronary artery surgery. Br Heart J 1988; 59: 304–308

Guyton RA, Arcidil JM, Langford DA, Morris DC, Liberman HA, Hatcher CR. Emergency coronary bypass for cardiogenic shock. Circulation 1987; 76 (suppl V): 22–27

Johnston JB, Lamb AC, Wright JS. Ventricular aneurysm after infarction. Pathological and surgical features. J Thorac Cardiovasc Surg 1969; 58: 14–19

Lytle BW, Loop FD, Cosgrove DM, et al. Fifteen hundred coronary reoperations. Results and determinants of early and late survival. J Thorac Cardiovasc Surg 1987; 93: 847–859

Wheatley DJ (ed.). Surgery of coronary artery disease. Chapman and Hall, London, 1986

Chapter 9

Miscellaneous Heart Disease

Most of the conditions included in this section are acquired lesions of the heart, but they may occur in the context of a congenital anomaly or their precise aetiology may be uncertain.

Constrictive Pericarditis

In the classic condition, the heart is encased in a thick, often calcified, inelastic pericardial sac that restricts its ability to relax in diastole. More recently, it has been recognised that a rigid pericardium in combination with a variable amount of pericardial fluid may produce the same haemodynamic consequences.

Anatomy and Pathology. The great majority of cases result from tuberculous infection of the pericardial sac, which is no longer common in Western countries. The active inflammation is converted into a mass of tuberculous granulation tissue that heals by dense fibrous scarring and often with calcification. There may be collections of caseous material. The heart is embedded in this dense tissue which is often a centimetre or more thick but irregularly distributed. In addition, one or the other pleural cavity may be similarly affected.

Rheumatic fever and a number of other conditions (viral infection, uraemia, radiation, malignancy) can also produce a dense adherent pericardial sac, but the constriction in these cases is rarely as marked as after tuberculosis. The pericardium becomes inelastic, however, and accumulation of fluid causes a more subacute compression of the heart than the chronic constrictive form.

Haemodynamics. There is interference with venous return to the heart, which, encased in rigid fibrous tissue, cannot relax to accept the venous blood ('inflow stasis'). The brunt of the increased intrapericardial pressure is born by the more compliant cardiac chambers, particularly the right atrium and right ventricle. Characteristically, the end-diastolic pressure equilibrates at the same level in all the cardiac chambers, usually between 15 and 25 mmHg. Cardiac filling is brisk in early diastole and then suddenly halted, giving the 'square root' sign in the ventricular pressure trace. With this restricted filling of the ventricles, there is a resultant diminution of cardiac output.

Clinical Features. Patients with chronic pericardial constriction may have a past history of vague chest pain or may reveal evidence of old tuberculous infection of the lungs or pleura. In other cases, the history may point to rheumatic or viral pericarditis. Patients are likely to present with peripheral oedema, which may be gross and associated with a large liver and ascites. Dyspnoea, although usually present, is not marked, and the patient is generally comfortable lying down, but becomes congested on bending over. The complextion may have a heather-blue tinge.

The pulse is small and, with critical cardiac constriction, characteristically illustrates the phenomenon of pulsus paradoxus; ('paradoxus' refers to the fact that a heartbeat can be heard on the precordium but the peripheral pulse, paradoxically, cannot be felt when the patient takes a breath.) The neck veins are usually markedly distended. On inspiration, the venous pressure tends to rise rather than fall, because the restricted heart cannot accommodate increased venous return (Kussmaul's sign). Late in the disease, patients show signs of malnourishment and wasting. A pericardial 'knock' may be present.

Special Investigations. The lateral chest radiograph may reveal calcification of the pericardium, but the overall cardiac shadow is not greatly enlarged and the lung fields are clear. The ECG is non-specific.

Echocardiography will demonstrate features of restrictive filling and any pericardial fluid which may be present. Computerised tomography also shows the pericardial thickening, calcification and fluid. While cardiac catheterisation confirms elevation of the venous pressure, rapid diastole filling and elevation of the end-diastolic pressures, these findings are not specific.

Differential Diagnosis. The association of ascites and an enlarged liver may lead to a mistaken diagnosis of primary liver disease. Also, these features in combination with the distended neck veins, are likely to be confused with tricuspid valve disease. The most difficult distinction may be between pericardial restriction and endomyocardial fibrosis or restrictive cardiomyopathy.

Indications for Operation. A diagnosis of constrictive pericarditis and the presence of impaired venous filling are sufficient indications for operation, as the disease is progressive and there is no effective medical treatment.

Principles of Treatment. The cardiac chambers are freed by removal of the thickened pericardial sac. Care must be taken to avoid injury to the coronary arteries while removing adherent pericardium. Calcification may extend into the myocardium, and cardiopulmonary bypass may facilitate dissection around the back of the heart.

Results. The relief of symptoms is often dramatic, and improvement tends to be sustained, despite the fact that cardiac movement rarely returns completely to normal. In patients with recent active disease, treatment for tuberculosis must be continued postoperatively. Operation does, however, carry a significant risk, with 5%–10% early mortality.

Cardiomyopathy

These conditions affect the heart muscle primarily. The changes are thus not secondary to coronary artery disease or valvar heart lesions. The possibility of treatment by transplantation of the heart has brought them within the realm of surgical interest.

Anatomy. Several types of cardiomyopathy are recognised on the basis of haemodynamic and clinical features. In dilated or congestive cardiomyopathy, the heart is enlarged with poor contractility. The myocardium shows extensive fibrosis and may have calcification. Restrictive cardiomyopathy is characterised by endocardial fibrosis and hypertrophy with fibrosis of the myocardium. The heart is thus 'stiff'.

Cardiomyopathy may be associated with amyloid disease or scleroderma. Hypertrophic (obstructive) cardiomyopathy (HOCM) produces extensive hypertrophy of ventricular muscle, particularly the ventricular septum. This too leads to a decrease in left ventricular compliance and may cause functional obstruction to the left or right ventricle. It has also been called 'idiopathic hypertrophic subaortic stenosis' and 'asymmetric left ventricular hypertrophy'.

In no type of cardiomyopathy has a definite aetiology been found, although hypertension, viral infection, systemic disorders and toxic myocardial damage have been implicated.

Haemodynamics. The restrictive cardiomyopathy may be extremely difficult to differentiate from pericardial constriction, as the end-diastolic pressure is elevated in all cardiac chambers in both conditions. The loss of ventricular compliance leads to elevation of venous pressures, and there is usually some increase in pulmonary arterial pressure. In dilated types, the volume of the heart is greatly increased, with an abnormally low ejection fraction and raised venous pressures. Obstructive cardiomyopathy, as might be expected, produces outflow obstruction to the left or right side of the heart with ventricular hypertension. The obstruction is typically made worse by administration of isoprenaline or amyl nitrate and may be relieved by phenylephrine.

Clinical Features. The onset may be insidious and non-specific, with vague symptoms of chest pain, dypsnoea and fatigue. In obstructive cases, a systolic heart murmur may be present. Signs of cardiac failure, restriction or obstruction soon develop, and the patient may become incapacitated by congestive heart failure, oedema and pleural or pericardial effusions.

Special Investigations. These are generally non-specific, but cardiac enlargement, arrythmias and conduction defects are common on the chest X-ray and ECG, respectively. Cardiac catheterisation is generally performed, to exclude other types of cardiac disease and to measure haemodynamics. In obstructive cardiomyopathy, ventricular angiography may show obliteration of the cavity during ventricular systole, while patients with dilated cardiomyopathy tend to have mitral and tricuspid valve regurgitation.

Differential Diagnosis. Other types of valvar heart disease causing obstruction must be excluded. Functional or muscular subaortic stenosis should be suspected in any adult with symptoms and signs of aortic stenosis but without an ejection click or a calcified valve on radiographic examination. Similarly, ischaemic heart disease must be considered in cases of dilated cardiomyopathy, and chronic constrictive pericarditis in the restrictive type.

Indications for Operation. Relief of the obstruction does not necessarily prolong life or maintain an unobstructed outflow; operation is undertaken, therefore, to relieve symptoms of syncope and chest pain. The prognosis for patients with dilated cardiomyopathy is poor, with about eight out of ten dying within 10 years. This becomes more likely in the presence of arrythmias and right heart failure, which are thus an indication to consider cardiac transplantation. More recently, there has been evidence that cardiomyoplasty may benefit these patients. The restrictive myopathies run a more protracted and chronic course, and survival may depend ultimately upon any associated disease.

Principles of Treatment. Surgery is reserved for cases that can no longer be managed on medical treatment. Hypertrophied muscle bundles may be excised to relieve right or left ventricular outflow obstruction, and mitral valve replacement has also been advocated for subaortic obstruction. When endocardial fibrosis is present, peeling this away from the inner layer of the myocardium may be beneficial. Cardiac transplantation offers a good possibility of survival, with greatly improved exercise capacity for patients with end-stage disease.

Results. Survival is greatly improved by cardiac transplantation, which currently carries a risk of less than 10%, and functional status is also markedly improved. The late results depend upon rejection of the transplanted heart. Conservative operations for obstructive and restrictive endocardial fibrosis also tend to bring about good functional improvement, albeit with an operative risk of 10%–20%.

Cardiac Tumours

Tumours of the heart or myocardium occur infrequently. They may be malignant or benign, primary or metastatic. About two-thirds are benign.

Anatomy and Pathology. Cardiac tumours may arise from any of the cell types within the heart and also may extend directly into the heart from abdominal organs by way of the systemic venous system. Myxomas are by far the most common cardiac tumour. They usually arise from the atrial septum as a pedunculated mass within the atrial cavity. Although generally benign, myxomas can recur locally with invasion of the myocardium; they rarely metastasise distally. The tumour is a soft, gelatenous polypoid mass with a greyish white colour.

In children, rhabdomyoma is the most common cardiac neoplasm. It tends to occur in siblings in association with tuberous sclerosis. The yellowish grey mass is found in either ventricle attached by a broad base. It is a benign neoplasm.

Fibromas are also benign lesions, occurring in the ventricles, often attached to the septum. The tumour resembles fibromas in other parts of the body and is not invasive. Lipomas tend to be incidental findings of encapsulated fat cells, usually attached to the atrial septum.

Tumours of the sarcoma group are malignant and tend to have distal metastases. They may involve any cardiac structure and present at any age. The gross appearances are variable, depending upon the dominant cell types.

Rarely, tumours grow up the inferior vena cava from abdominal organs. Such tumours are usually of renal origin and may become established in the right atrium.

Haemodynamics. Many tumours cause no alteration in haemodynamics. Left atrial myxomas may mimic mitral stenosis by intermittent obstruction of the mitral valve. Fibromas and rhabdomyomas may cause inlet or outlet obstruction of the ventricle.

Clinical Features. The presentation will depend upon the location and type of neoplasm. Atrial myxomas may present with signs and symptoms of mitral stenosis or tricuspid valve obstruction, but they also frequently embolise to peripheral or pulmonary vessels. Systemic symptoms, such as fever, are not uncommon. There is likely to be a diastolic murmur if the lesion is in the left atrium, while a right atrial myxoma is said to cause a loud sound early in systole when the mass regurgitates back from the ventricle into the atrium.

Rhabdomyomas and fibromas present with signs of ventricular obstruction – that is, a systolic murmur. The diagnosis is nearly always made early in childhood. Lipomas do not tend to produce clinical signs or symptoms. Sarcomas may present at any age in a variety of ways, depending upon the structures which are involved.

Special Investigations. Echocardiography is the investigation of choice and will usually show the size and attachment of the neoplasm. In some cases, the appearances are sufficiently characteristic to establish a diagnosis. Computed tomography or magnetic resonance imaging may also be useful.

Differential Diagnosis. Valvar cardiac disease (mitral or tricuspid stenosis) and subaortic or subpulmonary stenosis can be excluded by real-time echocardiography. It may be difficult to differentiate blood clot in the left atrium or mural thrombus in the ventricle from a neoplasm.

Indications for Operation. Myxomas are removed upon diagnosis to prevent cardiac obstruction and embolic complications. Fibromas are also removed to relieve or prevent obstruction of the heart, which is nearly always present. Lipomas are excised to confirm the diagnosis. Operation is also indicated to obtain a histological diagnosis for sarcomas, even though complete excision may not be possible. In cases of rhabdomyoma, surgery is undertaken to relieve obstruction. However, multiple tumours have been discovered without symptoms, particularly where cerebral lesions have caused severe mental retardation.

Principles of Treatment. Excision of the neoplasm is done as completely as possible, respecting vital cardiac structures and replacing those which can be sacrificed, such as the atrial septum. Recently, techniques of cardiomyoplasty have been applied to permit more extensive excision of ventricular malignancies. In this procedure, the lattissimus dorsi muscle is 'trained' for approximately 6 weeks with a pacemaker, after which it can assist or replace the cardiac muscle.

Results. Survival after removal of a benign tumour is generally good, although a small number of patients with myxoma suffer recurrence of the tumour, and overall survival after 10 years is about 70%. The prognosis for sarcomas tends to be poor, and most cases have little, if any, response to radiation or chemotherapy.

Bacterial Endocarditis

It is now generally recognised that infection within the heart may be caused by a variety of organisms, hence the term 'infective endocarditis' is often applied to this condition.

Anatomy and Pathology. It is likely that bacteria enter the blood stream periodically from a variety of sources, but it is probably necessary to have an area of turbulence and irregularity for them to become established upon the cardiovascular endothelium. When the normal immunological defences cannot clear the infection, organisms proliferate forming a 'vegetation' which consists of fibrin and cells mixed with the pathogens. This may go on to cause destruction of underlying tissues, such as valve cusps, or break off and embolise to the systemic or pulmonary arteries.

Patients who are particularly at risk for endocarditis are those with a ventricular septal defect, persistent ductus arteriosus, bicuspid or rheumatic aortic valve, mitral valve prolapse or coronary artery fistulae. The aortic valve remains more susceptible to infection than other cardiac valves. Since the advent of cardiac surgery, most cases of endocarditis occur in patients who have undergone cardiac operations, particularly the creation of a systemic–pulmonary anastomosis or the implantation of a cardiac valve. Endocarditis may, however, arise on a structurally normal valve. Another group likely to develop cardiac infection are drug addicts who habitually load the circulation with contaminated products.

Whereas endocarditis was formerly caused most often by *Streptococcus viridans*, this organism now only accounts for about one-third of the cases.

Staphylococcus aureus, Streptococcus faecalis and fungi are also found frequently, while viruses, rickettsiae or parasites may occasionally be identified as the causative organism. *Staphylococcus epidermis* is the usual organism in postoperative prosthetic endocarditis.

Haemodynamics. Haemodynamic alterations come about as the result of systemic effects of the infection (fever, tachycardia, anaemia), or direct involvement of cardiac structures. Destruction of an aortic or mitral valve cusp causes severe insufficiency and cardiac failure. From the aortic valve, infection may penetrate into the ventricular septum causing heart block or rupture into the right ventricle. Occasionally the area of aortic–mitral fibrous continuity is perforated, and this results in acute cardiac tamponade from haemorrhage into the pericardial sac or a root abscess. In some cases, cardiac failure occurs after the infection has been brought under control as the result of valve scarring during healing.

Clinical Features. The presentation and clinical course tend to be either subacute or acute.

In the more prevalent subacute disease, the onset is insidious and early symptoms are non-specific. There is frequently fever after some type of dental or surgical procedure, followed by malaise and loss of weight. A murmur is often present from the underlying cardiac anomaly and this may change in character. More importantly, the patient may develop a new murmur as the the result of tissue destruction. Embolisation of vegetations produces many of the clinical signs: painful nodules on the hands or feet (Osler's nodes), splinter haemorrhages and haematuria. Septic abscesses may also result in the brain, kidney or lung. After some weeks, enlargement of the spleen and clubbing of the fingers may appear.

Acute endocarditis is usually caused by the more aggessive *Staphylococcus aureus* and tends to present with sudden fever and chills. Abscess formation is early and widespread, often involving the heart muscle, the brain or the kidneys. It is more likely to affect structurally normal valves, such that the presentation of a murmur is of greater significance and the onset of congestive heart failure is often dramatic, due to perforation of a valve cusp.

Special Investigations. The diagnosis is based upon culturing organisms from the blood, and several specimens should be taken over a period of days (or hours in acute cases) prior to the administration of antibiotics. Once antibiotics have been given, they may suppress growth of the organism in cultures despite not controlling the intracardiac infection. Other laboratory investigation results suggestive of infection include elevation of the white blood count and erythrocyte sedimentation rate, high levels of serum c-reactive protein and anaemia. The ECG may demonstrate conduction defects if an abscess has penetrated the ventricular septum, or there may be changes of ischaemia when vegetations have embolised to a coronary artery. The chest X-ray is not diagnostic but may suggest septic pulmonary emboli with abscess formation, pericardial effusion or cardiac enlargement due to haemodynamic decompensation. Computed tomographic scanning should be carried out if there is any suggestion of abscess formation in distal organs.

Real-time echocardiography has proved invaluable in the diagnosis of infective endocarditis and circumvents cardiac catheterisation, with its attendant risk of dislodging vegetations into the circulation. Vegetations can be visualised, and some idea of the causative agent (fungi versus bacteria) may be obtained. Equally important, the response to treatment can be monitored directly, as well as any damage to valve mechanisms or formation of pericardial fluid. Abscesses can be visualised occasionally.

Differential Diagnosis. Other causes of fever must be excluded, including neoplasm, other types of infection and systemic connective tissue diseases. Atrial myxoma may closely mimic endocarditis, with fever, changing murmurs and systemic emboli. The diagnosis is usually clarified by echocardiography.

Indications for Operation. Cardiac surgery in the presence of active infection carries a very high mortality (30%–50%), therefore, every effort is made to control the infection with the appropriate antimicrobial agents. When this is not successful, operation is undertaken to remove the mass of vegetations (usually complicated by abscesses that must be cleared out), so that the antimicrobial drugs may reach and control residual organisms. Other indications for surgery include uncontrollable heart failure due to valve destruction, blockage of a systemic – pulmonary shunt by vegetations and perforation of the heart. Elective valve replacement may be necessary after the infection has been eradicated if the patient has significant residual aortic or mitral incompetence.

Results. Infective endocarditis continues to carry a substantial mortality, about 20% in subacute cases and as high as 50% in acute cases. This can be reduced by early diagnosis and aggressive treatment, particularly in the high-risk group of patients who have undergone previous cardiac surgery. Equally important is an active programme of prevention by antibiotic prophylaxis for patients with known cardiac disease who are undergoing dental treatment or other surgical procedures.

Trauma

Damage may be inflicted upon the heart by either blunt (non-penetrating) or sharp (penetrating) trauma. It is of interest that the repair of stab wounds probably represented the first successful cardiac operations.

Anatomy and Pathology. Sharp or penetrating wounds may be caused by a sharp weapon (knife, knitting needle, ice pick) being thrust through the chest wall into the heart or by a high velocity missile (bullet, shrapnel). The former tends to lacerate the right ventricle or right atrium, although a stab in the back may occasionally reach the left heart chambers. There may be transection of a coronary artery followed by production of an arteriovenous fistula, or penetration of the ventricular septum may result in a traumatic ventricular septal defect. Missile injuries usually cause widespread destruction of the heart.

Blunt trauma may result from compression of the thorax (crush injury), sudden deceleration, or a direct blow to the anterior chest wall (contusion injury). These are most commonly the result of road traffic accidents in which the patient is thrown forward against the steering wheel or the vehicle comes to a sudden stop. A sudden increase in intracardiac pressure may cause rupture of mitral chordae, the ventricular septum or the right ventricle. Contusion injuries tend to cause bruising of the myocardium (usually the right ventricle) and damage to the left anterior descending coronary artery or rupture of the aorta.

A new type of trauma is occurring with increasing frequency in the cardiac catheterisation laboratory as a complication of interventional procedures to dilate stenosed valves or vessels. Catheters or guide-wires may perforate the ventricle with little, if any, consequence; but atrial perforation or disruption of a valve annulus by balloon dilation may produce tears several millimetres in length.

Haemodynamics. Rupture of the mitral valve or ventricular septum leads to acute cardiac failure, while damage to the left anterior descending coronary may mimic acute myocardial infarction. Penetrating injuries usually cause haemorrhage into the pericardial sac with rapid development of cardiac tamponade.

Clinical Features. There will invariably be a history of trauma, although in sophisticated 'gang wars', the use of a concealed, stabbing instrument may make this difficult to obtain, and careful examination may be necessary to identify the point of penetration. Usually, there is external evidence of trauma, with a skin laceration or bruising. When there has been rupture of the ventricular septum or a cardiac valve, characteristic murmurs appear, usually followed by heart failure. Rupture of the tricuspid valve, however, may remain 'silent' for several weeks, until the gradual onset of right heart failure.

Special Investigations. In blunt trauma, the ECG may be the only indication of cardiac injury. The changes of pericardial inflammation or myocardial necrosis may be seen in ST and T wave changes. Chest X-ray may show cardiac or mediastinal enlargement due to haemorrhage into the pericardium, or other evidence of trauma such as sternal or rib fractures. Echocardiography may be useful in demonstrating pericardial fluid, mitral or tricuspid valve dysfunction, or impaired motion in a segment of contused myocardium.

Differential Diagnosis. Late presentation of a contusion injury may be confused with pericarditis or acute myocardial infarction. Usually, the problem is to recognise the presence of cardiac trauma in the midst of multiple injuries.

Indications for Operation. A penetrating wound virtually always requires emergency operation to relieve tamponade and to control haemorrhage. Contusion itself does not require surgical intervention, but operation may be required to repair or replace damaged valves or to relieve pericardial compression. Rupture of the heart and traumatic ventricular septal defect also necessitate operation.

Results. A surprising number of cases can be salvaged by prompt diagnosis and treatment, probably because trauma tends to occur in young, otherwise healthy individuals who have sufficient cardiovascular reserve to tolerate an episode of haemorrhage or tamponade. About 70% of patients recover from stab wounds of the heart, and similar salvage rates have been achieved for cardiac rupture after blunt trauma. Missile wounds, however, are nearly always fatal.

Arrythmias

Conduction defects and arrythmias produce abnormally slow or fast heart rates which may lead to impaired cardiac function. Their investigation and management traditionally lie within the physician's domain, now extended by sophisticated techniques of electrophysiological measurement at cardiac catheterisation, catheter ablation of conduction pathways, and an extended pharmacological armamentarium.

Surgical participation in this area is rapidly developing, however, in a variety of situations. Slow heart rates (bradycardias) may require implantation of a pacemaker system. This may be a simple 'demand' pacemaker which stimulates the ventricle after a certain period, or a more complicated device which senses the patient's movements and increases its rate to compensate for exercise. Sequential pacing of the atria and ventricles is also possible to achieve a more physiological situation.

The control of fast rhythms (tachycardias) may involve surgical ablation of accessory conducting pathways (the Kent's bundle in Wolff–Parkinson–White Syndrome) or one of several procedures to manage ventricular tachycardia unresponsive to drug therapy. The ventricular arrythmia usually arises from a focus of ischaemic myocardium. Thus, coronary artery bypass grafting or resection of a ventricular aneurysm may be beneficial. More complicated procedures involve resection of the subendocardial region where the arrythmia originates, as defined by intraoperative or preoperative mapping, or an 'encircling' ventriculotomy to isolate the irritable focus. Automatic implantable defibrillators or pacemakers may also have a role to play in some patients with life-threatening arrythmias.

Further Reading

Bisno Al (ed.). Treatment of infective endocarditis. Grune & Stratton, New York, 1981

Cox JL. The status of surgery for cardiac arrythmias. Circulation 1985; 71: 413–417

Donaldson RM, Ross DN. Homograft aortic root replacement for complicated prosthetic valve endocarditis. Circulation 1984; 70 (suppl II): 178–181

McAllister HA. Primary tumours and cysts of the heart and pericardium. Curr Prob Cardiol 1979; IV: 1–15

Report of the WHO/ISFC task force on the definition and classification of cardiomyopathies. Br Heart J 1980; 44: 672–673

Sawyer CG, Burwell CS, Dexter L, Eppinger EC, Goodale WT, Gorlin R, Harken DE, Haynes FW. Chronic constrictive pericarditis: Further consideration of the pathologic physiology of the disease. Am Heart J 1952; 44: 207–230

Wood P. Chronic constrictive pericarditis. Am J Cardiol 1961; 8: 48–52

Chapter 10

Acquired Lesions of Major Blood Vessels

The thoracic aorta, passing from its intrapericardial ascending portion to the descending aorta in the posterior chest, falls within the realm of thoracic and vascular surgery as well as cardiac surgery. Similarly, the management of massive pulmonary embolus or peripheral vascular occlusion may fall to the physician or general surgeon, as well as the vascular, thoracic or cardiac specialist. This is largely because cardiopulmonary bypass is absolutely necessary only for lesions of the ascending aorta or transverse aortic arch.

Aneurysm of the Thoracic Aorta

Aneurysms of the thoracic aorta may result from aortitis, degenerative arteriosclerotic changes or annulo-aortic ectasia. In a true aneurysm, there is a dilatation of the vessels which involves all the normal vascular layers. The aneurysm may be 'fusiform' with a long area of enlargement, or 'saccular' with a small neck. False aneurysms, in contrast, have walled off an extravasation of blood, usually with a single layer of aortic wall or organised fibrous tissue. Lesions arise predominantly in the ascending and descending portions of the aorta, a smaller number being found in the transverse aortic arch or thoracoabdominal regions.

Patients may be asymptomatic or complain of pain. Superior vena caval obstruction is sometimes seen from compression by a large aneurysm of the ascending aorta, while those in the region of the ligamentum produce hoarseness in some cases by pressure upon the recurrent laryngeal nerve.

The pulsating anterior chest wall mass of the syphilitic aneurysm is now rarely seen. The diagnosis of thoracic aneurysm in most patients is suggested by widening of the mediastinum on chest X-ray. This can be confirmed by an aortogram or computed axial tomography (CAT scan).

Most aneurysms will rupture sooner or later: in cases with chest pain or a very large blow-out, this tends to happen within about two years of the diagnosis. Therefore, surgery is advised in all but the most debilitated patients.

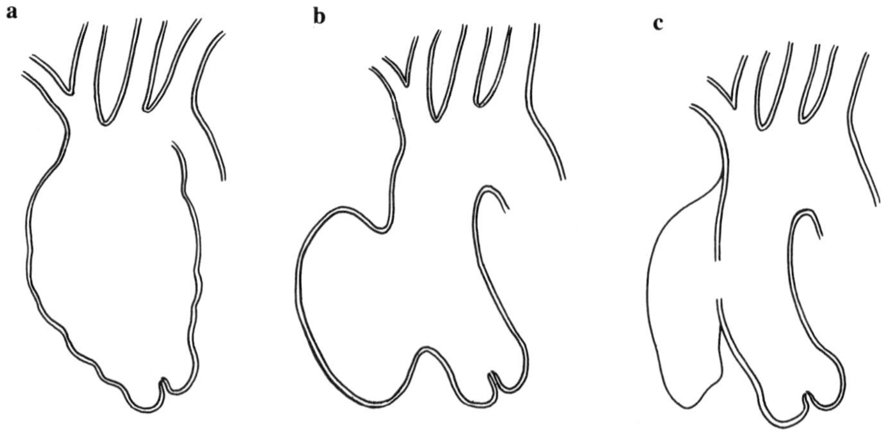

Fig. 10.1. Types of aortic aneurysm: fusiform (**a**); saccular (**b**); false (**c**).

Aneurysms of the ascending aorta are resected on cardiopulmonary bypass and replaced with a prosthetic graft. If dilatation of the aortic root has resulted in an incompetent aortic valve, replacement of the valve is also necessary. In the descending aorta, repair may be done without the heart–lung machine, taking

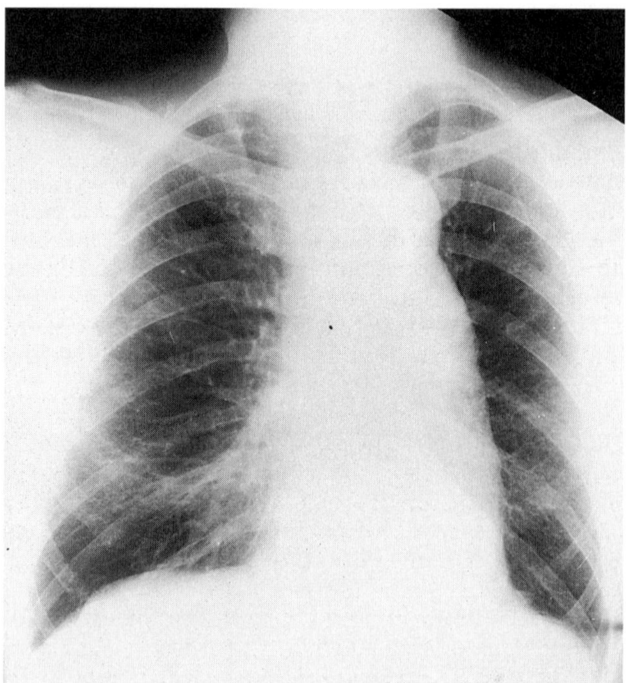

Fig. 10.2. Chest X-ray of descending aortic aneurysm.

care to control hypertension and to minimise the risk of spinal cord injury during the period of aortic cross-clamping. The diseased segment may be excised and replaced with a tube graft, or the neck of a saccular aneurysm may be closed with a patch. The walls of the aneurysm sac are often wrapped around the prosthetic graft for added haemostasis.

Thoracic aneurysms seen in Marfan's syndrome ('annulo-aortic ectasia') deserve special mention. This lesion tends to be found in younger patients, due to an inherited or spontaneously occurring abnormality in connective tissue metabolism. The resulting weakness in the medial layer of the aorta leads to generalised distension with loss of the aortic sinuses, giving the typical appearance of a flask seen on angiography. Aortic valve incompetence is frequently present as the result of the dilated aortic root, and dissection also occurs in about 15%–25% of cases. Patients who survive treatment of pathology in the ascending aorta tend to develop aneurysms more distally in the descending thoracic and abdominal aorta.

Because the patient population is heterogeneous the results of surgery for thoracic aneurysms are highly variable, as are the underlying pathological mechanisms and morphological types of aneurysms. A technically successful operation may be complicated by renal failure or spinal cord injury. However, most cases will survive at least 5 years after operation, which represents a considerable improvement over the natural history of the malformation.

Aortic Dissection

In this condition the aorta is split into two layers by blood 'dissecting' within the media. It is said to be acute when the dissection appears to be less than about a fortnight old, and chronic if the process has been going on for a longer time. There is an intimal tear which allows blood to pass from the normal ('true') aortic lumen into the wall ('false') lumen. The false lumen then spirals around the aorta, until a second intimal defect allows blood to re-enter the true lumen. Based upon the sites of the communications between true and false lumens, dissections have been divided into various types.

While dissection occurs more frequently in cases with Marfan's syndrome, it is also seen in patients with no obvious vascular disease although systemic hypertension is a definite predisposing factor.

The presentation of acute dissection is often catastrophic, with shock and sudden death due to aortic rupture, cardiac tamponade or acute aortic regurgitation. In less dramatic cases, the patient feels a severe tearing pain in the chest, and occasionally, dissection will have taken place with only mild discomfort. In addition to aortic incompetence, when the ascending aorta is involved, dissection may exclude branches from the circulation, such that a carotid or radial pulse is lost.

Widening of the mediastinum is usually present on the chest radiograph, and the ECG may show signs of ischaemia if blood flow to a coronary artery is impaired (usually the right). Echocardiography may demonstrate the double vascular channels, while the aortogram may also identify the points of entry and exit of the false lumen. Computed tomography is especially useful.

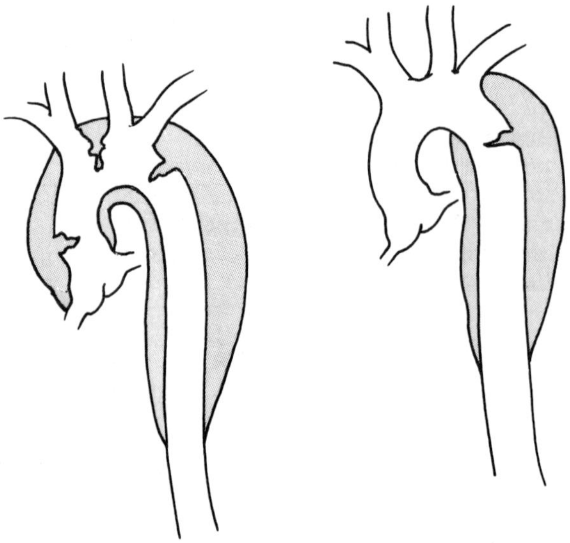

Fig. 10.3. Types of aortic dissection. *Left*: proximal (type I). *Right*: distal (type II).

Dissection of the ascending aorta is usually fatal within a few hours or days, and emergency operation should be carried out immediately to replace the diseased segment with a tube graft and, if necessary, to repair or replace the aortic valve. By obliterating the site of entry into the false lumen, blood remains in the true aortic lumen, and this permits compression and healing of the false channel. In dissections confined to the descending aorta, the chances of rupture are much lower and the benefits of surgery are less certain. These patients are, accordingly, often treated with bed rest and control of the blood pressure, which permits healing of the dissection. Although the patient may be left with a 'double-barrelled' aorta, this does not cause any disability provided there is no compromise of the branches. When there is evidence of spinal cord ischaemia or vascular occlusion or rupture, descending aortic dissections should be treated by operation as well.

Traumatic Rupture of the Aorta

Acute traumatic rupture of the aorta usually occurs at the level of the ligamentum arteriosum as the result of a severe deceleration injury. The upper thoracic aorta, held fast to the chest wall by the brachiocephalic branches and ligamentum, is sheered off the more mobile descending aorta. Depending upon the force of the injury, the pleura and all the layers of the aorta may be completely disrupted, or the adventitia and anterior wall may remain intact. In patients who survive the acute injury, a false aneurysm may develop. Occasionally direct penetrating trauma or a fractured spine will cause injury to the aorta lower in the chest. Usually aortic transection is seen in the context of multiple injuries that may dominate the clinical picture. The patient often is shocked, and chest radiography may show mediastinal widening or a pleural effusion.

Surgical treatment aims to restore continuity of the aorta, usually by excision of the damaged area and interposition of a prosthetic tube graft. Unlike coarctation, these patients do not have a well-developed collateral circulation, so cross-clamping the aorta carries a significant risk of paraplegia unless this can be accomplished within 20 min. This may be prevented by establishing a temporary heparinised shunt from above the laceration to the lower thoracic aorta, prior to dealing with the aortic repair.

Massive Pulmonary Embolism

The finding of embolic material in the lungs at post-mortem examination of cardiac cases is by no means uncommon, although their importance is less certain. Probably, small clots form in the right heart of patients with poor cardiac function, and periodically pass into the pulmonary circulation. This is the rationale for anticoagulating patients after a Fontan operation, where even a small rise in pulmonary arterial pressure may severely compromise cardiac output.

Massive pulmonary embolism, however, tends to occur in patients who have been confined to bed for a more-or-less minor surgical procedure, such as repair of a hernia or delivery of a baby. Soft clot formed in the deep veins of the legs and in the pelvis, suddenly become dislodged into the blood stream. Classically, this happens during straining at stool, and the patient collapses as the result of

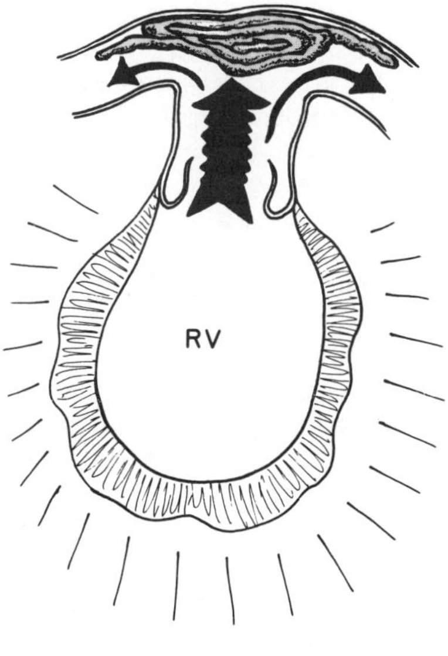

Fig. 10.4. Massive pulmonary embolism obstructing the outflow of the right ventricle.

the clot lodging at the pulmonary arterial bifurcation. Should the clot move distally, cyanosis, dyspnoea and right heart failure supervene, permitting the possibility of survival. The chest X-ray and ECG may be suggestive, and the patients condition permitting, lung scan will confirm the diagnosis.

Formerly, surgical extraction of the embolus from the pulmonary arterial tree was the only hope of survival for many of these patients, and this depended upon the diagnosis being made in circumstances where it was possible to open the chest. However, treatment with thrombolytic agents is now preferred in those cases whose haemodynamic situation will tolerate this and who are not at major risk of haemorrhage as a result of other recent surgical procedures. Otherwise, emergency embolectomy may still need to be carried out.

This is one condition for which prophylaxis, by the administration of low-dose subcutaneous heparin, has been shown to reduce morbidity and mortality and such therapy should be considered in any adult surgical patient.

Arterial Embolism

Obstruction of an artery by an embolus is a surgical emergency. This is likely to result in permanent loss of function of the tissues supplied, particularly if this is the brain, or it may result in loss of function of a limb or loss of the limb itself. Even after 'successful' conservative management, the function and nutrition of a limb which is dependent upon the collateral circulation is likely to be deficient, especially when exposed to cold, trauma or exercise.

The most common cause of arterial embolism is atrial fibrillation in association with mitral stenosis or a prosthetic heart valve. Emboli may also result from the dissemination of atherosclerotic or calcific plaques or infective material in bacterial endocarditis. Rarely, a left atrial myxoma may result in widespread embolisation.

Diagnosis usually depends upon the loss of a peripheral pulse. In a patient in whom there is reason to suspect embolism, the loss of a pulse is all that is necessary to justify an exploratory operation. Above the block, there may be an accentuation of the pulsation, giving it a pistol-shot quality. Associated features of arterial embolism which may be present are a reduction in the temperature of the limb, sometimes a change in colour and a slow capillary return after compression of the digits. There may also be sensory loss and some motor weakness. A useful sign in the early postoperative period is a rise in blood pressure. In the case of postoperative cerebral emboli, there may be abnormal restlessness. Pain may be felt in the limb involved but this may be entirely absent, particularly in a patient under the influence of an anaesthetic or analgesia.

Once a diagnosis has been made, operation should be carried out without delay. Emboli generally lodge at arterial bifurcations. Where one or the other femoral pulse is absent, the blockage is likely to be at the iliac or aortic bifurcation. After removal of the embolus, usually with balloon-tipped catheters, there should be free bleeding from the proximal and distal limbs of the

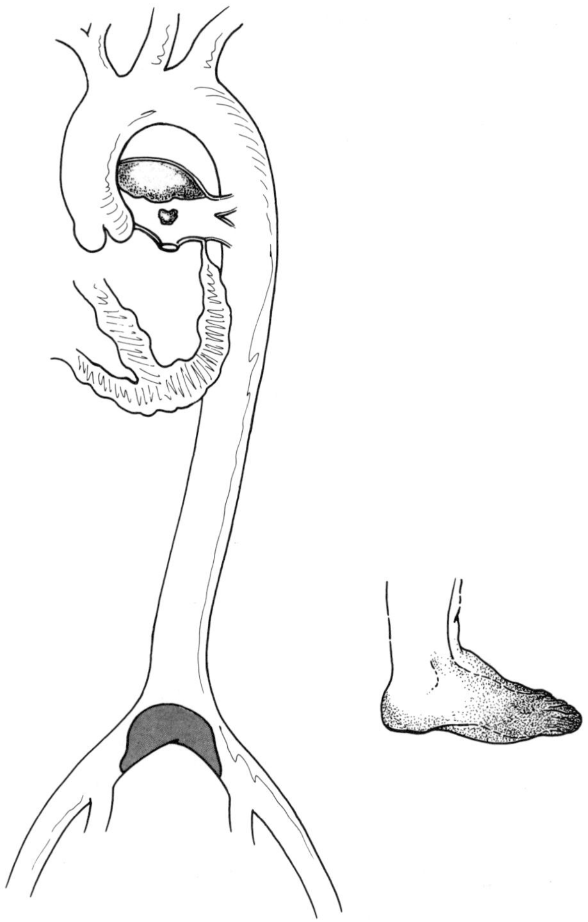

Fig. 10.5. Common sites of embolism in the pulmonary and aortic bifurcations. The latter may present as ischaemia of the foot.

artery. The opposite leg pulse should also be felt, as clot from a saddle embolus may be dislodged into the other extremity. An alternative to surgical treatment in some cases may be treatment with thrombolytic agents.

Further Reading

Bergen JJ, Yao JST (eds). Aneurysms: diagnosis and treatment. Grune & Stratton, New York, 1983
Bounameaux H, Vermylen J, Collen D. Thrombolytic treatment with recombinant tissue-type plasminogen activator with massive pulmonary embolism. Ann Intern Med 1985; 103: 64–65
Crawford ES, Svensson LG, Coselli JS, Safi HJ, Hess KR. Surgical treatment of aneurysm and/or dissection of the ascending aorta, transverse aortic arch, and ascending aorta and transverse aortic arch. Factors influencing survival in 717 patients. J Thorac Cardiovasc Surg 1989; 98: 659–674

Davies MJ. Pathology of the aorta. Curr Opin Cardiol 1986; 1: 643–645
Eastcott HHG. Arterial surgery, 2nd edn. Pitman Medical, London, 1973
International Multicentre Trial. Prevention of fatal postoperative pulmonary embolism by low dose heparin. Lancet 1975; ii: 45–51
Kerr IH, Simon G, Sutton GC. The value of the plain radiograph in acute massive pulmonary embolism. Br J Radiol 1971; 44: 751–717
Lindsey J Jr, Hurst JW (eds). The aorta. Grune & Stratton, New York, 1979
McIntyre KM, Sasahara AA. The haemodynamic response to pulmonary embolism in patients without prior cardiopulmonary disease. Am J Cardiol 1971; 28: 288–294

Subject Index